W0043768

ULTRASOUND IN CORONARY ARTERY DISEASE

Developments in Cardiovascular Medicine

VOLUME 113

The titles published in this series are listed at the end of this volume.

Ultrasound in Coronary Artery Disease

Present Role and Future Perspectives

edited by

Sabino Iliceto
Department of Cardiology, University of Bari, Bari, Italy

Paolo Rizzon
Department of Cardiology, University of Bari, Bari, Italy

and

Jos R. T. C. Roelandt
Thorax Center, Erasmus University, Rotterdam, The Netherlands

Kluwer Academic Publishers

Dordrecht / Boston / London

Library of Congress Cataloging-in-Publication Data

Ultrasound in coronary artery disease : present role and future perspectives / edited by
   Sabino Iliceto, Paolo Rizzon, and Jos R. T. C. Roelandt.
         p.   cm. – (Developments in cardiovascular medicine: v. 113)
      ISBN-13:978-94-010-6762-1   e-ISBN-13:978-94-009-0611-2
      DOI:10.1007/978-94-009-0611-2

   1. Coronary heart disease – Ultrasonic imaging.
   2. Echocardiography. I. Iliceto, Sabino. II. Rizzon, Paolo. III. Roelandt, Jos. IV. Series.
      [DNLM: 1. Coronary Diseases – diagnosis. 2. Echocardiography. 3. Myocardial Dis-
   eases – diagnosis. W1 DE997VME v. 113 / WG 141.5.E2 U47]
   RC685.C6U46 1990
   616.1'2307543 – dc20
   DLC
   for Library of Congress   90–4496

ISBN-13:978-94-010-6762-1

Published by Kluwer Academic Publishers,
P.O. Box 17, 3300 AA Dordrecht, The Netherlands

Kluwer Academic Publishers incorporates
the publishing programmes of
D. Reidel, Martinus Nijhoff, Dr W. Junk and MTP Press.

Sold and distributed in the U.S.A. and Canada
by Kluwer Academic Publishers,
101 Philip Drive, Norwell, MA 02061, U.S.A.

In all other countries, sold and distributed
by Kluwer Academic Publishers Group,
P.O. Box 322, 3300 AH Dordrecht, The Netherlands.

All rights reserved

© 1991 Kluwer Academic Publishers
Softcover reprint of the hardcover 1st edition 1991

No part of the material protected by this copyright notice may be reproduced or utilized in any
form or by any means, electronic or mechanical, including photocopying, recording or by any
information storage and retrieval system, without written permission from the copyright owner.

*This book is dedicated to
my father, Nicola Iliceto*

Table of contents

PART TWO: Evaluation of myocardial infarction

List of first contributors

Luciano Agati, 1 Cattedra di Cardiologia, Univ. La Sapienza, Policlinico Umberto 1, I-00161, Roma, Italy

Antonio F. Amico, Division of Cardiology, University of Bari, I-70124 Bari, Italy

N. Bom, Thorax Center, Erasmus University, P.O. Box 1738, 3000 DR Rotterdam, The Netherlands

Raimund Erbel, II Medical Clinic, Johannes Gutenberg University, Langenbeckstrasse 1, D-6500 Mainz, FRG

Harvey Feigenbaum, Hemodynamic Lab., Indianapolis University, School of Medicine, 926 West Michigan Street, Indianapolis, IN 46223, USA

Alan G. Fraser, Department of Cardiology, University of Wales, College of Medicine, Heath Park, Cardiff CF4 4XN, Wales, UK

M. García-Fernández, Lab. Cardiologia No Invasiva, Escuela Nacional del Thorax, Ciudad Universitaria, 28040 Madrid, Spain

Sabino Iliceto, Division of Cardiology, University of Bari, I-70124 Bari, Italy

Joseph Kisslo, Cardiac Diagnostic Unit, Duke University Medical Center, Box 3818, Durham, NC 27710, USA

Vito Marangelli, Division of Cardiology, University of Bari, I-70124 Bari, Italy

Paolo Marino, Division of Cardiology, University of Verona, Centro Ospedaliero di Borgo Trento, P. le A. Stefani 1, I-37126 Verona, Italy

David D. McPherson, Dir. Echocardiography Lab., Northwestern Memorial Hospital, Suite 586, Wesley Pazalian-Superior and Farbacks Court, Chicago, IL 60611, USA

Richard S. Meltzer, University of Rochester Medical Center, Cardiology Box 679, 601 Elmwood Ave., Rochester, NY 14642, USA

Navin C. Nanda, Heart Station SWB-W001, University of Alabama School of Medicine, Spain Wallace Building, Birmingham, AL 35294, USA

Natesa G. Pandian, Tufts University School of Medicine, Non Invasive Cardiac Lab., New England Med. Center Hospitals, 750 Washington Street, Box 32, Boston, MA 02111, USA

Eugenio Picano, Ist. di Fisiologia Clinica del C.N.R., Via Savi 8, I-56100 Pisa, Italy

Shimon A. Reisner, Department of Cardiology, Rambam Medical Center, Haifa 31096, Israel

Paolo Rizzon, Division of Cardiology, University of Bari, I-70124 Bari, Italy

Jos R. T. C. Roelandt, Thorax Center, Erasmus University, P.O. Box 1738, 3000 DR Rotterdam, The Netherlands

Daniele Rovai, CNR Clinical Physiology Inst., V. Savi 8, I-56100 Pisa, Italy

Patrick W. Serruys, Thorax Center, Erasmus University, P.O. Box 1738, 3000 DR Rotterdam, The Netherlands

Janine R. Shapiro, Box 604, University of Rochester Medical Center, Rochester, NY 14642, USA

John H. Smyllie, Thorax Center, Erasmus University, P.O. Box 1738, 3000 DR, The Netherlands

Giuseppe Specchia, Div. di Cardiologia, Univ. degli Studi, Policlinico S. Matteo, 27100 Pavia, Italy

Marc van Daele, Thorax Center, Erasmus University, P.O. Box 1738, 3000 DR, The Netherlands

Cees A. Visser, Dept. of Cardiology, Academisch Medisch Centrum, Meibergdreef 9, 1105 AZ Amsterdam, The Netherlands

Introduction

Today, coronary artery disease is one of the major causes of mortality and morbidity in the Western World. In the last decade many major diagnostic and therapeutic advances have been made, considerably furthering our potential in the management of coronary artery disease. At the same time, a new generation of cardiac tools has appeared. The field which has, perhaps, undergone the most important technological innovations is echocardiography. Nowadays, in fact, the world of ultrasounds offers the cardiologist a wide range of technical applicatons: two-dimensional real-time imaging, intra- and extra-cardiac Doppler flow measurements, real-time imaging of cardiac structure and flow by 2D color Doppler, high resolution cardiac imaging by transesophageal echocardiography, tissue characterization by analysis of ultrasound wave characteristics, information on myocardial perfusion by contrast echocardiography, etc. Thanks to these technical improvements and to its consequent increased potentiality, echocardiography now plays an important and irreplaceable role in the management of all cardiac diseases. In the field of coronary artery disease, echocardiography can reliably be used not only in the acute phases of the disease to derive useful functional and prognostic information but also as a stress diagnostic procedure (thanks to new stress modalities and the continuing improvement of reviewing digital systems) for the diagnosis of coronary artery disease and for the evaluation of various therapeutic interventions. Furthermore, other promising applications of ultrasounds in this disease are currently being investigated: tissue characterization, myocardial contrast echocardiography, coronary artery anatomy and flow evaluation by specially-designed ultrasound catheters.

This book evaluates the current situation and future potential of echocardiography in the management of patients with coronary artery disease.

PART ONE

Evaluation of wall motion abnormalities and stress echocardiography

1. Quantitative analysis of wall motion abnormalities

ANTONIO F. AMICO, SABINO ILICETO, VITO MARANGELLI,
GIOVANNI PICCINNI, FRANCESCO TOTA, LUCIA SUBLIMI
SAPONETTI, GAETANO D'AMBROSIO and PAOLO RIZZON

Introduction

Two-dimensional echocardiography has emerged as being an ideal non-invasive technique for studying the mechanical consequences of acute and chronic ischemia: because of its high spatial resolution, its sampling frequency and its safety, wall motion abnormalities can be identified within seconds of the onset of the ischemia and be monitored sequentially [1]. The clinical significance of the capability of the technique is demonstrated by the close relationship between the extent of the mechanical impairment as evaluated by echocardiography and the prognosis for the patients in whom spontaneous or induced ischemia is present [2–4].

In the light of such ideal characteristics, great efforts have been made to achieve quantitative, and therefore accurate, evaluations of the mechanical anomalies visualized by echocardiography. Some quantitative data could be better correlated to other important parameters in studying myocardial ischemia, as for example coronary blood flow and the histological extent of the infarct. This chapter sets out to revise the techniques put forward in echocardiography for quantitating wall motion abnormalities: although there are numerous studies on this subject, the ultimate aim of rapid and simple quantitative measurement of the regional function of the left ventricle has still not been definitively achieved.

Preliminary notions

Since two-dimensional echocardiography allows tomographic scanning of the heart in a theoretically unlimited number of planes, the sections to be used for quantitative readings need to be standardized, in order for them to be also reproducible. In research studies the parasternal sections in short axis are the ones commonly used: in fact, they provide anatomic landmarks which are sufficiently constant (mitral valve and papillary muscles) so that these sections can be comparable in different cases or with each other over time; moreover,

S. Iliceto et al. (eds.), Ultrasound in Coronary Artery Disease, 3–13.
© 1991 *Kluwer Academic Publishers.*

in the sections thus obtained, most of the endocardial points are visualized by using the axial resolution of the echocardiographic system which is much more accurate than the lateral resolution. A third advantage is that in order to obtain such sections a lower scansion depth than that required for the apical imaging planes is sufficient: thus the transducer scan rate can be proportionally higher on account of the shorter time required for the transit of the ultrasound impulses. Hence the parasternal planes show a better 'temporal resolution' than the deeper planes: however this resolution, of the utmost importance when analyzing the pattern of moving structures like the heart, is strongly affected by several technical factors linked partly to the echocardiographic system and partly to the system of image representation. The echocardiographic scan converter (Figure 1), which transforms the analogue signal from the transducer into a digital signal, has its own operative speed which varies from system to system, as well as its own speed for updating the image: this means that in any given time unit a part of the image collected in the converter is being continually updated, with the result that the overall data making up the single image are never really contemporaneous. Moreover, the video representation of the image picked up in the converter causes it to be produced by a vertical scanning of the screen with its own frequency, which will ultimately be the one that determines the system's actual temporal resolution. If the image is recorded on to a solid support, such as a video recorder or video disc, the final representation of the recorded image will be affected in its turn by the temporal resolution of this final link in the chain. Since the operative speeds of the single components of the system of representation (analogic-digital converter, video screen video, videorecorder) are not consistent with each other, it means that the final image, upon which the quantitative determinations are to be made, will show a certain heterogeneity of contraction which is not actually the case, but is related to the manipulations undergone along the representation chain.

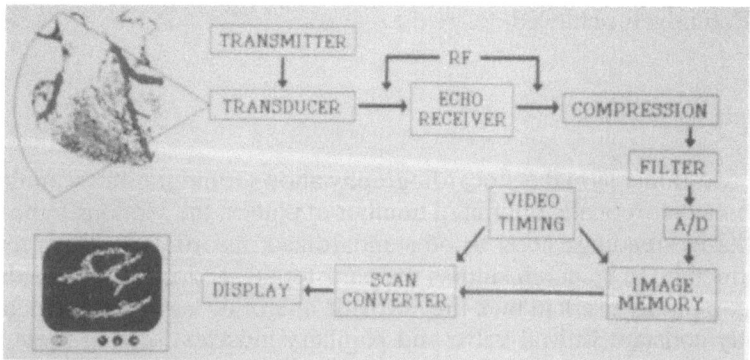

Figure 1. Schematic representation of the steps necessary to obtain an echocardiographic image from the reflected ultrasound beams. The manipulation of the image at each step could affect the quantitative analysis of the cardiac wall motion.

Apart from the technical problems summarized above, which must be borne in mind because of their affect on the accuracy of quantitative measurements, there are also other factors of a more anatomo-physiological nature which could create problems in analysing the images. The heart, in contracting, makes movements in space (partly rotating on one of its three axes, partly shortening on its longitudinal axis and partly totally translating) which could bring about the same echocardiographic section visualizing different anatomic sections during the course of the contraction. If during the contraction the base of the heart approaches the apex, in the short axis plane an apparent reduction of contractility will be recorded due to the magnifying of the section area.

Analysis of wall movement

The echocardiographic image of a short axis plane in the course of normal contraction shows the pattern briefly described as follows: the single points of the endocardium approach the centre of the ventricle, the perimeter bounded by the endocardium and the circular area within the ventricle are reduced in accordance; at the same time the wall thickness increases (Figure 2). Each of these patterns can in theory be 'measured' but for each of them a hypothetical 'measurement' creates different technical problems.

The first is common to all and is the identification of the endocardium: it can be produced by the operator or automatized [5, 6–9] by means of a process which is made up essentially of 4 steps:
- image enhancement;
- utilization of an algorithm called 'edge operator' which settles pixel by pixel whether it belongs to the endocardium image;

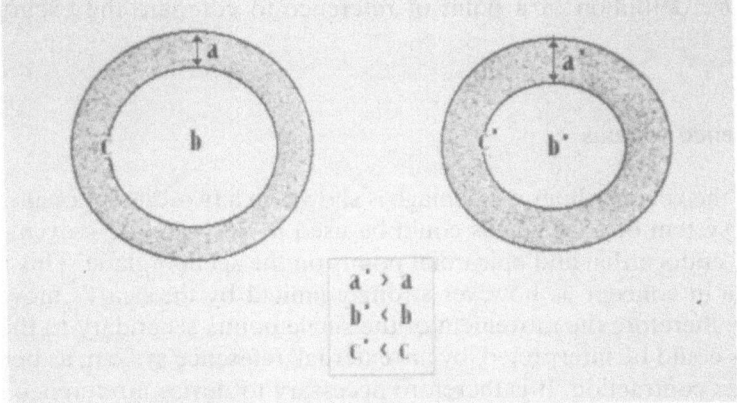

Figure 2. Schematic representation of the echocardiographic findings susceptible to quantitative evaluation during the cardiac contraction (see text).

- elimination of the pixels individually and wrongly attributed to the endocardium;
- filling of the spaces between the pixels definitively attributed to the endocardium to construct its continuous edge.

The greatest problem is obviously connected to the definition of the 'edge operator' algorithm for reducing the artefacts to a minimum: to this end 'interactive' algorithms have also been proposed in which computer definition occurred after a manual definition of a single frame on the part of the opera-tor [6].

After the endocardium has been identified it is necessary to record the position of the single points: these two steps, conceptually distinct, tend to be identified in most procedures utilized which envisage the continuous or dis-creet digitilization of the endocardial points by means of electronic cursor or automatic algorithms. The digital recording of the single endocardial points is essential since it is precisely on this data (made up of a pair of coordinates which identify on the plane the endocardial point in question) that all the calculations for the quantitative definition of the kinesis will subsequently be made.

The analysis of regional function in quantitative terms can utilize one or more of the contractile patterns described at the beginning of this paragraph, in other words the reduction of the ventricular cavity area, endocardial excur-sion [11] and wall thickening [12]. The two latter have been more extensively studied; for both endocardial definition is necessary, but to assess the thicken-ing, definition of the epicardium is also necessary. This type of definition is more problematic because of the reduced resolution in correspondence to the medial and lateral walls. Moreover wall thickening, being expressed in terms of percentage, can show great numerical variations even for small movements in absolute value of the endocardial and epicardial interfaces. In practice the endocardial excursion is mainly used for quantitative analysis. As pointed out previously, it is however affected by heart movements and requires the pre-liminary definition of a point of reference to compare the excursion itself with.

Reference systems

Since the echocardiographic image is shown on a two-dimentional screen, the same system of coordinates could be used to describe the movement of the single endocardial and epicardial points on the section plane. This approach, simple in concept, is however strongly limited by the heart's movements in space; therefore the movement of the single points secondary to these move-ments could be interpreted, by an 'external' reference system, as being due to cardiac contraction. It is therefore necessary to devise a reference system to move together with the heart so that only those movements which really express the contraction are recorded. It is in this direction that most studies have moved, since it should be extremely difficult to devise an 'internal' reference system which is able to identify and thus eliminate from the final computation all those movements caused by heart movements; moreover, even if such a system were to be set up, its accuracy could be affected by the type of echocardiographic plane being examined [10, 13–17].

Bearing in mind the circular configuration of the echocardiographic planes, all the internal reference systems devised are based on the hypothetical calculation of the ventricular mass, termed 'centroid'. Since no anatomic centroid exists, the calculation of such a centroid should be based in any case on the strict correlation with reproducible anatomic points. The mid-point on a line between the posterior junction of the right and left ventricle has been suggested [12] or the mid-point between the interventricular septum [10] and the respective endocardial surfaces opposite. Even though such centroids are theoretically reliable in examining a homogenous circular contraction, they may be less so where there are marked alterations of the segmentary contraction, especially if these abnormalities involve the above-mentioned anatomical reference points. A more complex, but more accurate, approach is to mathematically calculate the centre of the echocardiographic image using the largest possible number of points of the endocardial or epicardial profile. Numerous algorithms have been suggested, including those which calculate the centre of the ventricular cavity area or else the centre of the coordinates of the single endocardial points for each frame: the improved calculating capacity of modern computers can overcome the limitation of the greater number of operations necessary for a calculation of this type as compared to the approach using single anatomical reference points.

Once the reference point within the left ventricle has been decided, it is used for subdividing the ventricular walls into segments with rays starting from the centroid and intersecting the endocardial and epicardial profiles. Obviously these rays can number up to 360; the difficulty of manipulating too large a number of data forces a compromise between a sufficiently high number for achieving accurate measurements and a sufficiently low one to be of practical use (for example to correlate the wall segments deriving from the radial subdivision with the coronary distribution zones or with those which are most frequently affected by ischemic events in clinical practice). In an experimental study [18] it has been shown that wall movement anomalies induced by ischemia in the ventricle of a dog must have an angular extension of at least 5.5° to be significant; it is probable that in clinical echocardiography such an interval would be higher. Therefore the number of rays commonly used (from 8 to 12) is justified.

Once the ventricular centroid required for wall segmentation has been obtained, the movement of the single segments has to be compared image by image in order to check for any abnormalities of contraction. Such a comparison can be made using only one reference centroid (which can be the end-diastolic image or obtained mathematically as the average centroid of all the frames analyzed) onto which, during the course of the contraction, the shor-

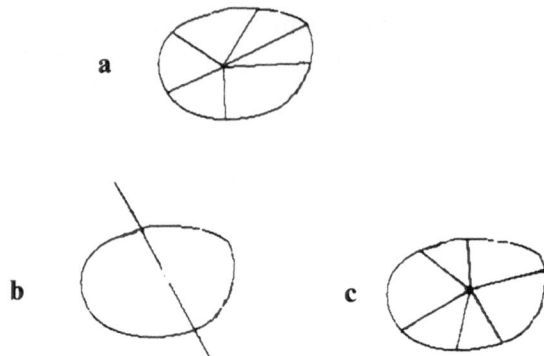

Figure 3. Comparison of the 'fixed axis' and 'floating axis' reference systems. The thin line represents the diastolic silhouette and the thick line the systolic silhouette of a left ventricle short axis. Radial shortening is, for each ray, the difference between the diastolic and systolic lengths of each ray divided by the diastolic length. *(a)* In the fixed axis system the centroid is obtained from the end-diastolic frame. *(b)* and *(c)* In the floating axis system the end-systolic centroid is superimposed to the end-diastolic centroid, thus avoiding the artifactual elongation of the rays due to heart translation.

tening of the preselected rays is measured: this system is termed 'fixed axis'. Alternatively the single centroids calculated in successive frames are superimposed onto those of the reference image ('floating axis' system) (Figure 3). The floating axis system appears to be the more attractive because it will be able to eliminate the effect of heart movements on the evaluation of wall movement. For example, if in a fixed axis system the systolic radium of a wall which has undergone a translation movement is compared with the diastolic radium, it will seem to have a lower excursion than the other rays, while the ray of the opposing wall will appear to have an increased excursion: therefore a hypokinesia and hyperkinesia will be evaluated which do not actually exist; in the floating axis system the superimposition of the systolic and diastolic centroids will lead to the correct evaluation of the contraction movements. However, if a dyskinesia is present, the systolic centroid calculated will appear to be shifted towards the asynergic area; when this centroid is superimposed onto the diastolic, the anomalous wall excursion will appear to be partially 'normalized', while the opposite wall will appear to be artificially hypokinetic, since the systolic rays calculated will have been 'lengthened' by the shifting of the centroid towards the asynergic area. The same situation, analyzed by the fixed axis system, would on the other hand be correctly interpreted. If, finally, the same wall shows a dyskinesia together with a translation movement, the effects of the two reference systems on the quantitative evaluations are more complex: the fixed axis system will overestimate both the wall anomaly as well as the normal function of the opposite wall; the floating axis system will identify the presence of a contraction anomaly but will underestimate and erroneously indicate the presence of a kinetic anomaly in relation to the opposite wall.

In conclusion, neither of the two systems is theoretically optimal; it is to be presumed from what has been said that a floating axis system could be more accurate in the case of significant translation movements, while the fixed axis system would be preferable in conditions in which heart movement in toto is less 'significant' compared to the wall motion. In closed chest experiments on dogs [17] it has been observed that the fixed axis system is more accurate than the floating axis in correlating wall motion abnormalities with reduction in coronary flow assessed with microspheres. Another experimental study [19], in which the quantitative echocardiographic assessment was correlated with the determination of wall thickening by means of Doppler probes implanted on the epicardium, concluded that the most accurate system was the floating axis with calculation of the epicardial centroid. The question therefore can still be considered open since no definite conclusions emerge for clinical echocardiographic application.

Identification of wall motion abnormalities and their quantitation

When the reference system to be used has been defined, the successive steps towards verifying the presence of wall motion abnormalities and determining their extent can thus be schematized:
- choice of cardiac cycle point in which the frames to be analyzed are to be acquired;
- choice of parameter to measure in the preselected frames;
- determination of normal and pathological values of the parameter.

If the ventricle contraction were perfectly symmetrical each endocardial point would shift by the same space in the same given time; unfortunately it has been shown that this is not so, even in perfectly normal hearts [12] and therefore the degree of shortening of the single rays can vary according to the cardiac cycle point being analyzed. Even the simple determination of end-diastole and end-systole creates problems; if for end-diastole the frame selected was the one in which the ventricular area is largest, and that for end-systole it was where it was smallest, in actual fact such frames would not be the equivalent of the corresponding moments of the cardiac cycle. For example the choice of frame with the smallest area (end-systole) also includes the isovolumetric relaxation period which strictly speaking belongs to the diastole. Alternatively, to mark end-diastole and end-systole, the maximum and minimum length of each ray could be chosen independently of the cardiac cycle phase; in doing so, since this type of analysis should be carried out frame by frame, it would make it possible to demonstrate more precisely the temporal heterogeneity of ventricle contraction along the preselected rays. However, the data obtained with this procedure would be very numerous: for a single cardiac cycle, shown in at least 8 frames, and for a single echocardiographic section divided into 36 rays (corresponding to an angular separation of 10 degrees), this would mean 288 numbers would be obtained. Even allowing for the measurements obtained not undergoing significant variations in different cycles, so that the analysis of a single cycle can be considered sufficient, such a figure would in any case be multiplied by the sections to be analyzed; the definitive number of data would therefore be high and difficult to handle.

The example given above refers to the measurement of a single parameter, namely the endocardial excursion. Obviously the whole procedure would have to be repeated for any other parameters such as the reduction of the cavity area, the reduction of the endocardial shortening and wall thickening. The analysis of radial endocardial shift and of area reduction does not seem to differ significantly as regards accuracy [17], although area determination should avoid excessive variability of data connected to irregularity of the endocardial profile. The endocardial perimeter between the two rays delimiting an ischemic area should, theoretically, reduce less than in the normal areas; however, it has been proved in experimental conditions [20] that this parameter, in normal areas, shows greater systolic reduction in the ventricle partially made ischemic as compared to non-ischemic conditions. Consequently, during ischemia, the actual ischemic area in percentage is overestimated since the whole endocardial perimeter will be reduced in comparison to the non-ischemic conditions. The final decisive step lies in determining the normality or abnormality of the parameters evaluated. From the general point of view, the definition of normality of a parameter may be obtained by fixing an interval of normality by means of statistical analysis in a normal population. Alternatively, the behaviour of this parameter is correlated to a condition of abnormality established independently.

The first approach has produced discouraging results: even in normal subjects there are important differences in local contraction [19, 21] both along the perimeter of the ventricle and along the base to apex axis [22]. Probably only wall thinning and dyskinesia show such a low frequency in normal subjects as to be considered certainly abnormal findings. In several experimental studies in which the ischemic area has been defined by means of histology or echocontrastography it has been observed that radial shortening in such an area can be lessened in a way which is not constant quantitatively: in one study, radial shortening of less than 10% was sufficient for accurately defining an ischemic area [23], in others this value reached 15% [18] or 20% [24].

Therefore such an approach does not provide conclusive results for accurately identifying the areas definable as ischemic on the basis of a change in motion. In one study [24], a modified method for calculating the centroid was suggested which gave better results. However, the high number of rays utilized renders it unfeasible for clinical purposes.

Other more complex methods have been put forward: in one study [25], a calculation was made of the *mean* radial shortening for all the rays chosen in an echocardiographic plane and for each frame of the systolic contraction. Then the shortening of each ray was compared with these mean values and the correlation coefficient was calculated between the relative values of the chosen ray and the mean values of the rays. If the ray chosen showed a shortening in keeping with the total mean then obviously the correlation coefficient approached unity while on the other hand it moved away as much from this value as the radial shortening, frame by frame, moved away from the behaviour of the total number of rays. The discriminating correlation coefficient value between normal and abnormal rays was calculated using 95% confidence limits of the correlation coefficients obtained in normal conditions. The delimitation of 'abnormal' wall segments with this method showed excellent correlation with the histological delimitation of the infarcted area.

Conclusions

The quantitation of wall motion abnormalities shown by two-dimensional echocardiography is an attractive topic because of its potential clinical applications. The possibility of measuring a mechanical parameter would make it possible to accurately and at the same time easily evaluate the effects of therapeutic interventions such as thrombolysis and angioplasty. The correlation of mechanical quantitative data with perfusional data would open up new possibilities of clinical research with regard to problems until now only experimentally compared. However, even today, it has not been proved that quantitative evaluations are better than semi-quantitative subjective ones: the capacity of the human eye to integrate in time and space can be emulated by means of complex algorithms which require the use of a very high number of data, a procedure which is still not applicable to routine purposes. The resolution of the mean clinical examinations is still today not sufficiently high to obtain reliable results with quantitative methods used for research. However, when particular operative conditions produce better quality images quantitative evaluations provide physiopathological information which is very refined [26]. The ever-improving resolution of echocardiographic instruments, the increasing adoption of methods like transesophageal and intraoperatory echocardiography, the development of digital echocardiography and of ever more powerful computers for processing images should all contribute to fulfilling expectations of a more quantitative approach to echocardiography in clinical practice.

References

1. Pandian NG, Kerber RE (1982) Two dimensional echocardiography in experimental coronary stenosis. I. Sensitivity and specificity in detecting transient myocardial dyskinesis: Comparison with sonomicrometers. *Circulation* 66: 597–602.
2. Gibson RS, Bishop HL, Stamm RB, Crampton RS, Beller GA, Martin RP (1982) Value of early two-dimensional echocardiography in patients with acute myocardial infarction. *Am J Cardiol* 49: 1110–1119.
3. Kan G, Visser CA, Koolen JJ, Dunning AJ (1986) Short and long term predictive value of

admission wall motion score in acute myocardial infarction: A cross sectional echocardiographic study of 345 patients. *Br. Heart J* 56: 422–7.

4. Iliceto S, Gaiati C, Ricci A, Amico A, Biasco G, Rizzon P (1988) Prognostic stratification of patients with recent uncomplicated myocardial infarction by transesophageal atrial pacing 2D Echo. *Circulation* 78, 4(II): 1094.

5. Garcia E, Gueret P, Bennett M, Corday E, Zwehl W, Meerbaum S, Corday S, Swan HJC, Berman D (1981) Real time computerization of two dimensional echocardiography. *Am Heart J* 101: 783–792.

6. Robinson EP, Pryor TA, Wellard SJ, Jones DS, Ridges JD (1976) Recognition of left ventricular borders using two dimensional echocardiograms: Identification of the endocardium. *Comput Biomed Res* 9: 247.

7. Skorton DJ, McNary CA, Child JS, Newton FC, Shah PM (1981) Digital image processing of two-dimensional echocardiograms: Identification of the endocardium. *Am J Cardiol* 48: 479.

8. Zhang L, Geiser EA (1984) An effective algorithm for extracting serial endocardial borders from two-dimensional echocardiograms. *IEEE TRans Bio Eng BME* 31: 441.

9. Collins SM, Skorton DJ, Geiser EA, Nichols JA, Conetta DA, Pandian NG, Kerber RE (1984) Computer-assisted edge detection in two-dimensional echocardiography: Comparison to anatomical data. *Am J Cardiol* 53: 1380.

10. Moynihan PF, Parisi AF, Feldman CL (1981) Quantitative detection of regional left ventricular contraction abnormalities by two-dimensional echocardiography. I. Analysis of methods. *Circulation* 63: 752–60.

11. Garrison JB, Weiss JL, Maughan WL, Tuck OM, Guier WH, Fortuin NJ (1977) Quantifying regional wall motion and thickening in two-dimensional echocardiography with a computer-aided contouring system. *Computers in Cardiology*, pp 25–35. Los Angeles, CA, IEEE Computer Society.

12. Pandian NG, Skorton DJ, Collins SM, Falsetti HL, Burke ER, Kerber RE (1985) Heterogeneity of left ventricular segmental wall thickening and excursion in 2-dimensional echocardiograms of normal human subjects. *Am J Cardiol* 51: 1667–73.

13. Parisi AF, Moyniham P, Folland ED, Feldman CL (1981) Quantitative detection of regional left ventricular contraction abnormalities by two-dimensional echocardiography. II. Accuracy in coronary artery disease. *Circulation* 63: 761–7.

14. Force T, Bloomfield P, O'Boyle JE, Pietro DA, Dunlap RW, Khuri SF, Parisi AF (1983) Quantitative two-dimensional echocardiographic analysis of motion and thickening of the interventricular septum after cardiac surgery. *Circulation* 68: 1013–20.

15. Force T, Bloomfield P, O'Boyle JE, Khuri SF, Josa M, Parisi AF (1984) Quantitative two-dimensional echocardiographic analysis of regional wall motion in patients with perioperative myocardial infarction. *Circulation* 70: 233–31.

16. Schnittger I, Fitzgerald PJ, Gordon EP, Alderman EL, Popp RL (1984) Computerized quantitative analysis of left ventricular wall motion by two-dimensional echocardiography. *Circulation* 70: 242–254.

17. Force TL, Parisi AF (1988) Quantitative Methods for Analyzing Regional Systolic Function with Two-Dimentional Echocardiography, in: Kerber RE (ed), *Echocardiography in Coronary Artery Disease*. Mount Kisco, New York: Futura Publishing Company.

18. Mann DL, Foale RA, Ascah KJ, Newell JB, Gillam LD, Weyman AE (1985) Persistence of abnormal wall motion in the canine ventricle after subacute infarction: Implications for reperfusion therapy. *J Am Coll Cardiol* 5: 425.

19. Zoghbi WA, Charlat ML, Bolli R, Zhu WX, Hartley CJ, Quinones MA (1980) Quantitative assessment of left ventricular wall motion by two-dimensional echocardiography: Validation during reversible ischemia in the conscious dog. *J Am Coll Cardiol* 11: 851–60.

20. Force T, Kemper A, Perkins L, Gilfoil M, Cohen C, Parisi AF (1980) Overestimation of infarct size by quantitative two-dimensional echocardiography: The role of tethering and of nalytic procedures. *Circulation* 73: 1360–68.

21. Franklin TD, Wiske PS, Clendenon JL et al. (1980) Variation in cross sectional echocardiographic radial target motion relative to a calculated mean centroid of the left ventricle. *Circulation* 62: 132.

22. Weyman AE, Franklin, TD, Hogan RD, Gillam LD, Wiske PS, Newell J, Gibbons EF, Foale RA (1984) Importance of temporal heterogenity in assessing the contraction abnormalities associated with acute myocardial ischemia. *Circulation* 70: 102–112.

23. Kaul S, Pandian NG, Gillam LD, Newell BA, Okada RD, Weyman AE (1986) Contrast echocardiography in acute myocardial ischemia. III. An in-vivo comparison of the extent of abnormal wall motion with the area at risk for necrosis. *J Am Coll Cardiol* 7: 383–92.

24. Mc Gillem MJ, Mancini GBJ, DeBoe SF, Buda AJ (1988) Modification of the centerline method for assessment of echocardiographic wall thickening and motion: A comparison with areas of risk. *J Am Coll Cardiol* 11: 861–6.

25. Gillam LD, Hogan RD, Foale RA, Franklin TD, Newell JB, Guyer DE, Weyman AE (1984) A comparison of quantitative echocardiographic methods for delineating infarct-induced abnormal wall motion. *Circulation* 70: 112–122.

26. Nicolosi AC, Spotnitz HM (1988) Quantitative analysis of regional systolic function with left ventricular aneurysm. *Circulation* 78: 856–62.

2. Assessment of wall motion by two-dimensional echocardiography
Should it be qualitative?

JOSEPH KISSLO and KHALID H. SHEIKH

Introduction

One common result of ischemia or infarction in patients with coronary artery disease is the development of segmental wall motion abnormalities of the left ventricle. In the desire to quantitate such abnormalities multiple computer based models for wall motion quantitation have been developed.

Quantitation of wall motion

Quantitative assessment of left ventricular wall motion requires comparison of spatial anatomic information in diastole with that in the subsequent systolic beat. Such quantitative methods require the assistance of computer based programs where endocardial borders are identified and digitized (by hand or automated). the computer than compares the traced border in diastole to that in systole and derives a number for any given area along the ventricular border.

Figure 1 demonstrates the principal of such quantitative approaches in schematic form superimposed on the left ventricular parasternal short axis. When images are of good quality and adequate endocardial and epicardial borders are identified. On the left is a diastolic image. Following digitization, the computer determines a mathematic centroid from which multiple radial lines are derived. Any number of equidistant radial lines may be determined around the circumference of the ventricle. Some programs may have as many as 360 such lines. In this example, however, only three such lines are shown for the purposes of simplicity.

The process is repeated in systole (right hand panel) and the center of the ventricle is calculated once again. For purposes of deriving a wall motion number, the computer than superimposes the diastolic and systolic centers of the ventricle and compares the position of the endocardium between the two cardiac cycles along each of the radial lines. The resultant number may be

S. Iliceto et al. (eds.), Ultrasound in Coronary Artery Disease, 15–20.
© 1991 *Kluwer Academic Publishers.*

Regional Abnormality

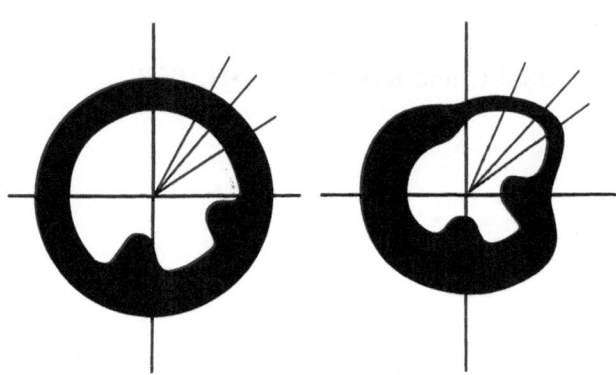

Figure 1. Overall principal for quantitative assessment of left ventricular wall motion. Diastole is on the left and systole is on the right (see text).

expressed as an absolute distance. More commonly, such numbers are expressed as percent shortening.

Quantitation of wall motion abnormalities

Figure 2 shows an ideal example of how such methods might be used to quantitate a specific wall motion abnormality. The left panel demonstrates the determination of the center of the left ventricle in diastole as before. The right panel, however, shows a discrete area of systolic wall thinning and dyskinesis.

In such an ideal model, the center of the ventricle remains the same in systole (right panel) so that the percent wall motion in the affected segment becomes negative (or away from the center). Data derived in such a way is than compared to normals and descriptive indices derived.

Problems in quantitation

This example is, however, only ideal. In reality, there are complex spatial differences between the position of the left ventricle in diastole compared to its position in systole. In normals, the ventricle moves somewhat anteriorly as the whole heart empties. At the same time, there are various rotations about the theoretic centroid of the ventricle making spatial determination of the true center difficult.

This problem is confounds the ability to easily quantify wall movement in individuals with severe wall motion abnormalities induced by ischemic heart disease. Figure 3 demonstrates one such significant limitation. The left panel

Quantitative Models

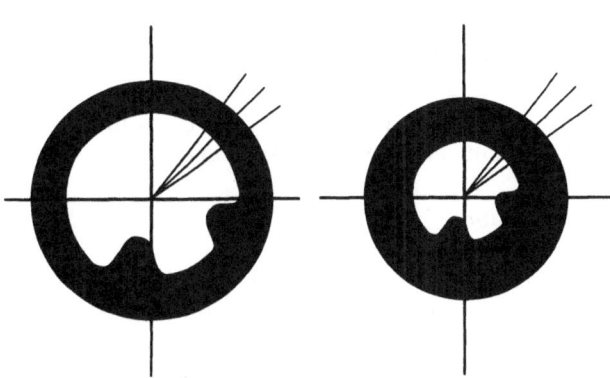

Figure 2. Schematic diagram of the left ventricular short axis demonstrating a severe left ventricular wall motion abnormality (see text).

shows the position of the short axis of the ventricle as before. In this computer model of quantitation of wall motion abnormalities the center of the ventricle is mathematically calculated from the circumference of the endocardial border. The right hand panel shows the problem. Calculation of the center of

Quantitative Limitation

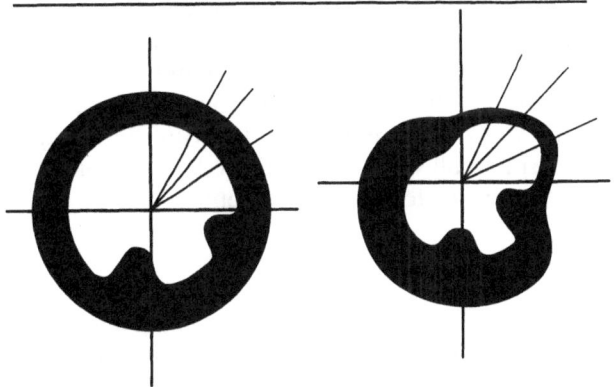

Figure 3. Schematic diagram of the left ventricular short axis demonstrating a severe limitation of any quantitative model. The centroid of the ventricle has moved making quantitation unreliable (see text).

the ventricle is profoundly affected by the severe wall motion abnormality at the upper right. The ventricular centroid is, in effect, moved upwards and to the right.

Any computer derived index of wall motion is then distorted by the abnormality in the systolic configuration of the ventricle. In this case, abnormal percent thickening would be identified by the computer around the entire circumference of the ventricle and the specific and discrete abnormality missed.

Models for quantitation

Almost all models for derivation of such quantitative data are highly dependent upon determination of the center of the left ventricle. As previously mentioned, the simplest models determine the diastolic and systolic center of the ventricle from a mathematic computation from the traced endocardial border. This approach is wholly inadequate because of the reasons previously cited. Any derived numbers are significantly distorted by the regional abnormality. The more discrete and severe the abnormality, the worse the distortion. This model is only applicable to very diffusely and symmetrically dilated left ventricles where there is little movement about any axis from the calculated diastolic ventricular center.

Recognition of these limitations has led to the development of other methods for determination of the ventricular center. One such method depends upon tracing both the diastolic and systolic endocardial and epicardial borders. Left ventricular spatial mass is then calculated and a center of mass derived. While spatial distortions are somewhat reduced with this approach they still exist to such a degree to deem this method unacceptable.

Other models have been developed in an attempt to overcome these problems. The center of the ventricle has been calculated spatially relating the position of the ventricule in diastole and systole to that of the chest wall and correcting these positions by the distance of the aorta from the chest wall at the same time in the cardiac cycle. Still other methods are dependent upon determination of the position of the papillary muscles in diastole and systole and then assuming a ventricular center from these positions. All methods derived from the ventricular centroid suffer from the complex spatial movements of the heart and all should be criticized in the context of their inability to adequately compensate for such movements.

Wall motion vs. wall thickness

Given these limitations other models of wall thickening, rather than percent shortening, have been developed. One such method with some appeal is the 'center line' method. Here, endocardial and epicardial boders are traced in diastole. Rather than calculate the center of the ventricle, hundreds of wall thicknesses are then calculated around the ventricular wall at equidistant points. The computer then calculates the center of the wall thickness along each equidistant point and each point is connected by a line, thus the name 'center-line'.

The same thing is done in systole and the same number of equidistant lines of thickness calculated. A systolic center line is calculated by connecting the mid point of each line. This method attempts to overcome severe spatial distortions but is not completely free of such problems.

The problem with quantitation

It can thus be concluded that all models for development of quantitative indices of wall motion are distorted to greater or lesser degrees by the spatial movement of the heart. In addition, such methods require superior quality images of both endocardium and epicardium at diastole and systole. Images of sufficient quality are difficult to acquire from the chest wall in older patients with ischemic heart disease. Further compounding quantitative methods is that they are very time consuming and require tedious identification of target information from recorded images.

It is understandable that practitioners desire quantitative indices. Such indices would provide practical estimates of infarct healing or extension when obtained at multiple points in time. Despite this desirability for deriving 'numbers' from echocardiographic images practicioners must keep in mind the limitations of any quantitative method. When the numbers are subject to distortions induced by complex three-dimensional spatial targets an unwarranted sense of security may result.

Subjective assessment of wall motion

To date, subjective interpretation of wall motion abnormalities remains the most practical method to approach. It is true that any subjective approach is inherently limited by inter and intra-observer variability. While this approach requires interpreter experience, it is likely that most individuals who use echocardiography in the evaluation of wall motion abnormalities can acquire such experience over time.

It appears that adequate physician interaction with angiographic images has been derived over time for the assessment of wall motion. When wall motion abnormalities occur they result in hypokinesis, akinesis or dyskinesis over a given wall segment. While such subjective interpretation of wall motion abnormalities is not precise, the ability of the human eye to integrate the complex spatial movements of the left ventricle helps to readily define the area of abnormality and assess its severity. Such methods are practised daily in most catheterization laboratories and have allowed for accurate communication of findings between physicians and have provided the basis for everyday clinical decision making.

Such methods can also be practiced based upon two-dimensional echocardiographic images. Various subjective wall scoring indices have been derived and most have been shown to be reproducable between various observers. The heart can roughly be divided into five major wall segments: septal, anterior, inferior, posterior and apical. Wall motion may be rated as normal, hypokinetic, akinetic, dyskinetic or aneurysmal at any of the segments with normal being given one point and aneurysmal five points. Using such subjectively based criteria, a normal ventricle then receives a total score of five with increasing scores implying more severe degrees of wall motion abnormality.

Continued experience with patients with coronary artery disease indicates that patients with normal, or near normal, wall motion have a better prognosis (for medical or surgical treatment) than those with severe wall motion abnormalities. Patients with massive infarctions and diffusely impaired wall motion abnormalities are likely to have an undesirable outcome when compared to those with small infarctions and consequently mild wall motion abnormalities.

A serious question remains whether the level of precision for determination and indexing wall motion abnormalities by computer aided methods has been achieved at present. For the basic clinical questions faced in everyday practice, subjective interpretation may provide the same (or even better) information more quickly and at lower cost. Once adequate quantitative models are developed it is likely that new, and more complex, clinical questions may be asked and perhaps answered. Until such time, however, the use of subjective and roughly qualitative assessments of wall motion serve to remind the practioner of the limitations of the results of any method.

3. Real-time, three-dimensional echocardiography
Feasibility and its potential use in evaluation of coronary artery disease

JOSEPH KISSLO and OLAF VON RAMM

Introduction

It has long been desirable to acquire as much spatial anatomic data about the heart as possible. Two-dimensional echocardiography offered considerable advantages over M-mode echocardiography because of the ability to provide real-time tomographic images of the heart and it extended the ability of practicioners to make complex diagnostic decisions. In the beginning, there were questions by some whether two-dimensional approaches were worth the time and expense. Continued experience with these methods provided an opportunity for clinicians to ask new questions. Similarly, three-dimensional echocardiography appears to be a desirable goal as it would likely provide a method for deriving new anatomic, functional and flow indices of the human heart.

Two-dimensional limitations

Despite the obvious advantages of two-dimensional echo methods over M-mode, serious limitations remain. Cardiac structures are spatially complex and a mental picture of the heart must be acquired from a series of two-dimensional interrogations. For example, calculation of ventricular volume by echocardiography must be performed based upon complex geometric assumptions such as whether a ventricle is elliptical or not. In the setting of a severe regional wall motion abnormality the ventricle may not conform to any geometric assumption and the resultant quantitative volume information is, therefore, limited.

Likewise, quantitative assessment of wall motion data derived from two-dimensional echocardiography is subject to limitations imposed by the complex spatial forward and rotational movements of the heart between diastole and systole. Almost all such computer based models are, therefore, inherently limited because it becomes spatially impossible to determine the same center geometric center of the ventricle between diastole and systolic for reliable determination of wall motion indices.

S. Iliceto et al. (eds.), Ultrasound in Coronary Artery Disease, 21–29.
© 1991 *Kluwer Academic Publishers.*

Three-dimensional reconstructions

Multiple attempts have been made to provide three-dimensional data from echocardiographic images. The most common the post acquisition three-dimensional reconstruction. Most echocardiographers are familiar with this approach where multiple two-dimensional views of the left ventricle are acquired. The transducer is equipped with a spark gap device that registers the spatial orientation of the transducer on x, y a z coordinates. The epicardial and endocardial borders of the left ventricle are then digitized 'off-line' and the coordinates entered into a computer. A three-dimensional image is then derived.

Such methods suffer from the fact that the derived data is collected at different times and are, therefore, not real-time. Accordingly, it is difficult to evaluate complex beat-to-beat changes of the heart as the final data is a composite of multiple beats collected over time.

In addition, such methods must necessarily reduce the highly resolved two-dimensional image data to a series of spatial points. For example, the entire circumference of the left ventricle is reduced to perhaps 20 points, connected by a series of lines to enable the computer to handle the detailed manipulations of reconstruction. The resultant image is the familiar 'birdcage' three-dimensional image of the left ventricle.

Three-dimensional echocardiography

Attempts to collect echo information in real-time have been in evolution for some time. Conventional two-dimensional images are the result of the transit

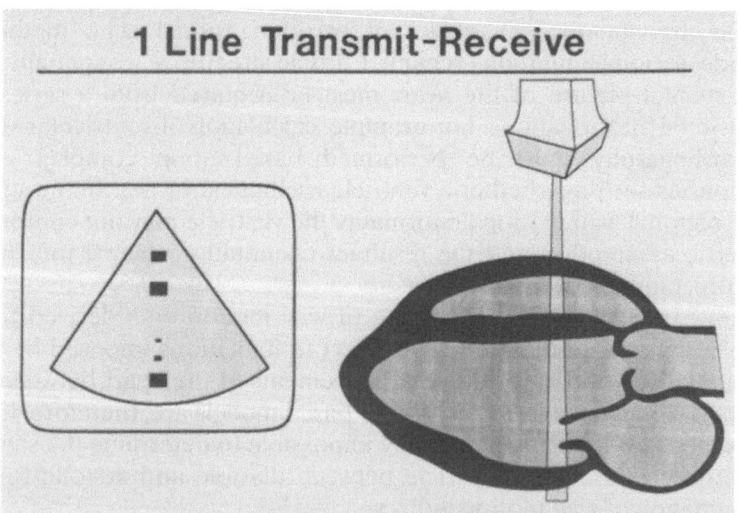

Figure 1. Schematic diagram of conventional 1 line transmit and receive sequence. For any single line (*right*) only a small amount of data is collected (*left*).

of ultrasound to and from a given target in space. Images of sufficient range and line density require conventional imaging systems to operate in single one line transmit and receive. Figure 1 demonstrates the fact that, for any single transmit-receive sequence, very little spatiel data is collected. Thus, there is little time available for a conventional system to interrogate in dimensions outside the primary plane of interest.

Methods to this point have involved the use of two imaging systems, one scanning in one plane and the alternate system in the other. Unless temporally sequenced, however, the ultrasound output of one system severly interferes with the other.

Other attempts have been made using one system but two alternating transducers. One scans in one dimension while the other scans in an alternate dimension or plane. Such systems are not 'real-time'.

Parallel processing

The key to real-time, three-dimensional echocardiography lies in the use of parallel processing techniques similiar to those common in computer processing. Here, multiple receive lines are collected for every single transmit sequence. When this can be done efficiently, more data returns to the transducer from any single transmit-receive sequence. Figure 2 demonstrates this point schematically.

Using this approach, images of low line density may be created that are of similiar quality to conventional scanning systems. Figure 3 shows successive parasternal short axis images from the Duke University phased array prototype scanning device. Panel *A* demonstrates an image operating in a conventional single line transmit-receive sequence comprised of 128 lines. Panel *B* shows the same system operating in a conventional 24 line scan. There is obvious image degradation.

Panel *C* demonstrates a 24 line scan with a 4:1 parallel process. Here 24 lines of transmit data are used to collect 96 lines of receive information. The resultant image is similiar in quality to Panel *A*. This achievement further demonstrates that the ultrasound system has time left over to operate at frame rates commensurate with cardiac dynamics while using other parallel processed transmit-receive sequences to scan in other planes.

Panel *D* shows the resultant image from such an initial trial. It is the resultant image of four real-time scan planes directed from the same transducer from four separate origins, each the result of a 4:1 parallel process. Note the wide origin of the ultrasound data at the skin surface. Here, the image is likely improved in data acquision over Panel A not only because of the increased data collection but because of the compounding effect of the four sector arcs.

Real-time orthogonal imaging

Using these methods, a transducer was then fabricated with the face plate cut

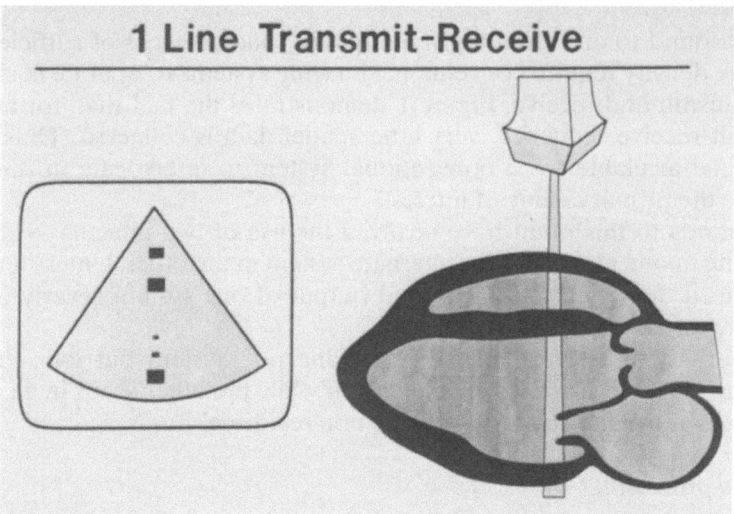

Figure 2. Schematic diagram showing the parallel processing principal. For any single transmit sequence (*right*), multiple lines are collected in receive resulting in more data in the image (*left*) and considerable system efficiency.

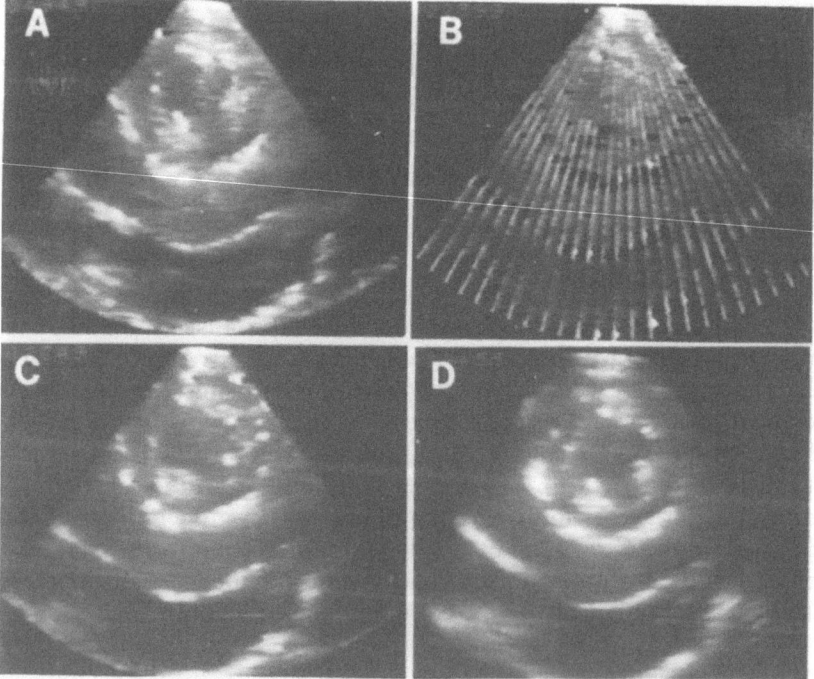

Figure 3. Parasternal short axes from a patient with a pericardial effusion demonstrating the effect of parallel processing. For explanation, see text.

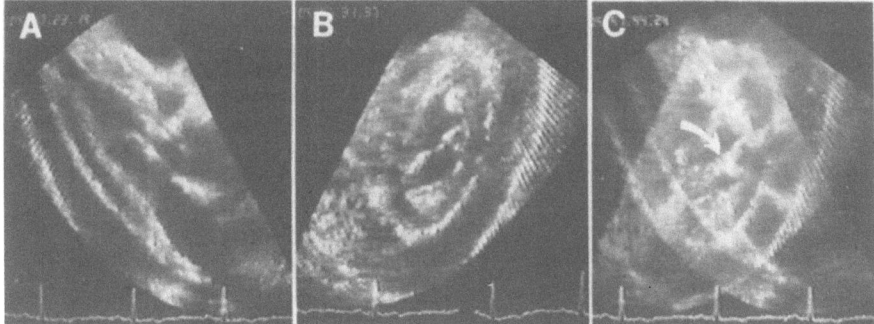

Figure 4. Still frame images derived from a real-time orthogonal mode scan (O-mode). Panel *A* shows a long axis; Panel *B* shows the short axis; Panel *C* shows simultaneous long and short. The arrow points to the intersection of both planes of the mitral valve (see text).

in a 'bow-tie' fashion. When operating in a parallel processed mode images could be simultaneously collected in true orthogonal planes. Figure 4 shows the result of such a manipulation within the Duke phased array prototype scanner. Panel *A* demonstrates a single parasternal long axis with the apex tilted toward the viewer and the scan plan electronically rotated to give the viewer perspective. Panel *B* shows the isolated short axis from the same subject. Panel *C* demonstrates the resultant simultaneous acquisition and presentation of both planes.

Such O-mode images are most confusing since there is so much data available to the viewer at any time. This accomplishment demonstrated, however, that a single ultrasound scanner could operate in two-dimensions simultaneously, a necessary precursor to real-time, three-dimensional echocardiography.

Real-time, three-dimensional echocardiography

Extension of these principals were then made toward acquiring data in three-dimensions. Further modifications were made to the Duke scanning system and transducers were fabricated to allow for true real-time, three-dimensional scanning within a pyramidal volume. Figure 5 demonstrates the volume within such a scanning system was able to interrogate.

Figure 6 shows the face of a conventional transducer as opposed to the three-dimensional configuration. The three-dimensional transducer face is comprised of rows of very small elements, able to interrogate in any plane within the pyramidal volume.

Data presentation from a real-time, three-dimensional scanning system requires special devices, not yet adapted for this purpose. In lieu of such systems, data is now presented in C-scans which are quadrangular images at any plane parallel to the transducer surface, rather than parallel as with conven-

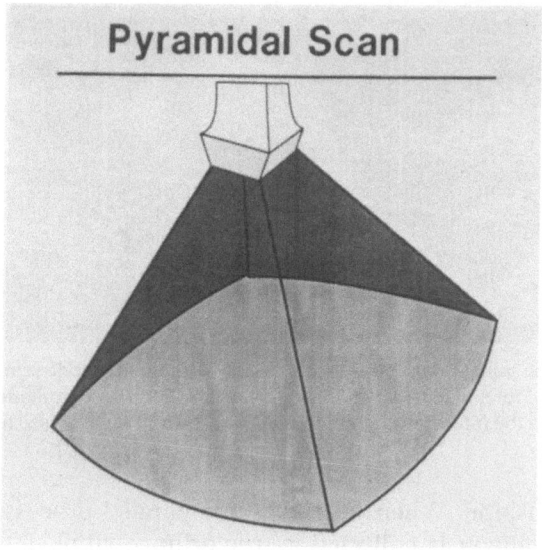

Figure 5. Schematic diagram of a pyramidal scan.

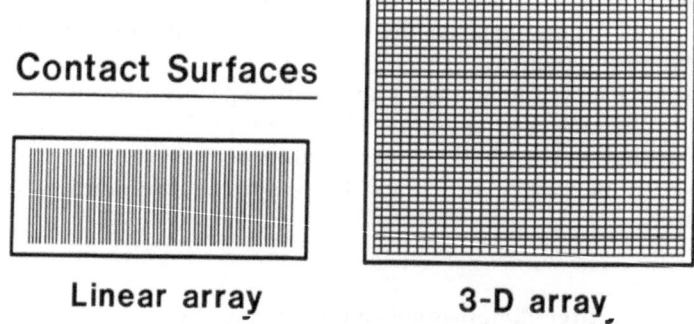

Figure 6. Schematic diagram of the face of a conventional linear array (*left*) and a three-dimensional array (*right*) (see text).

tional scanners. Figure 7 schematically demonstrates a series of C-scan planes.

Under current operating specifications, real-time, three-dimensional scanning within a water tank is now possible. Figure 8 shows a wrench presented in C-scan modified for perspective imaging. Perspective imaging shows objects closer to the transducer face as larger (left panel) than those held farther from the transducer face (right panel). Images are of 400 lines within the pyramidal volume and at frame rates of nearly 15 per second.

Because of the small transducer elements, significant problems with signal to noise remain. In addition, beam profiles are currently limited that, combined with signal to noise problems, limit application to human use. Such

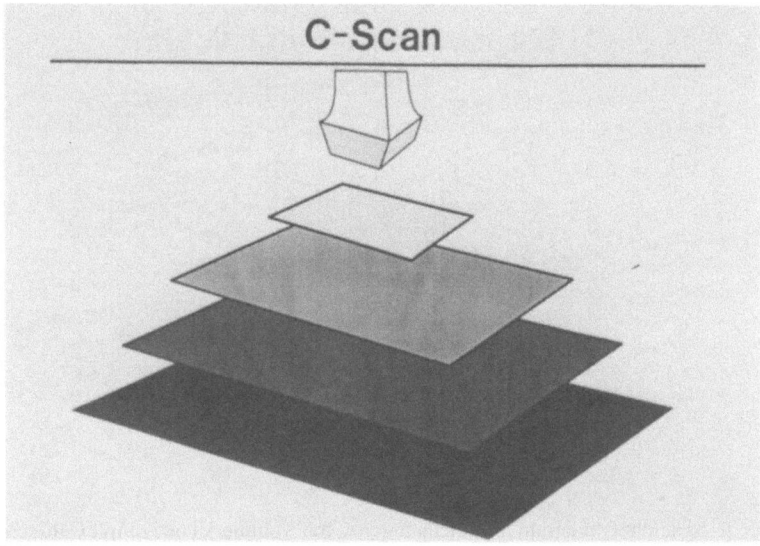

Figure 7. Schematic diagram of a C-scan presentation. Images are displayed with data parallel, rather than perpendicular as in a conventional sector arc format (see text).

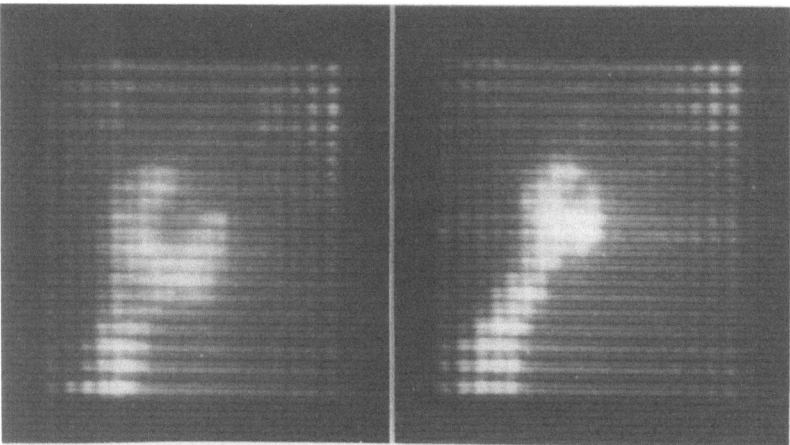

Figure 8. Still-frames from a real-time, three-dimensional C-scan scan of a wrench with perspective. The wrench is larger (left panel) when it is held close to the transducer and smaller (right panel) when it is held farther away.

advances do, however, demonstrate that real-time, three-dimensional echocardiography is a future probability.

Future use

When such images are possible, a host of new questions may be answered. For example, the volume of any complex structure may be calculated from a

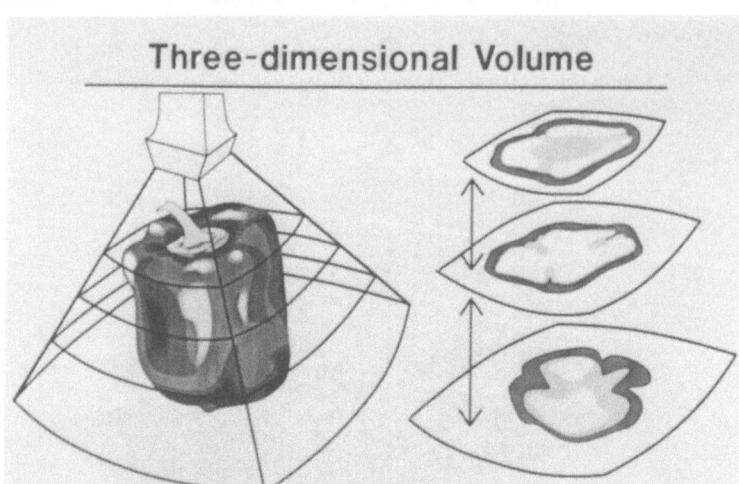

Three-dimensional Volume

Figure 9. Schematic diagram of calculation of the volume of a complex three-dimensional structure such as a green pepper. Volume may be calculated from the C-scan data independent of any geometric assumption.

series of C-scan planes free from any geometric assumption. Figure 9 shows a schematic rendition of calculation of the volume of a complex geometric object such as a green pepper. C-scan data could be planimetered by hand or by other automated device. Since the distance between C-scan planes is known, the volume could readily be determined.

These principals could then be used to collect beat-to-beat reliable volume data from any configuration left ventricle. With no geometric assumptions required, more reliable data would likely become available.

Now with direct ultrasound based myocardial perfusion techniques becoming more available. Real-time, three-dimensional studies into the volume of perfused and non perfused myocardium would provide a basis for more detailed studies of patients with coronary artery disease. Figure 10 shows a intraoperative epicardial injection of contrast into a saphenous vein bypass graft demonstrating the area of perfused myocardium.

the future possibility also exists for the adaptation of these methods to color flow imaging. When accomplished, the absolute volume of regurgitant flows can be calculated.

Such real-time methods based upon phased array devices hold great promise for the development of wholly new descriptors of left ventricular performance, myocardial perfusion and other indices in patients with coronary artery disease. Progress is, however, time-consuming and necessarily slow and several years remain before the ready adaptability of these approaches in humans.

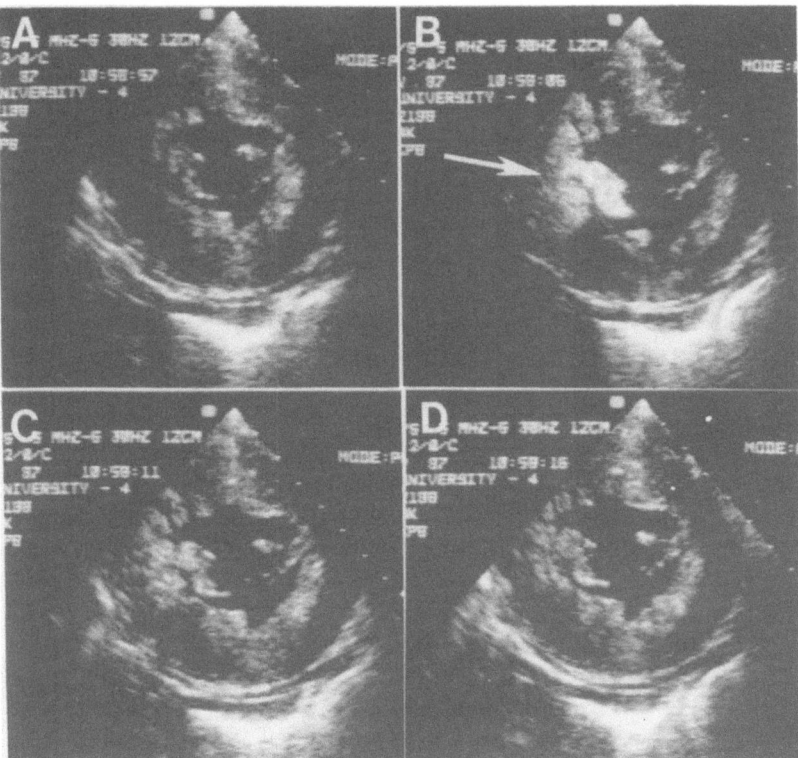

Figure 10. Sequential epicardial short axes demonstrating the baseline (Panel *A*) and inital uptake of contrast (arrow – Panel *B*) into the myocardium from a direct injection into a freshly placed saphenous vein graft. The contrast progressively disappears over a few seconds (Panels *C*, *D*).

4. Exercise 2D echocardiography
How reliable is it as a routine tool for the assessment of coronary artery disease?

HARVEY FEIGENBAUM

Introduction

One of the earliest and most fundamental consequences of myocardial ische-mia is alterations in systolic function of the affected myocardium. There are numerous experimental and clinical observations confirming that when coro-nary blood flow is impeded, reduced myocardial function is a reproducible consequence. There are many practical reasons why two-dimensional echo-cardiography is an ideal means for assessing regional ventricular function in the setting of coronary artery disease. The tomographic technique permits multiple views of the heart so that virtually every segment of the left ventricle can be assessed. The examination is obtained in real-time with excellent spa-tial and temporal resolution. Ventricular function can be judged with regard to wall thickening as well as wall motion. The fact that the examination is obtained with an instrument which is portable, permits the ultrasonic assess-ment to be performed in multiple settings, such as the coronary care unit or exercise laboratory. The examination is painless, as best we can determine harmless, avoids any ionizing radiation, and is truly non-invasive not even requiring an intravenous injection. The examination is also less costly than many other sophisticated imaging techniques.

Feasibility

Despite these many practical and theoretical advantages the use of two-dimensional echocardiography for evaluating ischemic myocardium is not nearly as widespread as one would anticipate. One of the major misconcep-tions is that two-dimensional echocardiography is technically demanding and that a large percentage of the patients, especially in the coronary disease population, are impossible to examine adequately. In addition, many feel that the expertise involved in obtaining and interpreting such an examination is so great that only a few 'experts' are able to obtain clinically useful information with this technique. This perception has been propagated for many years and

S. Iliceto et al. (eds.), Ultrasound in Coronary Artery Disease, 31–36.
© 1991 *Kluwer Academic Publishers.*

is erroneous. With only a modest amount of training and experience one should be able to use echocardiography as well in the setting of coronary artery disease as with any other form of heart disease. Many of the early misconceptions are based on limitations peculiar to M-mode echocardiography, most of which have been eliminated with the advent of two-dimensional echocardiography.

If two-dimensional echocardiography is an excellent and practical technique for detecting ischemia muscle, then the examination should be of value in noting changes in ischemic myocardium. For example one should be able to note improvement or deterioration in segmental function as a consequence of acute myocardial infarction. Furthermore one should be able to induce ischemia and detect the changes in ventricular function. The induction of ischemia could be a result of any stress which alters the supply and demand of coronary blood flow. Although there are many forms of stress which can induce ischemia, the most popular is exercise, either using a bicycle or a treadmill.

Practicality

Shortly after the introduction of two-dimensional echocardiography investigators began using this technique for evaluating patients with coronary artery disease and exercise testing. There were several early studies confirming the fact that two-dimensional echocardiography was in fact an excellent tool for detecting regional wall motion abnormalities resulting from of exercise-induced ischemia [1–7]. The sensitivity and specificity of these early studies were quite good and comparable to data being generated by other imaging technologies such as nuclear cardiology [8–11]. Despite these optimistic reports exercise echocardiography did not become an instantly popular technique. First of all there were many technical limitations that impeded its widespread use. The early studies utilized supine bicycle exercise. This approach was not ideal for echocardiographic studies. The echocardiographic window is not very good with the patient flat on his or her back. It is preferred that the patient be in the left lateral position to get the best quality images. In addition supine leg exercise may not always be adequate for producing ischemia since leg fatigue may be the limiting factor.

A significant advance in exercise echocardiography came about when some institutions demonstrated that one could obtain an echocardiogram immediately after treadmill exercise testing and still detect ischemic wall motion abnormalities [9, 11, 12]. These changes apparently persist long enough to be detected by a rapidly obtained two-dimensional echocardiographic examination. Several independent laboratories confirmed that the exercise-induced wall motion abnormalities persist for several minutes and that they can be detected with a post exercise echocardiogram. This observation greatly increased the success rate in performing exercise echocardiography since the patient could be examined in a more favorable setting for adequate images. Other investigators also noted that one could obtain clinically useful echocardiographic studies in patients undergoing upright bicycle exercise [13–15].

With this wealth of clinical and experimental data it was evidence that exercise echocardiography was a potentially viable technique for the clinical assessment of coronary artery disease. There was particularly impressive data on the value of exercise echocardiography for risk stratification following an acute myocardial infarction [16–18]. Despite these findings there still remained many practical difficulties which discouraged physicians from pursuing this test. The 2D examination was obviously done in real-time either during or immediately after the exercise. One can attempt to assess the wall motion while the examination is in progress. Such an approach can easily detect gross alterations in ventricular function. However it is unlikely that any subtle changes in wall motion could be detected with this method. Two-dimensional echocardiography is customarily recorded on videotape. Thus one could review the videotape for comparative evaluation of the resting and exercise echocardiogram. Although this type of analysis can be done at one's leisure, there are still technical difficulties in using videotape for analyzing exercise echocardiograms. The resting study is obviously not a major challenge; however interpreting the videotape of an exercise echocardiogram can be extremely difficult. There is respiratory artifact which causes the cardiac image to move in and out of view frequently. It is quite difficult trying to detect subtle wall motion changes with the heart moving in and out of the examining plane. One also must use ones memory to compare the resting images with the corresponding examination during or after exercise. Despite these difficulties most of the data in the literature was generated utilizing videotape recordings and the findings have been quite reasonable. Many of these studies however were performed for investigational purposes and exercise echocardiography was still not being obtained for routine clinical care.

The major development which has renewed interest and gained some popularity for exercise echocardiography is the introduction of digital recording and display of two-dimensional echocardiograms. By digitally recording the images one now has the ability to edit the examination so as to eliminate much of the respiratory artifact. By creating a continuous loop of a single cardiac cycle one can choose that cardiac cycle in which there is no respiratory artifact. Thus the exercising heart can be viewed without the nuisance of seeing lung artifact. Furthermore since the images are now in a digital form, the corresponding resting and exercising views can be displayed side-by-side for direct comparison. The advantages of this digital approach are numerous. The analysis of the study is much more convenient and sensitive. The examination is faster since only a few cardiac cycles are required rather than needing a twenty or thirty second recording of each cardiac view. Since the digital acquisition can now be done on-line, the speed with which the study can be done and analyzed is greatly enhanced. The examination can be retrieved and matched side-by-side before the patient leaves the laboratory. This digital recording and analysis technique has made exercise echocardiography a practical alternative to other forms of exercise testing. Much of the technical difficulty has been reduced with this development. In those institutions performing exercise echocardiography on a routine basis clinically useful interpretations can be obtained on over 90% of all patients [19–22].

Technical details

There is a variety of different protocols one can use with exercise echocardiography. The simplist protocol utilizes a four view examination before and immediately after treadmill exercise. The patient is examined in the left lateral position for both parts of the study. The post exercise examination can be followed with a recovery study several minutes later to see whether or not the wall motion abnormalities revert back to normal. If bicycle exercise either in the supine or upright positions is used, then one can also record the echocardiogram during exercise. The number of views one utilizes is also variable. When performing the study during exercise one probably will not want more than two views. The two views most commonly used would either be the apical four and two chamber views or the subcostal short-axis and four chamber views. The pre and post exercise examinations in the left lateral position can consist of more than two views.

The sensitivity and specificity of exercise echocardiography will naturally vary from institution to institution and from study to study largely dependent upon the type of patient being studied and the reference to which the echocardiogram is being compared. Almost every institution is claimining a sensitivity and specificity between 80% and 90% which is well within the same range as with comparable nuclear techniques. The ability to identify the regions supplied by individual arteries is also as good if not better than with a comparable nuclear approach. Thus it is safe to say that exercise echocardiography is a clinically viable and important technique and is very likely comparable to nuclear approaches. Unfortunately there is a small number of comparative studies with nuclear cardiology. There clearly is room for additional comparative evaluations.

Although exercise echocardiography is feasible in over 90% of all patients, the technical difficulties can't be ignored. There are technical details necessary in learning how to perform the test adequately. Possibly even more difficulty occurs with the interpretation of subtle wall motion changes which can occur with exercise. Despite these challenges the procedure is well worth the effort because of the valuable information it provides. The learning curve for both the person performing the examination and the one making the interpretations is not much different than with any other aspect of echocardiography. For many of us it probably took longer to learn the intricacies of Doppler echocardiography than it was to master the technique of two-dimensional exercise echocardiography.

Exercise echocardiography may not be ideal for every institution. If nuclear cardiology is well established and providing excellent results, the incentive or necessity to establish a competitive exercise echocardiographic laboratory may be fairly low. However if there is a desire for an alternative approach to evaluating patients with coronary artery disease, exercise echocardiography should be seriously considered.

References

1. Wann LS, Faris JV, Childress RH, Dillon JC, Weyman AE, Feigenbaum H (1979) Exercise cross-sectional echocardiography in ischemic heart disease. *Circulation* 60: 1300.
2. Paulsen WJ, Boughner DR, Friesen A, Persaud JA (1979) Ventricular response to isometric and isotonic exercise: Echocardiographic assessment. *Br Heart J* 42: 521.
3. Morganroth J, Chen CC, David D, Sawin HS, Natio M, Parrotto C, Meixell L (1981) Exercise cross-sectional echocardiographic diagnosis of coronary artery disease. *Am J Cardiol* 47: 20.
4. Naito H, Matsuzaki M, Takahashi Y, Natsuda Y, Ogawa H, Sasaki T, Kumada T, Kusukawa R, Takashiba K, Ikee Y (1981) Exercise echocardiography: Interventricular septal wall motion dynamics in patients with left anterior descending coronary disease during recovery (author's transl). *J Cardiogr* 11: 79.
5. Takahashi H, Koga Y, Itaya M, Nagata H, Itaya K, Ohkita Y, Bekki H, Jinnouchi J, Utsu F, Toshima H (1981) Detection of exercise induced left ventricular asynergy by two-dimensional echocardiography. *J Cardiogr* 11: 1193.
6. Fedele F, Arata L, Giannico S, Oastore LR, DiRenzi L, Penco M, Agati L, Dagianti A (1981) Echocardiography during ergometric tests in subjects with stable effort angina (author's transl). *G Ital Cardiol* 11: 310.
7. Crawford MH, Amon KW, Vance WS (1982) Exercise two-dimensional echocardiography: Quantitation of left ventricular performance in patients with severe angina pectoris. *Am J Cardiol* 51: 1.
8. Visser CA, Van der Wieken RL, Kan G et al. (1983) Comparison of two-dimensional echocardiography with radionuclide angiography during dynamic exercise for the detection of coronary artery disease. *Am Heart J* 106: 528.
9. Limacher MC, Quinones MA, Polner LR, Nelson JG, Wintters WL Jr, Waggoner AD (1983) Detection of coronary artery disease with exercise two-dimensional echocardiography. *Circulation* 67: 1211.
10. Crawford MH, Petru MA, Amon W, Sorensen SG, Vance WS (1984) Comparative value of two-dimensional echocardiography and radionuclide angiography for quantitating changes in left ventricular performance during exercise limited by angina pectoris. *Am J Cardiol* 53: 42.
11. Maurer G, Nanda NC (1981) Two-dimensional echocardiographic evaluation of exercise-induced left and right ventricular asynergy: Correlation with thallium scanning. *Am J Cardiol* 48: 720.
12. Robertson WS, Feigenbaum H, Armstrong WF, Dillon JC, O'Donnell J, McHenry PW (1983) Exercise echocardiography: A clinically practical addition in the evaluation of coronary artery disease. *J Am Coll Cardiol* 2: 1085.
13. Ginzton LE, Gonant R, Brizendine M, Lee F, Mena I, Laks MM (1984) Exercise subcostal two-dimensional echocardiography: A new method of segmental wall motion analysis. *Am J Cardiol* 53: 805.
14. Applegate RJ, Crawford MH (1985) Combined exercise stress testing and echocardiography in the diagnosis of coronary artery disease. *Practical Cardiology* 11: 73.
15. Presti CF, Armstrong WF, Feigenbaum H (1988) Comparison of echocardiography at peak

exercise and after bicycle exercise in evaluation of patients with known or suspected coronary artery disease. *J Am Society Echo*: 119.

16. Jaarsma W, Visser CA, Kupper AJF, Res JCJ, Van Eenige MJ, Ross JP (1986) Usefulness of two-dimensional exercise echocardiography shortly after myocardial infarction. *Am J Cardiol* 57: 86.
17. Ryan T, Armstrong WF, O'Donnell J, Feigenbaum H (1987) Risk stratification following myocardial infarction using exercise echocardiography. *Am Heart J* 114: 1305.
18. Applegate RJ, Dell'Italia LJ, Crawford MH (1987) Usefulness of two-dimensional echocardiography during low-level exercise testing early after uncomplicated myocardial infarction. *Am J Cardiol* 60: 10.
19. Armstrong WF, O'Donnell J, Dillon JC, McHenry PL, Morris SN, Feigenbaum H (1986) Complementary value of two-dimensional exercise echocardiography to routine treadmill testing. *Ann Intern Med* 105: 829.
20. Ryan T, Vasey CG, Presti CF, O'Donnell JA, Feigenbaum H, Armstrong WF (1988) Exercise echocardiography: Detection of coronary artery disease in patients with normal left ventricular wall motion at rest. *J Am Coll Cardiol* 11: 993.
21. Crouse LJ, Harbrecht JJ, Beauchamp GD, Kramer PH (1988) Exercise echocardiography: A new tool for assessing the functional impact of reperfusion therapy in acute myocardial infarction. *Circulation* 78: II-272.
22. Corday S, Martin S, Areeda J, Hajduczki I (1988) Prognostic value of treadmill echocardiography in patients with chest pain and positive stress ECG. *Circulation* 78: II-272, (abstract).

5. Echocardiography during transesophageal atrial pacing

SABINO ILICETO, ANTONIO F. AMICO, FRANCESCO TOTA, GIOVANNI PICCINNI, GAETANO D'AMBROSIO, GIULIA DE MARTINO and PAOLO RIZZON

Introduction

Echocardiographically detected wall motion abnormalities are a sensitive marker of coronary artery disease. However, even patients with severe coronary stenoses may have a normal ventricular wall motion at rest. Any stress which is able to induce myocardial ischemia may also induce mechanical alterations (i.e. wall motion abnormalities) whose onset is known to be an even earlier ischemic marker than electrical alterations and angina. Therefore, one can reasonably expect that by combining a suitable stress with an imaging technique such as echocardiography one has an efficient diagnostic means for coronary artery disease.

Unfortunately, echocardiography during physical exercise has some technical limitations which have prevented it being widely adopted. On the other hand, the physiopathological and technical bases of atrial pacing make it promising as a valid stress to be used in conjunction with echocardiography.

Experimental bases

The heart rate is one of the determinants of myocardial oxygen consumption [1]. Atrial pacing enables one to alter the heart rate in a way that can easily be controlled and reproduced. Several experimental studies have shown that increases in heart rate cause increases in coronary blood flow as long as there are no critical stenoses [2–3]. Studies done using radioactive microspheres have demonstrated that in the regions where there are coronaries with a critical stenosis, the overall perfusion remains virtually the same during rapid atrial pacing, though there is a redistribution of the flow with a reduction in subendocardial perfusion and a slight increase in the subepicardial one [4]. It is likely that this situation causes real ischemia in the region concerned because of the difference between the increased oxygen demands and the inadequate blood supply. Indeed, in this experimental situation, there is an increase in the partial pressure of CO_2 and a decrease in the partial pressure of O_2 in

S. Iliceto et al. (eds.), Ultrasound in Coronary Artery Disease, 37–48.
© 1991 Kluwer Academic Publishers.

the myocardial region distal to the coronary stenosis, thus leading to myocardial ischemia [5]. This ischemia can induce mechanical alterations [6]. The experimental findings have substantially been confirmed by studies on man carried out in the cardiac catheterization laboratory. Atrial pacing causes a reduction in regional myocardial perfusion, whether evaluated by Xenon 133 [7] or by Thallium 201 [8], in patients with coronary artery disease.

The quantity of experimental data leads one to conclude that atrial pacing is a good stress for inducing myocardial ischemia in patients with critical coronary stenoses. Consequently, the use of various cardiac imaging techniques in conjunction with atrial pacing has been suggested in order to show up the mechanical marker of ischemia during this stress. Wall motion abnormalities have actually been demonstrated by means of cine ventriculography [9], radionuclide ventriculography [10–11] and digital angiography [12–14].

Atrial pacing and cardiac imaging

The above experimental findings support the use of atrial pacing, combined with an imaging method such as echocardiography, for studying coronary artery disease. Atrial pacing can, nowadays, be done transesophageally. The technical possibility of doing this was suggested some time ago [15–18] but the pacing was excessively uncomfortable for the patient. In the last few years technological improvements have meant that transesophageal stimulation can now be better tolerated [19–20].

The joint use of transesophageal atrial pacing and two-dimensional echocardiography now satisfies most of the requirements for a diagnostic test: apart from the feasibility, safety and reproducibility of this type of stress there is also the high sensitivity of echocardiography in diagnosing abnormalities in myocardial contraction.

Two-dimensional echocardiography during transesophageal atrial pacing (TAP): Diagnosis of coronary artery disease

The diagnostic utility of such a test can only be ascertained by studying a sufficiently large series of patients with suspected coronary artery disease (CAD). An early study [21] was carried out on 85 consecutive patients admitted to our Institution because of chest pain but no signs of cardiomyopathy, mitral prolapse and/or valvular disease. The study protocol required continuous atrial pacing, started at 110 beats/min and increased every 2 min by 10 beats/min until severe chest pain occurred or a heart rate of 150 beats/min was achieved (Figure 1). The examination was performed with the patient in the supine or left lateral decubitus. 2D Echo images were obtained after introducing the transesophageal catheter but before beginning atrial pacing and then every 2 min thereafter throughout the stress test, the last recording being obtained after 3 min pacing at the highest rate reached (usually 150 beats/min). We chose 150 beats/min as the target rate since it reflects ap-

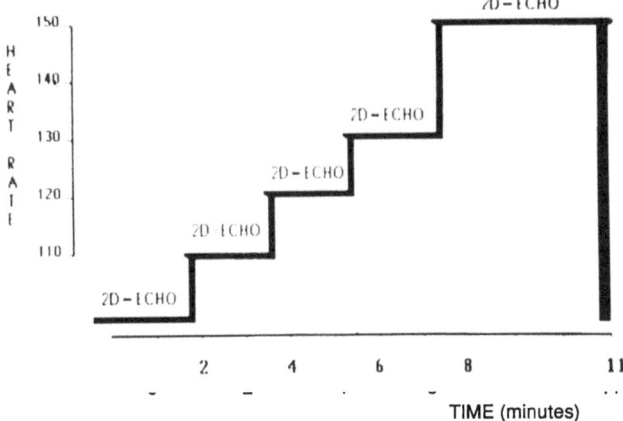

Figure 1. Pacing protocol. Atrial pacing is started at 110 min⁻¹ and increased every 2 min by 10 beats min⁻¹ until a heart rate of 150 beats min⁻¹ is achieved. Two-dimensional echocardiography (2D Echo) is performed at rest, during and after 3 min pacing at highest rate reached.

proximately 85 to 100% of the age-predicted heart rate of the majority of patients generally studied in our Institution. Evaluation of left ventricular wall motion abnormalities was based on the subjective impression of the endocardial echo inward motion toward the centre of the left ventricle and the degree of thickening of the myocardium. In 4 patients the test could not be

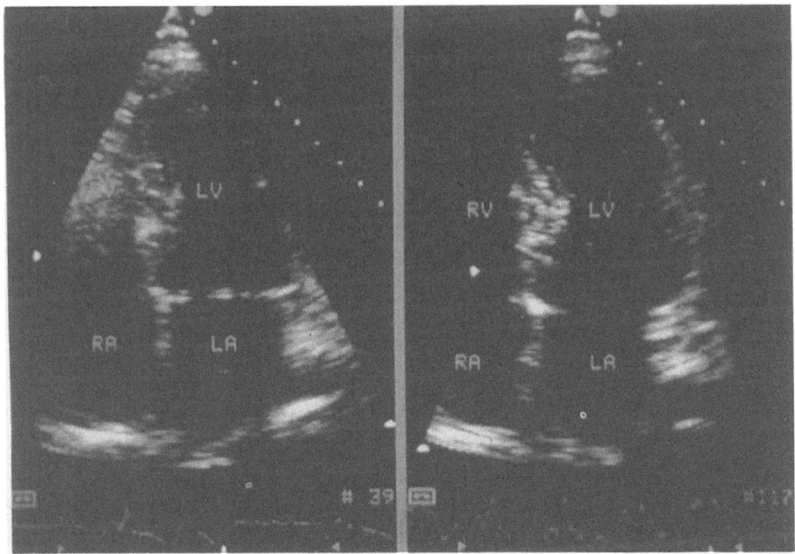

Figure 2. Two-dimensional echocardiography during transesophageal atrial pacing: on the left a systolic apical 4-chamber view at rest; on the right the same view during pacing at 150 min⁻¹; a large dyskinesis of the apex is evident.

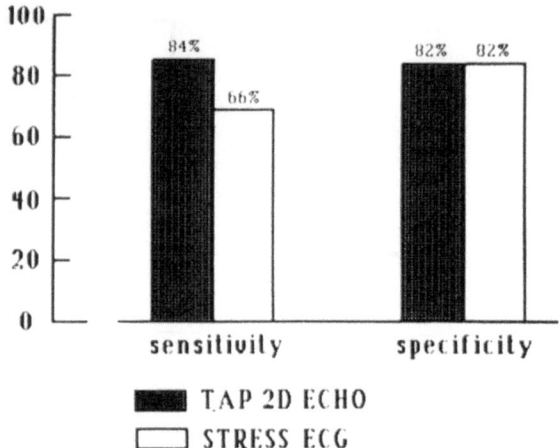

Figure 3. Comparison between ECG stress test and echocardiography during transesophageal atrial pacing (TAP 2D Echo) in a group of 117 patients: sensitivity and specificity.

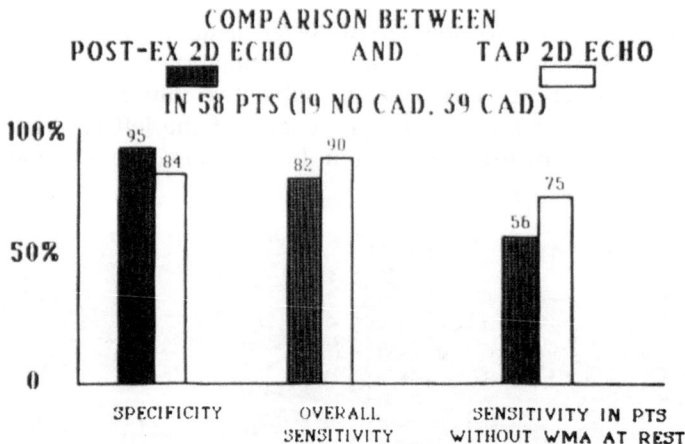

Figure 4. Comparison between post-exercise two-dimensional echocardiography (post-ex 2D Echo) and two-dimensional echocardiography during transesophageal atrial pacing (TAP 2D Echo) in a group of 58 patients. TAP 2D Echo was feasible in 95% of the cases, whereas post-ex 2D Echo in only 80%.

performed: in 2 because of lack of atrial capture and in 2 because of excessive discomfort caused by the pacing. In this series the sensitivity of the test was 91% and the specificity 88%.

Figure 2 shows an example of wall motion abnormalities induced by atrial pacing in a patient with significant coronary artery disease and normal wall motion at rest. These data were basically confirmed in a subsequent study of ours (22): in 176 patients the sensitivity was 89% while the specificity was 84%. In this second series, 117 patients also did a bicycle ergometer exercise test, giving a sensitivity and specificity of 66% and 82%, respectively (Figure 3). TAP 2D Echo has even proved to be diagnostically more accurate than exercise echocardiography. In 78 patients who did both tests (23), TAP 2D Echo showed a sensitivity of 90% and a specificity of 84% whereas exercise 2D Echo gave values of 82% and 95%, respectively (Figure 4). The feasibility of TAP 2D Echo was decidedly greater (95% as opposed to 80%). Indeed, in 16 patients (20%), the postexercise 2D Echo was inadequate for analysis. If one then also considers the considerable proportion of patients who are not able to do physical exercise for a variety of reasons (respiratory insufficiency, peripheral vascular disease, unfitness, etc.) TAP 2D Echo becomes even more valuable as it can widely be applied in the group of patients generally subjected to noninvasive diagnostic techniques because of suspected coronary artery disease.

Evaluation of the extent of the coronary disease

Patients with CAD are usually divided into those with single, two- and three-vessel disease, and it is established that the greater number of coronaries affected, then the worse the long-term prognosis [24]. This splitting of coronary angiographic findings into just three groups is, however, over-schematic as the area at risk can vary greatly in extent in any two patients with single-vessel disease, depending on the site and characteristics of the stenoses. In 46 patients who underwent coronary angiography [25] a coronary score was used which took the site, number and severity of stenoses into consideration. In the same patients, the results of TAP 2D Echo, expressed as a wall motion score, correlated inversely with the coronary score: in other words, patients with more extensive wall motion abnormalities, were more likely to have a

WALL MOTION ABNORMALITY
ONSET

CAD SEVERITY		< 120 b/m·	> 120 b/m·
	SVD	5	10
	MVD	19	3

Figure 5. Appearance of wall motion abnormalities during TAP 2D Echo and extent of the heart disease: in 19/22 patients with multi-vessel disease the onset of wall motion abnormalities occurs at a rate not higher than 120 beats/min, whereas in 10/15 patients with single vessel disease a frequency above 120 beats/min is required to induce wall motion abnormalities. SVD = single vessel disease; MVD = multivessel disease.

more serious CAD. We also analysed a group of 37 patients with normal ventricular wall motion at rest and a significant CAD (Figure 5). A large proportion of those who developed wall motion abnormalities at rates less than 130
beats/min had a serious coronary disease [26].

Evaluation of the extent of the CAD, and therefore the presence of areas at
risk, is an even more important decision-making factor in patients with previous myocardial infarction. In 62 patients with previous myocardial infarction, TAP 2D Echo showed up wall motion abnormalities in remote regions
in 75% of the patients with multivessel disease but also in 52% of those with
single vessel disease [22]. The specificity of this test is poor here. However, a
noninvasive test performed after myocardial infarction should principally aim
at identifying the patients with the worst prognosis and it does not matter if
the coronary angiography findings are totally predictive of future cardiac
events in the population of patients with infarction [27].

To test whether the information obtained with TAP 2D Echo could be
used to prognostically stratify patients with recent infarction, we examined
108 consecutive patients over a 30-month period. Eighteen patients were
excluded because of poor quality 2D echocardiographic images at rest or
unsatisfactory transesophageal atrial stimulation (patient intolerance, failure
to capture the atrium). Seven patients were lost at follow-up and were therefore subsequently excluded from the study; thus, the final study group consisted
of 83 patients. Transesophageal atrial pacing 2-dimensional echocardiography was performed within 3 weeks of the acute event. These patients were clinically followed up for 14 ± 5 months [28]. During TAP 2D Echo patients
were defined at high risk if wall motion abnormalities (WMA) were detected
in left ventricular regions remote from the infarcted area. On the other hand,
patients were considered to be low risk if they had no WMA during TAP in
remote regions. 21/83 patients had major cardiac events during the follow-
up. Cardiac events occurred in 15/23 (65%) and 5/60 (8%, $p < 0.001$)
patients assigned to the high and low risk groups, respectively, on the basis of
TAP 2D Echo results (Figure 6). Thus, the detection of atrial pacing induced
WMA in regions remote from the infarcted area is useful in identifying
patients at higher risk of future cardiac events after uncomplicated MI. What
is more its prognostic accuracy is superior to that of exercise stress testing: in
the same series major events occurred in only 6 out of the 19 patients with a
positive stress test (32%) and in 14 out of 64% patients with a negative exercise stress test (22%, p = NS vs. positive exercise stress test) (Figure 6).

Evaluation of the effects of therapy

The clinical cardiologist often requires noninvasive tests for the evaluation of
the efficacy of various therapeutic procedures. In a group of 15 patients [29]
the wall motion score at rest did not change after giving isosorbide-5 mono-
nitrate. On the other hand, this parameter showed marked improvement after
administering the drug at 130 beats/min and at 150 beats/min. At rest 131 of

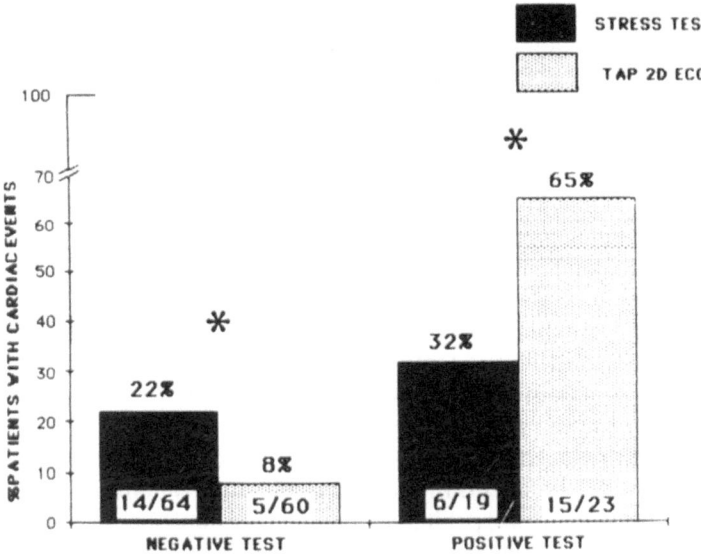

Figure 6. TAP 2D Echo and prognosis in patients with recent myocardial infarct: the incidence of cardiac events in the 2 years following the infarct is significantly greater in patients with positive test.

the 135 segments examined (nine segments for each of the 15 patients) remained unchanged, three improved and one worsened after therapy. During pacing at 130 beats/min 38 segments showed improvement in the postdrug study.

In patients who have undergone coronary artery bypass graft surgery it is also important to be able to assess with reasonable accuracy if the patient's clinical condition has actually benefitted. In 35 patients [30], 2-dimensional echocardiography during TAP was performed both before and after (28 ± 7 days) coronary artery bypass graft surgery. The wall motion score, evaluated excluding septal score, (since septal motion abnormalities can often be detected after heart surgery), was unchanged at rest before and after surgery but improved postoperatively. Comparison of pre and post-surgery data showed that atrial pacing WMS improved or remained normal in 27 patients (Group A), while it was unchanged or decreased in the remaining 8 (Group B). No patient in group A developed angina or ST depression during exercise, whereas in group B 5 cases had ischemic ECG changes and 2 had angina. Thus all the post-operative abnormal clinical and electrocardiographic responses to exercise were in group B.

Doppler echocardiography and atrial pacing: A new technique for studying left ventricular filling

The imaging techniques which are generally used to study left ventricular filling (cineventriculography, radionuclide ventriculography) only make it possible to analyse this phenomenon for just a few cardiac cycles. Further-more, like physical exercise, the stress which is usually used to induce ische-mia considerably alters the heart rate and, consequently, the ventricular filling modalities independently of the ischemia itself. By using Doppler echocardio-graphy to evaluate the transmitral flow the former problem is overcome: the parameters thus obtained accurately estimate the major determinants of left ventricular filling [31]. Atrial pacing, in turn, makes it possible to induce a myocardial ischemia which lasts for some time even after interrupting the pacing when the heart rate is comparable with the pre-stress one [32]. By using Doppler echocardiography to analyse the transmitral flow velocity after interrupting an ischemia-inducing atrial pacing, it is therefore possible to visualize and then follow the temporal evolution of filling alterations *exclu-sively* induced by ischemia (Figure 7). In 17 patients with CAD [33] the trans-mitral flow velocity was recorded at rest and immediately after stopping TAP. 8 patients developed ischemia, which was revealed by electrocardiographic alterations of the ST segment. In these patients, the transmitral flow velocity, as recorded on interrupting pacing, changed considerably, showing a marked reduction in the rapid filling rate and an increase in the velocity due to atrial contraction. Continuous monitoring after pacing showed a progressive re-adjustment of the flow velocity curves with a return to the resting morphology within one minute. In the 9 patients who did not develop ischemia, the ven-tricular filling remained the same as it was in the pre-stress conditions.

This approach to the study of left ventricular filling is limited by the follow-ing difficulties: Obtaining an adequate execution technique so as to have long Doppler tracings of consistently good quality; optimal acoustic penetration of

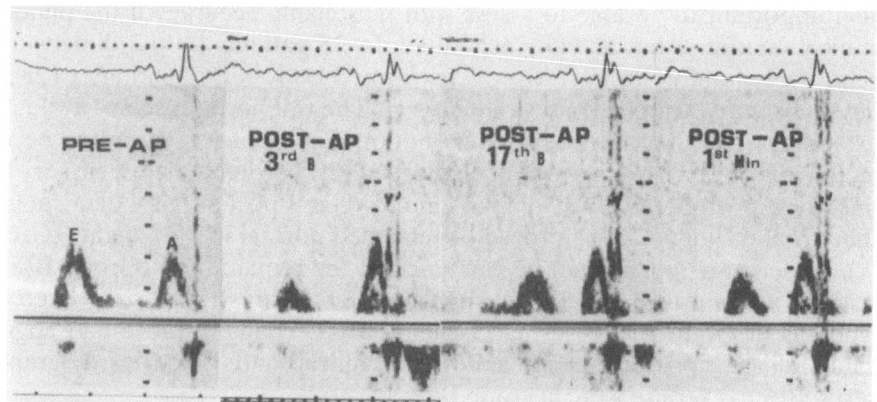

Figure 7. Effect on left ventricular filling (transmitral flow velocities) of atrial pacing-induced ischemia and recovery modalities: at rest before atrial pacing (PRE-AP) left ventricular charac-teristics are normal (first panel). Immediately after cessation of atrial pacing (third beat POST-AP) early peak flow velocity decreases whereas atrial peak flow velocity increases. A gradual tendency to return to pre-atrial pacing filling values is observed during recovery as shown in the third panel (17th post-atrial pacing beat). At 1 minute after pacing (fourth panel) transmitral flow velocities are very similar to those of the 17th beat. (With kind permission of *J Am Coll Car* 11: 953–61.)

the ultrasounds; the evaluation of overall filling must not be changed, even in the presence of ischemia, by compensatory segmentary 'improvements'. However, it does have the unique characteristic of enabling one to analyse the recovery modalities of the filling alterations, supplying new information on the physiopathology of diastole in CAD.

Color Doppler during transesophageal atrial pacing

Acute myocardial ischemia can induce acute mitral regurgitation [34–38]. Mitral regurgitation caused by myocardial ischemia is a well-known phenomenon that has been attributed to the development of an abnormal function in the mitral subvalvular-valvular apparatus. This malfunctioning seems to be caused by
– papillary muscle ischemia,
– by the ischemia, and consequent abnormal function, of the myocardial wall from which the papillary muscle arises and
– by a severe overall impairment of left ventricular function and a consequent malfunction of valve apparatus.
We have used color Doppler during transesophageal atrial pacing to investigate this phenomenon [39]. This approach seems to be particularly suitable for this. In fact, the 2D Echo color Doppler exam can monitor both left ventricular wall motion and normal and abnormal intracardiac flow, while atrial pacing is capable of safely inducing myocardial ischemia. We performed 2D Echo and color Doppler in 48 patients undergoing coronary angiography before and immediately after interrupting incremental atrial pacing. Performing the color Doppler exam immediately after atrial pacing interruption presents the advantage, as previously mentioned, of exploring ischemia effects at normal heart rates. If color Doppler is used this is a great advantage,

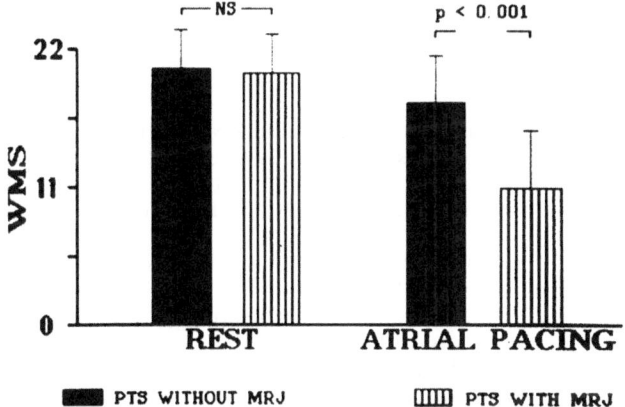

Figure 8. Relation between wall motion score (WMS) during TAP-2D Echo and appearance of mitral regurgitant jet (mrj) in patients with coronary artery disease: patients developing mrj have a significantly lower WMS during TAP 2D Echo than in patients who do not.

since the low frame of color Doppler display would make the evaluation of phenomena occurring at high heart rates decidedly troublesome. In the series of patients we studied, mitral regurgitation developed in 15. While there was a slight difference between resting wall motion score between patients developing and those not developing mitral regurgitation, there was a great and significant difference between wall motion scores obtained in the same group of patients during atrial pacing. In fact, left ventricular wall motion was more compromised in patients developing mitral regurgitation (Figure 8). Furthermore, the number of coronary vessels presenting a significant stenosis was greater in patients developing them than in those not developing mitral regurgitation. Thus, color Doppler during transesophageal atrial pacing is a useful tool for evaluating the phenomenon of acute mitral regurgitation induced by myocardial ischemia. Our data show that this is caused by a greater impairment of regional left ventricular function and is an expression of severer coronary artery disease.

Conclusions

Nowadays, clinicians not only require static information (coronary anatomy) when dealing with CAD but also an increasing amount of dynamic data (myocardium at risk, actual perfusion, coronary reserve). Non-invasive techniques must try to meet these needs. Stress echocardiography is now a reality which is becoming increasingly important as a part of the diagnostic routine of this common pathology. Echocardiography associated with TAP has resolved major problems of feasibility without compromising accuracy. The results obtained so far in the research laboratory are such that it could not only be proposed as a widely-used test in diagnosing coronary disease but also in perfecting the knowledge of its physio-pathological characteristics.

References

1. Laurent D, Bolene Williams C, Williams FL, Katz LN (1956) Effects of heart rate on coronary flow and cardiac oxygen consumption. *Am J Physiol* 185: 355–64.
2. Berglund E, Borst HG, Duff F, Schreiner GL (1958) Effect of heart rate on cardiac work, myocardial oxygen consumption and coronary blood flow in the dog. *Acta Physiol Scand* 42: 185–90.
3. Pitt B, Gregg DE (1968) Coronary hemodynamic effects of increasing ventricular rate in the unanesthetized dog. *Circ Res* 22: 753–59.
4. Becker L (1976) Effect of tachycardia on left ventricular blood flow distribution during coronary occlusion. *Am J Physiol* 230: 1072–77.
5. O'Riordan JB, Flaherty JT, Khuri SF, Brawley RK, Pitt B, Gott VL (1977) Effects of atrial pacing on regional myocardial gas tensions with critical coronary stenosis. *Am J Physiol* H49–H53.
6. Tomoike H, Franklin D, Ross J (1978) Detection of myocardial ischemia by regional dysfunction during and after rapid pacing in conscious dogs. *Circulation* 58: 48–56.

7. Schmidt DH, Weiss MB, Casarella WJ, Fowler DL, Sciacca RR, Cannon PJ (1976) Regional myocardial perfusion during atrial pacing in patients with coronary artery disease. *Circulation* 53: 807–19.
8. Heller GV, Aroesty JM, Parker JA, McKay RG, Silverman KJ, Als AV, Come PC, Kolodny GM, Grossman W (1984) The pacing stress test: Thallium-201 myocardial imaging after atrial pacing. Diagnostic value in detecting coronary artery disease compared with exercise testing. *J Am Coll Cardiol* 3: 1197–1204.
9. Pasternac A, Gorlin R, Sonnenblick EH, Haft JI, Kemp HG (1972) Abnormalities of ventricular motion induced by atrial pacing in coronary artery disease. *Circulation* 45: 1195–205.
10. Stone D, Dymond D, Elliott AT, Britton KE, Spurrell RAJ, Banim SO (1980) Use of first-pass radionuclide ventriculography in assessment of wall motion abnormalities induced by incremental atrial pacing in patients with coronary artery disease. *Br. Heart J* 43: 369–75.
11. Hecht HS, Chew CY, Burnam M, Schnugg SJ, Hopkins JM, Singh BN (1981) Radionuclide ejection fraction and wall motion during atrial pacing in stable angina pectoris: Comparison with metabolic and hemodynamic parameters. *Am Heart J* 101: 726–33.
12. Tobis J, Nalcioglu O, Johnston WD, Seibert A, Iseri LT, Werner R, Walter LH (1983) Digital angiography in assessment of ventricular function and wall motion during pacing in patients with coronary artery disease. *Am J Cardiol* 51: 668–75.
13. Johnson RA, Wassermann AG, Leiboff RH, Katz RJ, Bren GB, Varghese J, Ross AM (1983) Intravenous digital left ventriculography at rest and with atrial pacing as a screening procedure for coronary artery disease. *J Am Coll Cardiol* 2: 905–10.
14. Mancini GBJ, Peterson KL, Gregoratos G, Higgins CB (1984) Effects of atrial pacing on global and regional left ventricular function in coronary heart disease assessed by digital intravenous ventriculography. *Am J Cardiol* 53: 456–61.
15. Zoll PM (1952) Resuscitation of the heart in ventricular standstill by external electrical stimulation. *JAMA* 247: 768–71.
16. Burack B, Furman S (1969) Transesophageal cardiac pacing. *Am J Cardiol* 23: 469–72.
17. Rowe GG, Terry W, Neblett I (1969) Cardiac pacing with an esophageal electrode. *Am J Cardiol* 24: 548–50.
18. Lubell DL (1971) Cardiac pacing from the esophagus. *Am J Cardiol* 27: 641–644.
19. Gallagher JJ, Smith WM, Kasell J, Smith WM, Grant AO, Benson DW (1980) The use of esophageal lead in the diagnosis of mechanisms of reciprocating supraventricular tachycardia. *PACE* 3: 440–4.
20. Gallagher JJ, Smith WM, Kerr CR, Kasell J, Cook L, Reiter M, Sterba R, Harte M (1982) Esophageal pacing: A diagnostic and therapeutic tool. *Circulation* 65: 336–41.
21. Iliceto S, Sorino M, D'Ambrosio G, Papa A, Favale S, Biasco G, Rizzon P (1985) Detection of coronary artery disease by two-dimensional echocardiography and transesophageal atrial pacing. *J Am Coll Cardiol* 5: 1188–97.
22. Iliceto S, Sorino M, D'Ambrosio G, Lopriore V, Ricci A, Papa A, Amico A, Chiddo A, Rizzon P (1986) Atrial pacing in the detection and evaluation of coronary artery disease. *Eur Heart J* 7(C): 59–67.
23. Iliceto S, D'Ambrosio G, Sorino M, Papa A, Amico A, Ricci A, Rizzon P (1986) Comparison of postexercise and transesophageal atrial pacing two-dimensional echocardiography for detection of coronary artery disease. *Am J Cardiol.* 57: 547–53.
24. Bruschke AVG, Proudfit WL, Sones FM (1973) Progress study of 590 consecutive non surgical cases of coronary disease followed 5–9 years. I. Arteriographic correlations. *Circulation* 47: 1147–1153.
25. Iliceto S, Papa A, D'Ambrosio G, Amico A, Sorino M, Coluccia P, Rizzon P (1987) Prediction of the extent of coronary artery disease with the evaluation of left ventricular wall motion abnormalities during atrial pacing. A cross-sectional echocardiographic study. *Int J Cardiol* 14: 33–45.
26. Amico A, Iliceto S, D'Ambrosio G, Sorino M, Coluccia P, Rizzon P (1987) Evaluation of

timing of occurrence of wall motion abnormalities during incremental atrial pacing aids in the prediction of the severity of coronary artery disease. *Eur Heart J* 8 (suppl II): 190.

27. Gibson RS, Watson DD, Craddock GB, Crampton RS, Kaiser DL, Denny MJ, Beller GA (1983) Prediction of cardiac events after uncomplicated myocardial infarction: A prospective study comparing predischarge exercise thallium-201 scintigraphy and coronary arteriography. *Circulation* 68: 321–36.

28. Iliceto S, Caiati C, Ricci A, Amico A, Biasco G, Rizzon (1988) Prognostic stratification of patients with recent uncomplicated myocardial infarction by transesophageal atrial pacing 2D Echo. *Circulation* 78(4) (suppl II): 1094.

29. Iliceto S, Papa A, Ricci A, Lopriore V, D'Ambrosio G, Rizzon P (1986) Effects of Isosorbide-5-mononitrate on left ventricular wall motion abnormalities induced by atrial pacing. 2nd International Symposium on Mononitrates, Berlin, Dec 11–13, p 62, (abstracts).

30. Amico A, Ricci A, Lopriore V, Sorino M, D'Ambrosio G, Coluccia P, Iliceto S, Rizzon P (1987) Effects of coronary artery by-pass surgery on left ventricular wall motion at rest and during transesophageal atrial pacing. A two-dimensional echocardiographic study. *Cardiologia* 32(8): 699–706.

31. Rokey R, Kuo LC, Zoghbi WA, Limacher MC, Quinones MA (1985) Determination of parameters of left ventricular diastolic filling with pulsed Doppler echocardiography: comparison with cineangiography. *Circulation* 71: 543–50.

32. Markham RV, Winniford MD, Firth GB, Nicod P, Dehmer GJ, Lewis SE, Hillis LD (1983) Symptomatic, electrocardiographic, metabolic and hemodynamic alterations during pacing-induced myocardial ischemia. *Am J Cardiol* 51: 1589–94.

33. Iliceto, S, Amico A, Marangelli V, D'Ambrosio G, Rizzon (1988) Doppler echocardiographic evaluation of the effect of atrial pacing-induced ischemia on left ventricular filling in patients with coronary artery disease. *J Am Coll Car* 11: 953–61.

34. Finn MC, Bower PJ (1977) Severe papillary muscle dysfunction substantiated by atrial pacing during cardiac catheterization. *Am Heart J* 93(5): 626–628.

35. Burch GE, DePasquale N, Phillips JH (1968) The Papillary Muscle Syndrome. *JAMA* 204(3): 157–160.

36. Burch GE, DePasquale NP, Phillips JH (1968) The syndrome of papillary muscle dysfunction. *Am Heart J* (March): 399–415.

37. De Busk RF, Harrison DC (1969) The clinical spectrum of papillary-muscle disease. *New Engl J Med* 281: 1458–1467.

38. Bailas N (1965) Functional mitral insufficiency in acute myocardial ischemia. *Am J Card* 16: 807–812.

39. Iliceto S, Tota F, Selvaggi G, De Martino G, Piccinni G, D'Ambrosio G, Rizzon P (1989) Color Doppler evaluation of mitral regurgitation induced by acute myocardial ischemia. *Circulation* (suppl II) 90(4): 338.

6. Detection and assessment of the severity of coronary artery disease by dipyridamole echocardiography test

EUGENIO PICANO and FABIO LATTANZI

Rationale of the dipyridamole-echocardiography test

Dipyridamole is a potent coronary arteriolar vasodilator that has been employed in combination with thallium-201 imaging for the detection of coronary artery disease. Since a coronary stenosis may significantly reduce the regional coronary reserve without inducing ischemia, the presence of coronary artery disease can be documented by the different uptake of a flow tracer, such as thallium-201. Theoretically, myocardial ischemia is not required for the dipyridamole-thallium test to be positive. However, dipyridamole infusion can also induce myocardial ischemia in the presence of a coronary obstruction. This has been shown by a large amount of experimental and clinical evidence [1]. At a dosage of 0.75 mg/kg over 10 min, the electrocardiogram (ECG)-dipyridamole stress test has been proposed for the diagnosis of coronary artery disease, with a diagnostic accuracy comparable to the exercise stress test and an overall sensitivity (ECG changes and/or anginal pain) of about 80% (for a review, see ref [1]).

These data represented a solid rationale for proposing a new diagnostic test: the dipyridamole-echocardiography test [2]. Dipyridamole-induced ischemia might be detected through its mechanical marker, which is more sensitive and specific when compared with the conventional markers of ECG changes and pain. The development of a regional asynergy is the only criterion of positivity, and therefore myocardial ischemia is required, unlike with the thallium-201 scintigraphy test.

Mechanism of dipyridamole-induced ischemia

The regional transient asynergy occurring after dipyridamole infusion in a region supplied by a critically stenotic coronary artery can be reasonably accounted for by the ischemia resulting from a local imbalance between myocardial oxygen supply and demand [1].

S. Iliceto et al. (eds.), Ultrasound in Coronary Artery Disease, 49–57.
© 1991 *Kluwer Academic Publishers.*

Role of myocardial oxygen demand

The main determinant of myocardial oxygen consumption, i.e. the rate-pressure product (systolic arterial pressure × heart rate) is moderately increased (usually, less than 20%) at the onset of the asynergy occurring after dipyridamole infusion, when compared to a mean increase of more than 200% in the same patients during an exercise stress test [3]. Furthermore, in patients with a negative low dose and positive high dose test, the rate-pressure product at ischemic overlaps values reached during a negative low dose test. Consequently, the increase in myocardial oxygen consumption cannot by itself account for the ischemia following a high dose dipyridamole infusion. However, the rate-pressure product tends to increase in the presence of overt ischemia, possibly inducing more ischemia independently from the triggering event of flow maldistribution. Aminophylline antagonizes the effects of dipyridamole by blocking adenosine receptors. This may not always be sufficient to break the vicious circle of myocardial ischemia (ischemia – increase in oxygen demand – ischemia), once it has become independent from the initial event of flow maldistribution. In these patients, the administration of nitrates (which decrease demand and increase supply) readily abolishes the symptoms and signs of myocardial ischemia.

Role of oxygen supply

The mechanism responsible for dipyridamole-induced ischemia is likely to be flow reduction in the region supplied by the stenotic coronary artery. Five mechanisms possibly resulting in a decrease in myocardial oxygen supply have been suggested: passive collapse of the stenosis, vertical steal, horizontal steal, systemic steal and luxury perfusion [1].

Each of these mechanisms results from coronary arteriolar vasodilation induced by dipyridamole by means of the accumulation of adenosine. Adenosine is a by-product of adenine-nucleotide metabolism in myocardial tissue and is likely to play an active role in coronary flow regulation. Dipyridamole acts by inhibiting adenosine-deaminase and by preventing adenosine captation in myocardial tissue. Interestingly, a dipyridamole-like mechanism might also be responsible of effort-induced ischemia, at least in a subset of patients [4].

Passive coronary collapse
With dipyridamole, the arterioles dilate, thereby increasing flow across the stenotic lesion. This increased flow will lead to an increased pressure drop, the magnitude of which relates to the severity of the stenosis and to the increase in flow. Decreased aortic pressure following dipyridamole administration would also reduce the intraluminal pressure and thereby cause of further decrease in poststenotic intraluminal distending pressure.

This may predispose to collapse of the artery, thereby increasing the severity of the stenosis.

Unlike the 'vertical steal', this mechanism of passive coronary collapse necessarily postulates that the stenosis is severe but not fixed, i.e. it is able to undergo changes in size. It is known that approximately three fourths of all significant coronary stenoses contain a portion of normal wall within their circumference, and therefore have the potential for active or passive vasomotion.

In this regard, it is interesting to note that about one half of the patients with dipyridamole-induced ST-segment elevation also had spontaneous or ergonovine-induced ST-segment elevation. This might appear paradoxical. However, the presence of spontaneous or ergonovine-induced ST-segment elevation should imply that the coronary stenosis undergoes active vasoconstriction. This may represent an indirect evidence that diseased but pliable (not fixed) coronary artery is present, which is a theoretical prerequisite for the occurrence of a passive collapse of the stenosis.

In some patients with tight coronary stenosis, the angiographic findings during dipyridamole-induced ischemia were consistent with the phenomenon of passive collapse showing almost no poststenotic opacification of the vessel.

Vertical steal
One of the interesting aspects of atherosclerotic lesions is that even in the presence of a fixed anatomical stenosis, resistance is not fixed. Because myocardial oxygen demands of the endocardium are greater than those of epicardium, the resistance vessels of the endocardium are more dilated than those of the epicardium. A vasodilator stimulus may then decrease resistance in the subepicardial but not in the subendocardial vessels because the subendocardial vasodilator reserve is already exhausted. Even is total blood flow increases, the net effect is shunting of blood from the subendocardium to the subepicardium, ultimately resulting in myocardial ischemia.

This explanation has been substantiated by experimental and, more recently, clinical evidence. Patients with single vessel disease of the left anterior descending artery exhibited the mechanical manifestation of myocardial ischemia (regional asynergy after dipyridamole) associated with an increase in anterior coronary flow, although to a much lesser extent than in patients with normal coronary arteries or patients with coronary disease and a negative dipyridamole-echocardiography test.

Horizontal steal
In the presence of a coronary occlusion, it seems conceivable that arteriolar vasodilators might not have any effect. Actually, the hydraulics of the coronary tree are more complex for several reasons, one of which is the presence of collateral circulation. The administration of an arteriolar dilator may be detrimental. When dipyridamole is given, it can fully dilate the resistance

vessels of the unoccluded artery, thereby increasing the pressure gradient along the vessel. In the situation in which a partial stenosis of the vessel feeding the collaterals exists, the small pressure drop across the stenosis present under baseline conditions increases, thereby decreasing the pressure at the point of origin of the collateral vessels. Such a reduction in collateral perfusion pressure decreases collateral blood flow to the myocardium dependent upon the occluded artery.

In some patients with coronary occlusion, the angiographic findings during dipyridamole-induced ischemia were consistent with the hypothesized mechanism of horizontal steal, showing less opacification of the collateral circulation in the presence of myocardial ischemia.

Systemic steal
Dipyridamole has a peripheral arteriolar dilatory effect, although it is less pronounced in comparison with other drugs such as nifedipine or nitroprusside in the presence of severe coronary artery disease and decreased diastolic perfusion pressure, the lowering of arteriolar peripheral resistances can lead to a coronary steal diverting perfusion from an ischemic coronary vascular bed to a preferentially dilated peripheral vascular bed.

Luxury perfusion
After dipyridamole, a paradoxical situation takes place. The flow is regionally augmented, but it cannot be used by the metabolism of the myocardial cell, which then suffers oxygen 'hunger amidst affluency'. This can be due to the preferential opening of non nutritional pathways in the microcirculation. In addition, the increased flow velocity that is induced by dipyridamole reduces the vascular transit time, which limits oxygen cellular uptake. Consistent with this interpretation is the finding that the oxygen saturation in great cardiac vein is markedly augmented even in the presence of transient anterior myocardial ischemia induced by dipyridamole.

Final result

The final result of all these mechanisms is a drop in the subendocardial, rarely transmural, 'metabolically useful' flow. This is a prerequisite for the occurrence of the regional contractility dysfunction revealed as a transient asynergy by the dipyridamole-echocardiography test. Interestingly, even when dipyridamole infusion is not sufficient to provoke ischemia in the presence of coronary artery disease, it sensitizes the myocardium to the ischemic stress of exercise [5]. Each of the mechanisms determining ischemia during dipyridamole stress requires an 'organic' limitation of coronary reserve. This fact implies the conceptual allocation of this test in the spectrum of provocative testing as an unique means of exploring the pure organic component of coronary reserve. However, aminophylline termination of dipyridamole stress (which is routinely performed also in negative tests) can trigger coronary vasospasm, with ST segment elevation, in almost 30% of patients with variant angina [6]. The mechanism of vasospasm remains elusive. It is possible that aminophylline determines an abrupt withdrawal of the dipyridamole vaso- dilatory stimulus and this might trigger the coronary artery spasm. This hypothesized mechanism might be in some way similar – on a shorter time scale – to the coronary vasospasm due to nitrate exposure withdrawal. It is important to clearly separate this findings from the previously described ST segment elevation occurring after dipyridamole infusion and reversed by aminophylline.

Dipyridamole-echocardiography test

Patients are instructed to fast for at least 3h before the test and, specifically, to avoid tea or coffee, whose xanthine content can limit dipyridamole action.

Dipyridamole is administered intravenously (i.v.), 0.56 mg/kg in 4 min fol- lowed by 4 min of no dose and then by 0.28 mg/kg in 2 min. The cumulative dosage is therefore 0.84 mg/kg in 10 min [7].

During the procedure, the blood pressure is recorded each minute with a cuff sphygmomanometer. A 12-lead ECG is performed before and every min after the i.e. infusion is begun. Some leads (usually V_2 and V_4) are slightly dis- placed to avoid interfering with the positioning of the transducer.

Two-dimensional echocardiograms are continuously recorded during the dipyridamole infusion and up to 10 min after the end of the infusion. In the baseline studies, all standard echocardiographic views are obtained, if pos- sible. During the test, new asynergic areas of abnormal wall motion are identi- fied on multiple views by rapidly moving the ultrasound transducer through various positions. After an optimal position for the observation of abnormal wall motion is established, the transducer is held stationary throughout the remainder of the study and the recovery period.

Positivity of the test is linked to detection of a transient asynergy of con- traction that was absent or of lesser degree in the baseline examination (e.g. hypokinesia at rest becoming akinesia or dyskinesia after dipyridamole ad- ministration). Any region that was already dyskinetic in a rest condition was not considered for analysis. The development of the asynergy can be preced- ed by a transient hyperkinesia, which almost invariably accompanies negative tests. The hyperkinesia results from the decrease in afterload (systolic pres- sure), the increase in heart rate, and the increased contractility. The test protocol requires ready-to-use availability of
- Aminophylline (240 mg) (i.v. infusion in 2–3 min promptly abates dipyri- damole effects).
- Trinitrine (or sublingual isosorbide dinitrate), to be administered if aminophylline has failed to eliminate ischemia completely.

The time duration of the test is usually less than 30 min.

The dosage issue

We initially performed the dipyridamole-echo test adopting the same dosage employed in Thallium-201 scintigraphy testing [1]. At that dosage, the test had a sensitivity of 50–60% [2]. In order to further increase the sensitivity, and based upon the available clinical experience with dipyridamole – ECG stress, we gave, after the standard dose of 0.56 mg/kg over 4 min, and extra dose of 0.14 mg/kg/min for 2 min, up to the cumulative dose of 0.84 mg/kg over 10 min [7].

This attempt also stemmed from the obvious suspicion that a considerable inter patient variability existed, and a single dipyridamole dosage might not provide maximal vasodilation in all patients. In a study performed on 93 patients, the sensitivity rose from 53% to 74%, employing the higher dose of dipyridamole in patients with a negative lower dose test. There was no loss in specificity and no apparent increase in risk [7].

Recently, the assumption that the standard dose provides maximal and uniform vasodilation in all patients has been questioned. From the physiologic viewpoint, there is a considerable variation in flow response after dipyridamole, and the higher dose is often required to fully recruit the coronary reserve. This is also consistent with clinical experience with the dipyridamole-ECG test showing how the diagnostic sensitivity rises if one uses progressively higher doses [1].

In our opinion, such an approach represents a very reasonable trade-off between the need for diagnostic power and the priority of safety [8].

In our institution, in the first 4 years of experience, nine hundred fifty-two high-dose dipyridamole-echocardiography test were performed in 771 patients with history of chest pain and/or myocardial infarction. There were no death, myocardial infarction, malignant arrhythmias, severe hypotension. Out of the 771 study pts, a subset of 580 was studied without therapy, and underwent coronary arteriography; on this subset, the sensitivity and specificity were calculated. Patients were considered to have coronary artery disease if they had at least one stenotic lesion with 70% or greater diameter reduction in the coronary angiogram. The overall sensitivity of dipyridamole-echocardiography test was 75%; it was lower in single than in multivessel disease (54% vs 86%). The sensitivity was 84% in pts with a resting ventricular asynergy and 67% in pts with normal resting function. The overall specificity was 95%, with similar values in hypertensives and normotensives (92 vs 97%, p = ns) [9], males and females (96 vs 93%, p = ns) [10]. Thus, high dose Dipyridamole-echocardiography test is feasible and safe, with high specificity, and acceptable sensitivity – especially in pts with multivessel disease and/or resting asynergy – for non invasive detection of angiographically assessed coronary artery disease.

Stratification of ischemic response

The exercise stress test allows not simply a dichotomous evaluation (positive vs negative), but also a grading of the ischemic response, assessed through the work threshold at which ischemia occurs. The work threshold is sometimes poorly reproducible in the same patient, both for 'central' (modulations of coronary tone) and 'peripheral' (variations in cardiovascular efficiency) reasons. Despite such limitations, the intensivity of cardiac work at which ischemia occurs during exercise is even more important than its presence. The dipyridamole-echocardiography test can also stratify the ischemic response, with high reproducibility and independently from factors affecting work load that are not related to organic coronary reserve [11–14]. This stratification of positive response regards three different parameters or 'coordinates' of the ischemic process: 'vertical' spatial extension of ischemia (either subendocardial or transmural), 'horizontal' spatial extension of ischemia (area 'at risk' during ischemia), and 'temporal' location of ischemia (compared with the beginning of dipyridamole infusion).

Vertical spatial extension of ischemia

ST-segment depression (a marker of subendocardial ischemia) is by far the most common ECG finding in dipyridamole test results, but also ST-segment elevation can rarely accompany positive test results. When occurring in the absence of myocardial necrosis and/or left ventricular baseline regional asynergy, such a finding reflects a more severe degree of ischemia than ST-segment depression, i.e. transmural – not exclusively subendocardial – ischemia.

Unlike ST-segment depression, ST-segment elevation reliably predicts the presence and the site of a transient regional asynergy after dipyridamole [12].

Horizontal spatial extension of ischemia

The horizontal spatial extension of ischemia can be defined by the dipyridamole-echocardiography test and semiquantitatively expressed with a 'wall motion score'. A response 'positive for ischemia' in the area supplied by the left anterior descending coronary artery can affect, for instance, either the sole distal septum or the whole septum, the apex and lateral wall. The extent of the 'area at risk' is obviously quite different in the two cases, and this information has to be taken into account when considering individually tailored therapeutic approaches.

Temporal location of ischemia

To test the hypothesis as to whether dipyridamole echocardiography can also stratify different degrees of coronary reserve impairment, the test response of each patient was evaluated against a physiologic reference standard, i.e. the maximal or 'ischemic' rate-pressure product value on exercise stress test.

Three different levels of functionally impaired coronary reserve were defined on the basis of the timing of the onset of asynergy during the test [15]:
- 'Low threshold' coronary reserve (early low-dose positivity, i.e. onset of asynergy within 3 min after the end of the first infusion of 0.56 mg/kg).
- 'Intermediate threshold' coronary reserve (late low-dose positivity, i.e. after 3 min following the end of the first infusion).
- 'High threshold' coronary reserve (high-dose positivity).

Dipyridamole-Echocardiography: Back to the future

Much has been said on dipyridamole-echocardiography test, but still much abides. We believe that the research in this field in future years will focus on a series of clinical issues, namely:

- what is the clinical and pathophysiological meaning of 'echocardiographically silent' myocardial ischemia with ST segment depression and/or pain in the various models of 'microvascular angina', such as syndrome X [16], arterial hypertension [17], acute myocardial rejection [18]?
- Can the transmitral [19] and/or aortic Doppler monitoring expand the diagnostic information provided by dipyridamole-echocardiography test?
- Is there any role for combined testing – such as dipyridamole-exercise electrocardiography test [5] – to enlighten the diagnostic gray zone of patients with coronary artery disease and negative both exercise and dipyridamole stress tests?
- What is the prognostic meaning of dipyridamole-echocardiography test, especially when compared with other strong prognostic predictors, such as exercise stress test, ejection fraction and coronary angiography [20]?
- There is the possibility of the simultaneous representation of flow, function and electrical phenomena during a dipyridamole-echo-contrast-cardiography test?

The answer to these questions will assign the priority of dipyridamole-echocardiography test in the cardiology armamentarium of the nineties.

References

1. Picano E (1989) Dipyridamole-Echocardiography test: The historical background and the physiologic basis. *Eur Heart J* 10: 365–376.
2. Picano E, Distante A, Masini M, Morales MA, Lattanzi F, L'Abbate A (1985) Dipyridamole-echocardiography test in effort angina pectoris. *Am J Cardiol* 56: 452–56.
3. Picano, E, Simonetti I, Masini M, Lattanzi F, Marzilli M, Distante A, De Nes M, L'Abbate A (1986) Transient myocardial dysfunction during pharmacologic vasodilation as an index of reduced coronary reserve: a coronary hemodynamic and echocardiographic study. *J Am Coll Cardiol* 8: 84–90.

4. Picano, E, Pogliani M, Lattanzi F, Distante A, L'Abbate A (1989) Exercise capacity after acute aminophylline administration in angina pectoris. *Am J Cardiol* 63: 14–16.
5. Picano E, Lattanzi F, Masini M, Distante A, L'Abbate A (1988) Usefulness of the dipyridamole-exercise echocardiography test for diagnosis of coronary artery disease. *Am J Cardiol* 62: 67–71.
6. Picano E, Lattanzi F, Masini M, Distante A, L'Abbate A (1988) Aminophylline termination of dipyridamole stress as a trigger of coronary vasospasm in variant angina. *Am J Cardiol* 62: 694–98.
7. Picano E, Lattanzi F, Masini M, Distante A, L'Abbate (1986) High dose dipyridamole echocardiography test in effort angina pectoris. *J Am Cardiol Coll* 8: 848–54.
8. Lattanzi F, Picano E, Masini M (1988) Safety of high dose dipyridamole echocardiography test. *J Am Coll Cardiol* 11 February (suppl): 217A, (abstracts).
9. Picano E, Lucarini AR, Lattanzi F, Distante A, Di Legge V, Salvetti A, L'Abbate A (1988) Dipyridamole-echocardiography test in essential hypertensives with chest pain. *Hypertension* 12: 238–242.
10. Masini M, Picano E, Lattanzi F, Distante A, L'Abbate (1988) High dose dipyridamole-echocardiography test in women: Correlation with exercise electrocardiography test and coronary angiography. *J Am Coll Cardiol* 12: 682–685.
11. Picano E, Morales MA, Distante A, Lattanzi F, Moscarelli E, Masini M, L'Abbate (1984) Dipyridamole echocardiography test in angina at rest: Noninvasive assessment of coronary stenosis underlying spasm. *Am Heart J* 111: 688–691.
12. Picano E, Masini M, Distante A, Simonetti I, Lattanzi F, Marzilli M, L'Abbate (1986) Dipyridamole-Echocardiography test in patients with exercise-induced ST segment elevation. *Am J Cardiol* 57: 765–770.
13. Picano E, Marraccini P, Lattanzi F, Levantesi D, Masini M, Dalle Vacche M, Distante A, L'Abbate A (1987) Dipyridamole echocardiography test as a clue to assess the organic 'ceiling' of individual coronary reserve. *Eur Heart J* 8: 38–42.
14. Picano E, Masini M, Lattanzi F, Klassen GA, Distante A, Levantesi D, Marraccini P, L'Abbate A (1988) Short term reproducibility of exercise testing in patients with ST segment elevation and different responses to the dipyridamole test. *Br Heart J* 60: 281–86.
15. Picano E, Lattanzi F, Masini M, Distante A, L'Abbate A (1987) Different degrees of ischemic threshold stratified by dipyridamole-echocardiography test. *Am J Cardiol* 59: 71–73.
16. Picano E, Lattanzi F, Masini M, Distante A, L'Abbate A (1987) Usefulness of a high-dose dipyridamole-echocardiography test for diagnosis of syndrome X. *Am J Cardiol* 60: 508–512.
17. Picano E, Lucarini AR, Lattanzi F, Marini C, Distante A, Salvetti A, L'Abbate A (1890) ST segment depression elicited by dipyridamole infusion in asymptomatic hypertensive patients. *Hypertension* (in press).
18. Picano E, De Peri G, Salerno JA, Arbustini E, Distante A, Martinelli L, Pucci A, Montermartini C, Viganò M, Dorieto L (1990) Electrocardiographic changes suggestive of myocardial ischemic elicited by dipyridamole infusion in acute rejection only after heart transplantation. *Circulation* 81: 72–77.
19. Lattanzi F, Picano E, Masini M, De Prisco F, Distante A, L'Abbate A (1989) Transmitral flow changes during dipyridamole-induced ischemia: A doppler-echocardiographic study. *Chest* 95: 1037–1042.
20. Picano E, Severi S, Michelassi C, Lattanzi F, Masini M, Orsini E, Distante A, L'Abbate A (1989) Prognostic importance of dipyridamole-echocardiography test in coronary artery disease 80: 450–457.

7. The use of color Doppler ultrasound in exercise testing

JOHN W. COOPER and NAVIN C. NANDA

Introduction

Vigorous exercise of the large skeletal muscles produces an increase in myocyte oxygen demand which must be satisfied by an increase in cardiac output of up to, even exceeding, 500% in normal individuals. Since this is accomplished by a combination of increased heart rate and contractile force, myocardial oxygen demand also rises, and this demand, in turn, is satisfied by an increase in blood flow in the coronary arteries. In patients with ischemic heart disease, this increased flow produces a pressure drop distal to any narrowed coronary arterial segment. If this pressure drop is large enough, transient myocardial ischemia will result. Such ischemia causes changes in both electrical and functional properties of the heart muscle, and since these changes may be detected non-invasively in various ways, exercise stress testing has been useful in the detection and assessment of ischemic heart disease since 1931 [1].

Although a fairly wide variety of exercise modes have been employed, the two which are currently the most popular are the upright treadmill and the bicycle ergometer (usually with the patient supine). Each of these methods has its own set of advantages and limitations. With upright treadmill exercise, the oxygen demand is greater because more muscle groups are employed than with the bicycle, and ventilation is improved as well. Also, high work rates can be obtained with less active patient cooperation. This is a more important consideration in America than in other countries where bicycles are a common primary transportation source. On the other hand, the walking patient inherently has more movement artifact than the supine bicycling patient, and venous return is not quite as good, and the exercise induced increase in stroke volume may not be as prominent. In general, while upright treadmill exercise stresses the patient more and is therefore more likely to induce myocardial ischemia, movement artefact precludes intraexercise assessment of many parameters.

With the introduction of imaging ultrasound in the late 1960s came indices of cardiac performance which were a potential use in an exercise setting, although this was limited by the poor anatomic orientation of M-mode echo-

S. Iliceto et al. (eds.), Ultrasound in Coronary Artery Disease, 59–65.
© 1991 *Kluwer Academic Publishers.*

cardiography. With the advent of two-dimensional echocardiography, the use of ultrasound in conjunction with stress electrocardiography began in earnest, and the use of stress echocardiography was demonstrated to improve the rather low sensitivity of stress electrocardiography without interfering with its generally high specificity. Recently, Doppler analysis of blood flow during exercise has been used to supplement the stress ECG and/or echocardiographic findings, and more recently a few studies have been done in this setting using the new modality, color Doppler or Doppler color flow mapping.

Color Doppler

This is essentially a pulsed Doppler system, but shifts in phase rather than frequency of the reflected sound are considered, and auto-correlation rather than fast Fourier transform analysis is used to manage the phase shift data [2, 3]. This allows a large number of very small sample regions to be sampled, on the order of 256 for each scan line position. Thus, phase shift signals from moving blood cells can be displayed directly on the two-dimensional sector image. These signals are color coded for transducer-relative flow direction, blue representing flow away from and red, flow toward the probe.

A variety of other parameters are displayed along with the basic colors, and these alter flow display appearance in certain predictable ways under certain circumstances. The lighter the color, for example, the higher velocity below the Nyquist limit. Any region of a flow exceeding the Nyquist limit will be seen to alias, as in conventional pulsed Doppler, but this phenomenon appears as a reversal of color in the region exceeding the Nyquist limit. The amplitude, or intensity, of the signals is influenced by the number of reflectors (cells) passing through a sampling region and determines the brightness of the color signal. In most systems the color green is added in proportion to the 'variance' in the flow, which is essentially the same parameter as the degree of 'spectral broadening' in a conventional spectral trace Doppler display.

These elements combine to allow a virtually instantaneous appreciation of blood flow, its direction, its character (whether smooth and normal or disturbed), and within certain limits, its velocity as it moves around within the chambers and vessels of the cardiovascular system.

This aspect of color Doppler allows the potential variation and error in flow pattern sampling mentioned by several authors [4, 5] studying exercises conventional Doppler to be reduced by aiding in confident placement and then maintenance of a conventional Doppler sample volume in a discrete and well defined portion of the flow within a vessel (for example, the region of highest velocity near the center of the lumen in the ascending aorta), guaranteeing that all sampling done will be as consistent and as uniform as possible.

In addition to providing improved beam steering capability, color Doppler also allows flow parameters other than ejection acceleration and velocity to be used in an exercise setting. Color Doppler is an ideal means for both detecting and assessing the severity of the mitral regurgitation which can occur in the presence of acute myocardial ischemia. This was examined by our group in 1987 [6]. The mode of exercise chosen for this study was supine bicycle ergonometry using a specially designed bicycle table which could be tilted so that the subjects were effectively in 45 degree left decubitus position. Thirty-nine subjects (seventeen normal volunteers and twenty-two patients with angiographically demonstrated coronary disease, none of whom had mitral regurgitation at rest), were exercised to maximum tolerance through a series of increasing work stages. Prior to exercise, a complete cardiac ultrasound examination, including color Doppler, was done. Because of the relative stability of these patients due to the nature of the exercise, a two-dimensional structural and color Doppler examination from the apical position was possible throughout exercise and for three minutes after exercise in each subject, using alternating views of the apical 2 and 4 chamber planes.

Although there was no significant correspondence between the semi-quantitative degree of severity of any exercise induced mitral regurgitation and the severity of the subjects' coronary disease [7], the very occurrence of an exercise induced leak was seen to be a significant indicator of both the presence and the degree of severity of coronary artery disease (Figure 1). As an indication of the existence of disease, this parameter increased the sensitivity of the exercise test from 54% to 59% and the specificity from 88% to 100%. If the development of left ventricular wall motion abnormalities was also taken into consideration, the 100% specificity was retained and the sensitivity further improved to 82%. When the electrographic changes were used in combination with the color Doppler and echocardiographic criteria, the specificity declined to the original 88%, but the sensitivity increased to 91%. Thus, this combination of criteria not only resulted in very high sensitivity and specificity but also in near equality of those indices, an important consideration.

In addition, as mentioned, this study also suggested that the development of mitral regurgitation during exercise can aid in the assessment of disease severity as well. A mitral leak developed in 89% of subjects with 3 vessel disease, in 36% of those with 1 or 2 vessel disease, and in one of the normal subjects. Thus, just over 10% of those subjects with 2 vessel disease or less developed mitral regurgitation, while it was seen in nearly 90% of those with three vessel disease, and only those subjects with coronary artery disease developed it.

Color Doppler has helped to add another potential sampling site for use in Doppler exercise testing. Occasionally, the suprasternal window is unavailable due to reasons such as patient body habitus or unusual heart position, so the flow in the ascending aorta is difficult or impossible to interrogate. A study done at this center indicates that the common carotid arteries may be used as an alternative when changes in the parameters of volume and velocity are being considered [8].

In this study, twenty-two subjects (ten normal volunteers and twelve

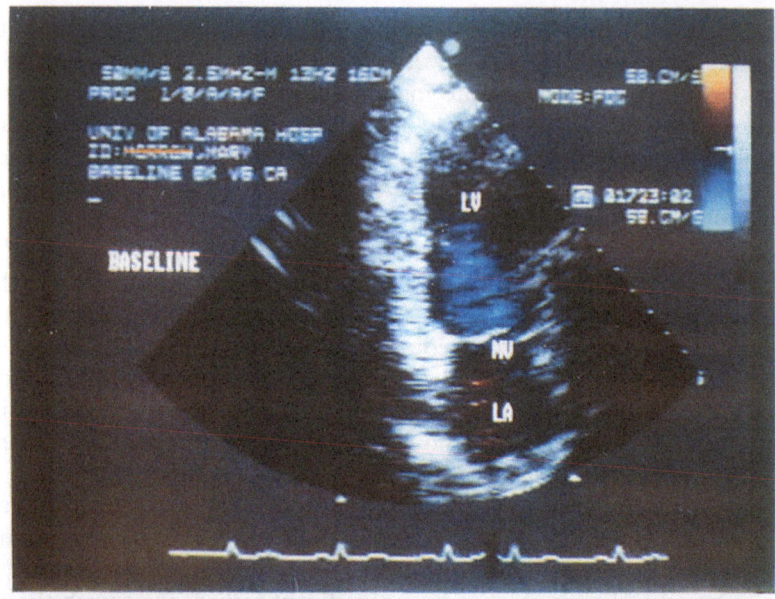

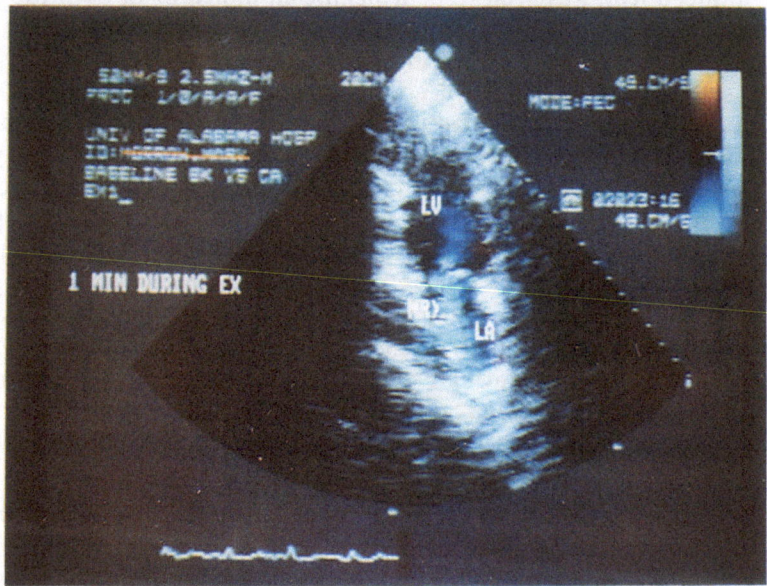

Figure 1. Color Doppler exercise echocardiography. *(A)* The apical four chamber view in an elderly female patient shows no evidence of mitral regurgitation at baseline. *(B)* One minute into the supine bicycle exercise, bluish green signals are visualized originating from the mitral valve (MV) and occupying a large area of the left atrium (LA) indicative of significant mitral regurgitation (MR) resulting from exercise induced myocardial ischemia. LV = left ventricle.

Reproduced with permission from: Cooper JW, Nanda NC (1990), The use of color Doppler ultrasound in exercise testing, in: Teague SM (ed) *Stress Doppler Echocardiography*, p. 258. Dordrecht, The Netherlands: Kluwer Academic Publishers.

patients with a previously established diagnosis of coronary artery disease) underwent staged exercise during which color guided conventional pulsed Doppler was used to interrogate both the right common carotid artery and left ventricular outflow tract (from the apical position). The mode of exercise used was again supine bicycle ergometry because of the inherently increased patient stability and ease in maintaining transducer position. The ten normal volunteers exhibited a proportional increase in flow velocity and calculated flow volume in both channels. This exercise-induced percentage change in the left ventricular outflow tract velocity was found to be similar to changes in the carotid flow velocity, making it possible to use Doppler interrogation of the carotid artery to monitor changes in stroke volume produced by exercise. An increase in velocity and volume occurred in those patients with documented disease but no resting wall motion abnormalities, but not to the extent seen in the normal cohort. The patients with contractile abnormalities at rest showed a decrease in both parameters in both channels. Since the common carotid artery and its flow is nearly universally available to two-dimensional structural and color Doppler interrogation because of the relative immobility of the neck region during exercise, the proximity of the artery to the transducer, and lack of interposition of obstacles to ultrasound such as lung or bone, it appears to be a viable alternative sampling position when changes in velocity or calculated flow volume are to be considered.

Limitations to the use of color Doppler

There are two major limitations to the use of color Doppler as a part of an exercise examination. In the first place, the learning curve is long and considerable operator experience is required before the modality can be used reliably in any setting. The relationships of the color settings to one another are more complex than in conventional Doppler equipment and until the effects of these relationships on the video display are fully understood, the examinations will not be of optimal quality and may be confusing and misleading. The second major limitation is the presence of 'ghosting', an artifact caused by the assignment of color values to moving structures. The resultant display appears as transient sheets or 'flashes' of color splashed across the screen, and although these bear no relation to chamber and vessel contours, they can cause confusion. This type of display is very common during exercise because the heart tends to be hyperdynamic. Adjusting filter, compression, frame rate and pulse repetition frequency settings can help, but experience and familiarity with the equipment and its display are the most important factor in circumventing this limitation.

Conclusion

The field of exercise color Doppler ultrasound is very new, and few studies have been done. These preliminary studies suggest that it can add important information to a conventional electrocardiographic stress test, and increase sensitivity and the ability to assess severity of coronary artery disease, although specificity may not be much improved. The parameters considered, primarily related to changes in ejection velocity and acceleration during exercise and to the development of mitral regurgitation, all appear useful. Changes in acceleration and the development of mitral regurgitation appear to add the most information. It is also worthy of note that the best results have been achieved using a combination of modalities, each supplementing the others. In the mitral regurgitation study by our group, high sensitivity and specificity were best achieved using a combination of electrocardiographic, echocardiographic and Doppler criteria. Ejection velocity and acceleration were not included in this study as parameters, so it is not known what affect consideration of these additional criteria might have had on overall sensitivity, specificity, and severity assessment. This might be a subject for future consideration.

The use of color Doppler appears to have the additional utility of allowing enhanced appreciation of these parameters by allowing visual guidance to flow interrogation using more conventional Doppler modalities. It also appears to allow quicker acquisition of potential sampling regions such as the left ventricular outflow tract, ascending aorta and the common carotid arteries, and time is an important consideration in an exercise examination.

The studies seem to indicate that while upright treadmill exercise produces the greater degree of work, both because of the larger amount of skeletal muscle involved and because of its increased familiarity (at least to Americans), supine bicycle exercise may also play an important role in the non-invasive evaluation of patients with suspected or proven coronary artery disease. This is not only because of the more stable transducer positions involved but because the use of the cycle allows employment of all of the ultrasound modalities throughout exercise, in addition to before and after. We have found that subjects respond well to encouragement as the work load increases, and are able to achieve and maintain a high degree of performance on the bicycle.

The studies which have been done suggest that color Doppler ultrasound can be a desirable addition to exercise testing in patients with ischemic heart disease.

References

1. Sheffield LT (1988) Exercise Stress Testing, in: Braunwald E (ed), *Heart Disease: A Textbook of Cardiovascular Medicine*, pp 223–242. Philadelphia: W.B. Saunders & Co., Harcourt, Brace-Jovanovich, Inc.
2. Nanda NC (ed) (1989) *Textbook of Color Doppler Echocardiography.* Philadelphia: Lea & Febiger.
3. Nanda NC (ed) (1989) *Atlas of Color Doppler Echocardiography.* Philadelphia: Lea & Febiger.

4. Fisher DC, Sahn DJ, Friedman MJ, Larson D, Valdez-Cruz L, Horowitz S, Goldberg S, Allen H (1983) The effects of variations on pulsed Doppler sampling site on calculations of cardiac output: An experimental study in open-chested dogs. *Circulation* 67: 370.

5. Louie EK, Maron BJ, Green KJ (1986) Variations in flow-velocity waveforms obtained by pulsed Doppler echocardiography in the normal human aorta. *Am J Cardiol* 58: 821–826.

6. Zachariah ZP, Hsiung MC, Nanda NC, Kan MN, Gatewood Jr RP (1987) Color Doppler assessment of mitral regurgitation induced by supine exercise in ischemic heart disease. *Am J Cardiol* 59: 1266–70.

7. Helmcke F, Nanda NC, Hsiung MC, Soto B, Adey C, Goyal RG, Gatewood R (1987) Color Doppler Assessment of mitral regurgitation with orthogonal planes. *Circulation* 75: 175.

8. Moos S, Fan P, Chopra HK, Kapur KK, Shah VK, Helmcke F, Oberman A, Nanda NC (1989) Exercise carotid artery Doppler: A new method to assess cardiac function in coronary artery disease. *Clin Res* 37: 280A. (University of Alabama at Birmingham, Al).

8. Identification of intraoperative myocardial ischemia by transesophageal echocardiography

MARC E.R.M. VAN DAELE, GEORGE R. SUTHERLAND
and JOS R.T.C. ROELANDT

Introduction

The perioperative management of patients who are at risk for cardiac complications has improved dramatically with both the introduction of invasive hemodynamic monitoring and the aggressive use of inotropic and vasoactive drugs [1]. Nevertheless myocardial ischemia and infarction remain the primary cause of perioperative morbidity and mortality in the increasing number of older patients undergoing major surgery [2–6]. This perioperative cardiac mortality could be further reduced if myocardial ischemia could reliably be detected early enough to allow therapeutical intervention before ischemia has progressed to infarction as perioperative infarction carries a mortality of 50–70%. In this respect previous studies have found both hemodynamic monitoring and the electrocardiogram to be insensitive detectors [5, 7, 8].

The body surface ECG remains the most commonly used method of monitoring intraoperative myocardial ischemia, although it often fails to reveal subendocardial ischemia and infarction [9–11], and interpretation of ST-segment changes may be impossible because of bundle branch block, rhythm disturbances or cardiac pacing. Moreover, as a standard 12-lead ECG is impractical during surgery, often only a single ECG lead is used. Then even severe transmural ischemia may go unnoticed [12].

Invasive hemodynamic monitoring cannot compensate for the limitations of the ECG or replace it, since the correlation between hemodynamic abnormalities and the onset of myocardial ischemia is poor [13–15]. Therefore a more sensitive monitoring technique for the early detection of myocardial ischemia in the anesthetized patient would be of great clinical value.

In 1935 Tennant and Wiggers [16] were the first to demonstrate, in open-chested dogs, that coronary occlusion is followed by hypokinesia in the affected myocardium within 10 to 15 seconds. This progressed within 30 to 60 seconds to akinesia and dyskinesia, whereby the myocardial wall moves outward and becomes thinner during systole. In early myocardial ischemia,

S. Iliceto et al. (eds.), Ultrasound in Coronary Artery Disease, 67–81.
© 1991 Kluwer Academic Publishers.

changes in diastolic and systolic myocardial function were found to preceed the electrical changes. Therefore wall motion abnormalities are an early and sensitive indicator of ischemia. The superiority of wall motion dynamics over ECG changes as an early indicator of myocardial ischemia has been confirmed in many subsequent animal studies [11, 17–19]. However, the real time monitoring of wall motion dynamics has remained inaccessible for intra-operative monitoring until the advent of transesophageal echocardiography (TEE). TEE offers high-resolution real time images of the beating heart. It can usually be performed without interfering with the surgical field and the transducer can stay for hours in the same position relative to the heart and, more particularly, to the left ventricle. Recent studies have demonstrated that the detection of new regional wall motion abnormalities (RWMA) by TEE correlates more closely with perioperative myocardial ischemia and infarction than do intraoperative ECG-changes [20]. Thus TEE can be used for early recognition of evolving myocardial ischemia and facilitates immediate and specific fluid and pharmacologic interventions [21]. In this chapter we will discuss some aspects of current applications and expected developments of monitoring of myocardial ischemia by TEE.

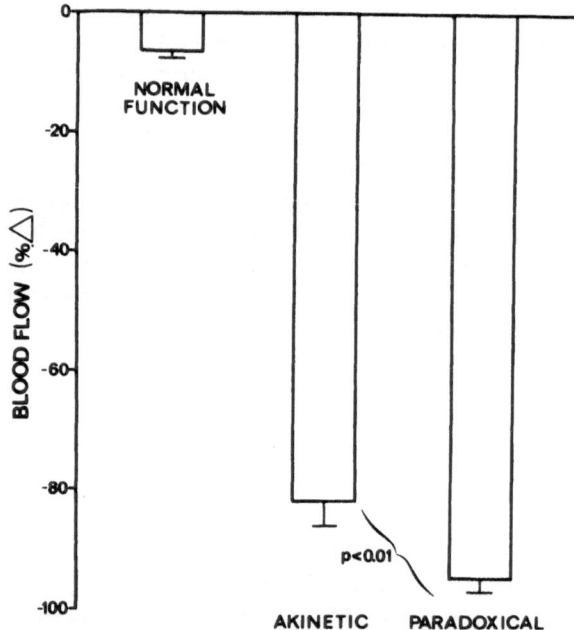

Figure 1. In the myocardium of open-chesed dogs, segments not demonstrating reduced shortening show only minimal decreases in blood flow. Segments characterized by paradoxical bulging show greater flow reductions than akinetic segments. (Reprinted, with permission, from Vatner [ref 18]).

Regional wall motion abnormalities (RWMA)

Regional wall motion abnormality is a nonspecific term applied to a segment of myocardium that demonstrates abnormal contraction or relaxation. The term does not specify the precise nature of the impaired wall motion dynamics, its timing in the cardiac cycle or the technique by which wall motion was studied.

After Tennant and Wiggers' initial demonstration of paradoxical motion in an ischemic area of myocardium, subsequent studies confirmed that wall motion abnormalities occur within seconds of the onset of ischemia [18, 23–24], simultaneously with lactate production [25, 26] and before, or even in the absence of changes on the surface ECG [11]. A constant sequence of changes in RWMA, going from hypokinesia through akinesia to dyskinesia was not only demonstrated as a sequence in time after total coronary occlusion; the same sequence was found in experimentally controlled progressive partial obstruction of the coronary arteries.

Vatner [18] demonstrated a sensitive coupling between coronary blood flow reduction and myocardial function in dogs. An acute reduction in coro-

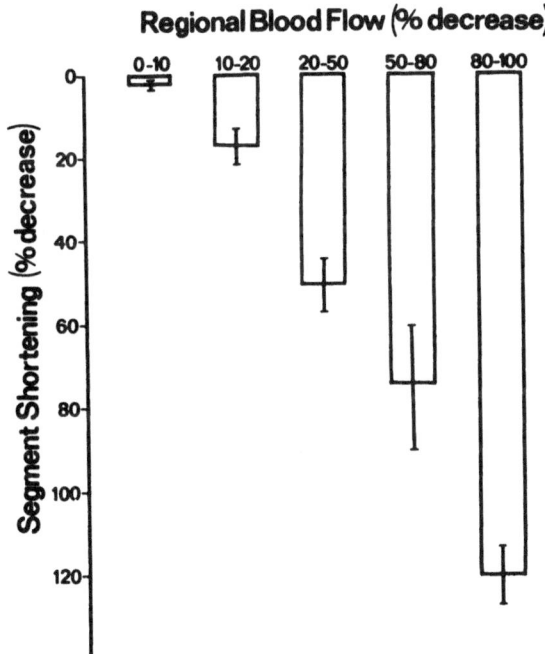

Figure 2. Controlled coronary blood flow reduction in dogs. Segments grouped according to % decrease in regional blood flow show progressive decreases in regional myocardial function. Segments with 10–20% decreases in regional blood flow show significant decreases in function. (Reprinted, with permission, from Vatner [ref 18]).

nary blood flow by 10–20% results in considerable hypokinesia, progressing to akinesia at a coronary blood flow reduction of $82 \pm 4\%$ and paradoxical motion to further reduction of $95 \pm 2\%$ (Figures 1, 2). Battler [11] studied the relationship between regional wall motion and ECGs during complete and partial coronary obstruction in conscious dogs. During mild coronary stenosis, RWMA were identified without changes in the surface ECG, while in moderate coronary stenosis the RWMAs preceded surface ECG alterations by several minutes. Only in acute total coronary occlusion changes in ST-segments of the ECG were present after 30–60 seconds, without an obvious delay to the RWMA.

The effects of coronary occlusion on wall motion, as documented in animal studies, were confirmed in humans during coronary balloon angioplasty. Visser et al. [27] used precordial echocardiography in 15 patients undergoing angioplasty and found regional wall motion abnormalities in all patients 8 ± 3 sec after balloon inflation, returning to baseline 19 ± 8 sec after balloon deflation. Only four patients in this study developed ST-segment changes in the extremity leads of the ECG, always preceded by the RWMAs.

Clements and de Bruyn [28] reviewed these and a series of similar studies and summarized the results in one diagram (Figure 3), concluding that the time of onset of ECG changes is highly dependent on the severity of ischemia, in contrast to wall motion abnormalities.

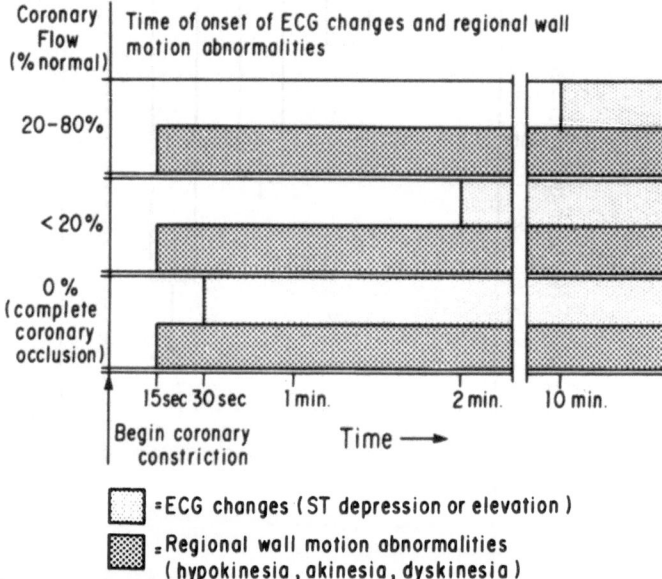

Figure 3. Temporal relationship between acute coronary constriction and onset of ECG and regional wall motion abnormalities. This Figure summarizes the data from several animal and human studies. (Reprinted, with permission, from Clements [ref 28]).

Transesophageal echocardiographic monitoring

The knowledge that ischemia induces RWMAs is not new, but gained little clinical interest as long as no method was available to detect and monitor these RWMAs in other than experimental circumstances. With the advent of two-dimensional TEE [29–31] a practical tool came available that allowed intraoperative wall motion analysis by real time imaging of the beating heart in the anesthetized patient.

Current equipment for TEE consists of multielement phased array 5 mHz ultrasound transducers, 10–12 min in diameter, mounted on the 9 mm shaft of a modified gastroscope (Figure 4). The wires for each element run through the gastroscope in the space that formerly contained the fiberoptics. Some types of transducers still contain fiberoptics, offering the potential advantage of visualising the throat and esophagus during introduction of the probe. A disadvantage is that they are stiffer and potentially more difficult to pass into the esophagus and stomach. With all recent instruments two-dimensional imaging, M-mode, pulsed Doppler and color flow mapping examinations can be performed. A horizontal cross-section with a 90 degrees width is produced. The controls of the gastroscope allow manipulation of the transducer along two axes; approximately 90 degrees forward and reverse mobility and approximately 70 degrees lateral mobility. In combination with advancement and rotation of the transducer, a variety of semihorizontal planes can be scanned within the constraints of the anatomy of the esophagus. A lock on the steering mechanism of the flexible tip is a standard feature enabling the transducer to remain in a stable position relative to the heart. The cardiac cross-sectional anatomy of standard obtainable views has been described [32].

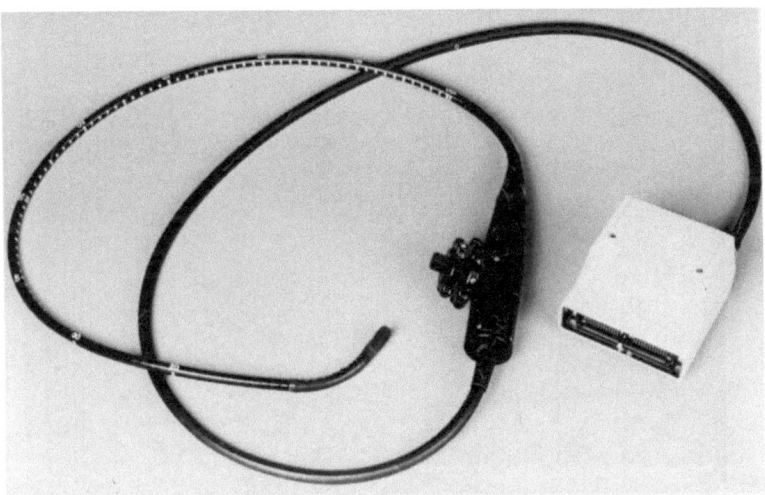

Figure 4. Transesophageal echocardiographic trasducer, mounted on a modified gastrocope.

Procedure

After some experience the transducer can be passed within a few seconds into the esophagus of the anesthetized, intubated patient. The steerable end of the transducer must be covered with lubricant and unlocked to follow the bends during its passage down into the esophagus and stomach. With the patient supine and the head in midline position the physician uses one hand to lift the mandible anteriorly and the other hand to pass the transducer. Using an adequate technique the transducer will slide into the esophagus with virtually no resistance. In rare cases, e.g. coexisting throat anomalies, a laryngoscope may be needed to visualize the esophagus directly. At a probe depth of approximately 40 cm from the incisors the tranducer usually is in the fundus of the stomach and a short axis view of the left ventricle can be obtained (Figure 5).

Myocardial contraction is best studied from short-axis views. Rankinn et al. [33] have shown, in the canine heart, that 87% of stroke volume is derived from shortening in the short axis of the left ventricle; very little contribution to cardiac output results from shortening of the long axis. For intraoperative monitoring purposes for ischemia-induced RWMAs the LV short axis view at midpapillary level (Figure 5) is the best single view to monitor, as this image includes segments of myocardium supplied by each of the 3 main coronary arteries (Figure 6). However, if the precise site of a critical coronary stenosis is known from angiography another view may be selected, imaging more of the myocardium at risk.

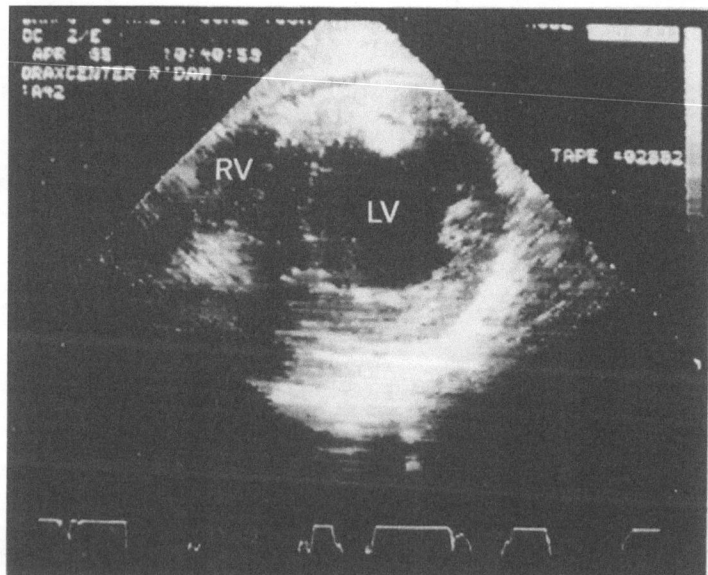

Figure 5. Transesophageal echo short-axis view of the left ventricle at the level of the papillary muscles.

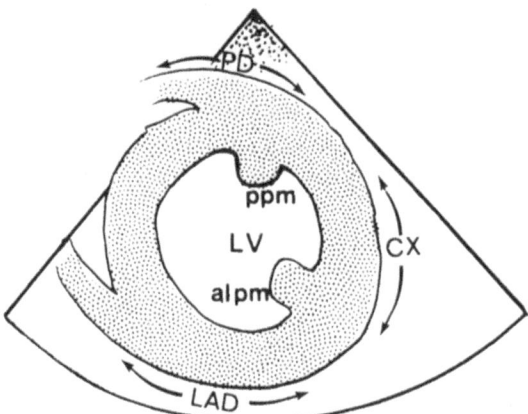

Figure 6. Schematic representation of the left ventricular short-axis view with an indication of the areas supplied by the main coronary arteries. alpm = anterolateral papillary muscle, ppm = posterior papillary muscle.

Risks and contraindications

Intraoperative TEE is a relatively safe procedure. At present the only complications reported in the literature are two cases of transient vocal cord paralysis in neurosurgical procedures conducted with extreme neck flexion against an endotracheal tube in whom TEE may have contributed to pressure on the laryngeal nerves [34]. Other risks are, (in theory):
- Abrasion of mucosa.
- Tracheal rather than esophageal introduction.
- Esophageal trauma and perforation or perforation of a Zenker's diverticulum.
- Rupture of esophageal varices.
- Stomach bleeding or rupture.
- Electrical or thermal hazards.

However, none of these have been reported so far, thus the risk is extremely low and comparable to upper gastro-intestinal endoscopy. Nevertheless esophageal varices, throat tumors and abcesses are considered to be serious contraindications, and coagulopathies and swallowing problems of any origin are relative contraindications. The airway of the anesthetized patient should always be protected by an endotracheal tube before introduction of the TEE transducer, so that accidental tracheal introduction of the probe cannot go unnoticed and eventual reflux of gastric contents will not result in aspiration. Good practise also requires that preexisting throat- and vocal cord anomalies are documented before TEE monitoring.

Conversion of electrical to ultrasonic energy in the transducer produces some heating, especially if Doppler measurements or color flow mapping (requiring more ultrasonic energy) are performed. Therefore all devices should have a temperature monitor, switching off transmittal power if the probe temperature exceeds 41°C. In case of cooling on cardiopulmonary bypass there may be an undesirable temperature gradient, even when the probe does not exceed it's maximum temperature. It is recommended to switch off transmittal power when TEE monitoring is not necessary, especially during cardiopulmonary bypass (when there is no use in monitoring wall motion anyway).

Clinical studies

The first report on a myocardial infarction occurring during TEE monitoring of the heart was published by Beaupré et al. [8]. A 57-year old woman with normal coronary arteries underwent mitral valve replacement. Prior to cardiopulmonary bypass TEE showed normal LV wall motion, but immediately after cardiopulmonary bypass LV anteroseptal akinesis was evident. The ECG did not indicate a myocardial infarction then. After surgery the 12-lead ECG revealed an anteroseptal transmural infarction and increased enzyme-levels suggested a large area of myocardial necrosis. The patient died subsequently of complications related to low cardiac output.

A high specificity of new and persistent RWMA for myocardial infarction was demonstrated by Kremer et al. [35]. In a series of 43 high-risk patients undergoing cardiac surgery they observed new, persistent RWMA in 7 patients. Five of them had a myocardial infarction, diagnosed by postoperative ECGs and enzymes. No infarctions were found in 8 patients of the same series who had transient RWMA during the procedure. The significance of these transient RWMAs was not clear, as none of these patients had ECG changes suggesting ischemia.

Smith et al. [20] compared sensitivity of surface ECG versus TEE for detection of perioperative ischemia in 50 patients with ischemic heart disease. New RWMAs were seen in 24 patients whereas only 6 of them developed ST-segment changes on a seven-lead ECG. All 6 patients with ECG changes also had new RWMAs: in three instances RWMAs occurred before ECG changes and in three instances they occurred simultaneously. This clinical study corroborated results from previous animal studies, demonstrating that RWMA monitored by TEE is more sensitive in detecting ischemia than is the body surface ECG.

In our own experience [36] we monitored for myocardial ischemia during and following induction of anesthesia in 68 patients with documented severe coronary artery disease. Simultaneous 12-lead ECG and TEE recordings were made and analysed independently. Wall motion analysis was performed by two investigators who were blinded to the ECG or other patient data. In 11 out of 68 patients a period of new RWMAs was diagnosed. In 8 of these 11 patients an ST-segment depression by one mm or more was apparent. There were no patients who had ST-segment changes and no RWMAs while the onset of ST-segment changes never preceded the RWMAs.

Wall motion analysis

In normal ventricular wall motion the myocardium thickens during systole and the endocardial border moves inward, reducing the ventricular cavity. Furthermore a translation and a small degree of rotation of the whole heart occur during systole. For immediate intraoperative analysis of wall motion, the investigator has to rely on a subjective impression of what is good or bad contraction, discounting myocardial movement that is not caused by contraction. Therefore the skill of the observer to detect, in real time, new RWMA may have great impact on the reliability of the method. Clements et al. [37] reported that this skill was readily acquired. They exposed a group of 53 clinicians to 20 min of instruction about transesophageal echocardiography and the recognition of regional wall motion abnormalities. With this background they were asked to grade regional wall motion in 12 videotaped recordings and their scores were compared to those of four trained observers. The 53 clinicians correctly identified 95% of the RWMAs. The incorrect responses most frequently were related to mild grades of abnormality.

For research purposes the LV short axis image is usually recorded on videotape and analysed off-line. Most investigators follow or modify the practise as described by Smith et al. [20, 38, 39]. The image of the myocardium is divided in four segments (inferior, lateral, anterior, septal) using the papillary muscles as a landmark (Figure 7). Each segment is subjectively scored by two independent observers on a scale of five classes (normal wall motion, mild and severe hypokinesia, akinesia, dyskinesia). The definition of myocardial ischemia in such semi-quantitative studies is a deterioration of wall motion in a myocardial segment by more than one class, noticed by both observers.

Such criteria for wall motion analysis may be quite satisfactory for clinical

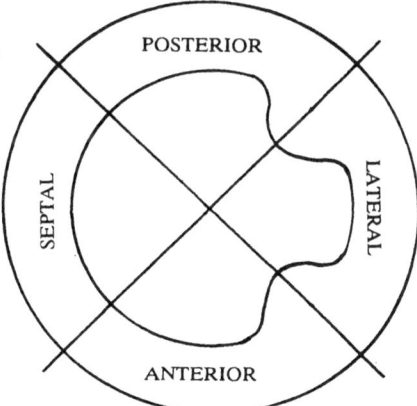

1. Normal * systolic shortening of the imaginary radius
   from the LV wall segment to the center of
   the LV cavity estimated more than 30%
   * considerable wall thickening
2. Mild hypokinesia
   * 10-30% systolic radial shortening
   * systolic wall thickening
3. Severe hypokinesia
   * less than 10% systolic radial shortening
   * minimal systolic wall thickening
4. Akinesia
   * no systolic radial shortening
   * no wall thickening
5. Dyskinesia
   * LV wall bulging out during systole

Figure 7. Schematic representation of the division of the short-axis view into four segments, and the criteria to grade wall motion per segment, as they are used in most studies in which regional wall is analysed by subjective grading.

studies, especially when inter-observer variability is low, but they reveal no gold-standard: both observers can be wrong. Therefore several systems for quantitative wall motion analysis are under development. Most of them currently are based on comparison of end diastolic versus end systolic images. After selection of these frames the endocardial border is traced, either by hand or by computer-supported contour detection, and fed into a computer analysis system. However, there are several problems which these quantitative analysis systems have to overcome, such as:

- How to select the end systolic frame; should that be defined as either the frame with the smallest intracavity area, the end of the T-wave on a synchronous ECG or the second heartsound, requiring a synchronous phonocardiogram?
- How to differentiate motion of the endocardial border, due to myocardial contraction, from motion due to translation and rotation of the whole heart? Both fixed and floating reference systems are being used in the analysis of wall motion [39].

Computer analysis of hand-drawn contours still contains subjective influences and it is not proven that the results are more accurate than those obtained by 'eyeballing' wall motion. Moreover it is uncertain whether quantitative analysis of RWMA from enddiastolic and endsystolic frames alone is reliable. Two new developments, currently in a preclinical state of technical development, appear to be promising adjuncts for quantitave wall motion analysis. These are automated (rather than manual) endocardial contour detection and frame-to-frame analysis within the cardiac cycle rather than analysis of enddiastolic and endsystolic frames only. However, implementation of such sophisticated computer software requires extremely good resolution of the endocardial border in every frozen frame image.

Problems and limitations

As stated before, analysis of LV wall motion from echocardiographic images remains subjective and qualitative rather than quantitative and meets several problems:

- The investigator must be able to distinguish myocardial contraction from motion that is due to translation and rotation of the whole heart. Akinetic regions, due to scar from previous infarctions, must be distinguished from new, ischemia-induced RWMAs and the assessment of changes over a longer period of time may be highly subjective, unless dual projection on the screen allows simultaneous projection of previous and actual wall motion.
- The contraction pattern of the normal left ventricle is not simply concentric and uniform. Myocardial systolic shortening and cross-sectional frac-

tional area change (FAC), as seen by echo, increase from the mitral valve (FAC $38.8 \pm 3.3\%$) to the lower left ventricular level (FAC $60.7 \pm 4.5\%$) [41]. Septal segments exhibit lowest contraction at the base, but the greatest increase from base to apex. Lateral regions do not show significant changes along the length of the left ventricle [41]. These regional differences may not be essential in assessing grossly abnormal contraction, but could be critical for interpretation of hypokinesis as frequently encountered in patients with coronary artery disease. It also implies that any system for quantitative wall motion analysis should not be compared to a model of concentric contraction but to regional myocardial contraction in a control-group of normals without cardiac disease.

– Quantification of RWMA is a complex problem in which the time course of the contraction is important to consider [42]. During the early onset of ischemia a temporal inhomogeneity in contraction may preceed real hypo-kinesia. This results in a 'wave-like' systolic contraction pattern which can be identified by accurate 'eye-ball' analysis but may be missed when quan-tifying regional wall motion from only end diastolic and endsystolic images. Zeiher et al. [43] found that in man ischemic injury first manifests itself as asynchronous polyphasic wall motion rather than as a change in the amplitude of wall excursion and that, if only enddiastolic and end systolic frames are analysed, up to 44% of ischemic episodes were missed when compared to integrative analysis of the entire contraction.

– Not all new RWMAs are necessarily due to myocardial ischemia or infarc-tion. Persistence of impaired contractile function after reperfusion ('stunned myocardium') can hamper the estimation of infarct size by echo-cardiography. In animal studies a lack of correlation was demonstrated between infarct size and the extent of wall motion abnormality during early reperfusion. Correlation improved again after myocardial edema and hyperemia had resolved [44]. So patients undergoing coronary angioplasty for acute myocardial infarction and patients undergoing coronary bypass grafting may exhibit reperfusion wall motion abnormalities. Estimates of viable and nonviable tissue made on the basis of echocardiographic images are not reliable in such patients [45].

– Following aortic and mitral valve replacement septal wall motion abnor-malities have been reported without any other indication that myocardial ischemia was apparent [46]. However, systolic myocardial thickening may be a useful criterium to assess the presence or absence of ischemia in these patients.

– Monitoring a single short-axis view during surgery one may miss myocar-dial ischemia localized outside the scanned plane. Although the short-axis view at midpapillary level provides images of segments of myocardium supplied by all three main coronary arteries, apical ischemia may go unno-ticed.

– As monitoring by TEE is uncomfortable for the awake patient, the technique is impractical for use before induction of anesthesia and in the postoperative period, both representing a high-risk period for the development of myocardial ischemia.

Early detection of ischemia by TEE requires a continuous and concentrated attention to the screen. As this is impractical, and interpretation remains subjective, increasingly sophisticated technology has prompted a trend toward instant automated and quantitative analysis of cross-sectional echocardiographic images.

Future perspectives

With further development of appropriate computer software, a system for on-line automated wall motion analysis and ischemia detection is rapidly coming into view. Ideally such a system should provide an integrated analysis of wall motion all through the cardiac cycle. The bottleneck in the development of such approach is the automated endocardial contour detection, for which several systems are under development [47–49].

A completely different approach to the identification of myocardial ischemia by echocardiography is tissue characterization by ultrasound integrated backscatter analysis [50–52]. Vital, non ischemic myocardium exhibits a diastolic to systolic cardiac cycle dependent variation of integrated backscatter in man. In infarcted segments the magnitude of cyclic variation is reduced or absent [53] and ultrasound tissue characterization therefore in theory is a potentially useful technique to differentiate various myopathic manifestations from normal myocardium.

Furthermore new sonicated microbubble echo-contrast agents, passing through the pulmonary capillary bed after intravenous injection, are currently subject of clinical research [54, 55]. In theory this may, in combination with TEE imaging, provide the surgeon with an intraoperative equivalent of perfusion scan and thereby contribute to a further expansion of the clinical application of TEE in monitoring intraoperative myocardial ischemia.

References

1. Rao TLK, Jacobs KH, El-etr AA (1983) Reinfarction following anesthesia in patients with myocardial infarction. *Anesthesiology* 59: 499–505.
2. Steen PA, Tinker JH, Tarhan S (1978) Myocardial reinfarction after anesthesia and surgery. *JAMA* 239: 2566.
3. Kennedy JW, Kaiser GC, Fisher LD (1981) Clinical and angiographica predictors of operative mortality from the collaborative study in coronary artery surgery (CASS). *Circulation* 63: 793–802.

4. Lunn JN, Mushin WW (1982) *Mortality Associated with Anesthesia*. London: Muffield Provincial Hospitals Trust.
5. Roizen MF, Beaupre PN, Alpert RA (1984) Monitoring with two-dimensional transesophageal echocardiography. *J Vasc Surg*: 300–305.
6. Jamieson WRF, Janusz MT, Miyagihima RT, Gerein AN (1982) Influence of ischemic heart disease on early and late mortality after surgery for peripheral occlusive vascular disease. *Circulation* 66: 92–7.
7. Roy WL, Edelist G, Gilbert B (1979) Ischemia during non-cardiac surgical procedures in patients with coronary artery disease. *Anesthesiology* 51: 393–397.
8. Beaupre PN, Kremer PF, Cahalan MK (1984) Intraoperative detection of changes of left ventricular segmental wall motion by transesophageal two-dimensional echocardiography. *Am Heart J* 107: 1021–1023.
9. Barnard RJ, Buckberg GD, Duncan HW (1980) Limitations of the standard transthoracic electrocardiogram in detecting subendocardial ischemia. *Am Heart J* 99: 476.
10. Sughishita Y, Koseki S, Matsuda M (1983) Dissociation between regional myocardial dysfunction and ECG changes during myocardial ischemia induced by exercise in patients with angina pectoris. *Am Heart J* 106: 1–8.
11. Battler A, Froelicher VF, Gallagher KP, Kemper WS, Ross J, Jr (1980) Dissociation between regional myocardial dysfunction and ECG changes during ischemia in the conscious dog. *Circulation* 62: 735.
12. Chaitman BR, Bourassa MG, Wagmans P (1978) Improved efficacy of treadmill exercise testing multiple lead ECG system and basic hemodynamic response. *Circulation* 57: 71.
13. Slogoff S, Keats AS (1985) Does perioperative myocardial ischemia lead to postoperative myocardial infarction? *Anesthesiology* 62(2): 107–114.
14. Leung J, O'Kelly MB, Browner W (1988) Are regional wall motion abnormalities detected by transesophageal echocardiography triggered by acute changes in supply and demand? *Anesthesiology* V69(3A): A801.
15. Häggmark S, Hohner P, Östman M (1989) Comparison of hemodynamic, electrocardiographic, mechanical and metabolic indicators of intraoperative myocardial ischemia in patients with coronary artery disease. *Anesthesiology* 70: 19–25.
16. Tennant R, Wiggers CJ (1935) The effect of coronary occlusion on myocardial contraction. *Am J Physiol* 112: 351–361.
17. Kerber RE, Marcus ML, Ehrhardt J (1975) Correlation between echocardiographically demonstrated segmental dyskinesis and regional myocardial perfusion. *Circulation* 52: 1097–1104.
18. Vatner SF (1980) Correlation between acute reductions in myocardial blood flow and function in conscious dogs. *Circ Res* 47: 201–207.
19. Wyatt HL, Forrester JS, Tyberg JV (1975) Effect of graded reductions in regional coronary perfusion on regional and total cardiac function. *Am J Cardiol* 36: 185–192.
20. Smith JS, Cahalan MK, Benefiel DJ (1985) Intraoperative detection of myocardial ischemia in high risk patients: Electrocardiography versus two-dimensional transesophageal echocardiography. *Circulation* 72: 1015–1021.
21. Gewertz BL, Kremer PC, Zarins CK (1987) Transesophageal echocardiographic monitoring of myocardial ischemia during vascular surgery. *J Vasc Surg* 5(4): 607–613.
22. Forrester JS, Wyatt HL, Protasio L (1976) Functional significance of regional ischemic contraction abnormalities. *circulation* 54: 64.
23. Gallagher KP, Kumada T, Koziol JA (1980) Significance of regional wall thickening relative to transmural myocardial perfusion in anesthetized dogs. *Circulation* 62: 1266.
24. Kerber RE, Marcus ML, Erhardt J, Wilson R, Abboud FM (1975) Correlation between echocardiographically demonstrated segmental dyskinesia and regional myocardial perfusion. *Circulation* 52: 1097.
25. Waters DP, Luz PD, Wyatt HL, Swan HJC, Forrester JS (1977) Early changes in regional and global left ventricular function induced by graded reductions in regional coronary perfusion. *am J Cardiol* 39: 537.

26. Massie BM, Botvinick EM, Brundage BR (1978) Relationship of regional myocardial perfusion to segmental wall motion: A physiological basis for understanding the presence of reversibility of asynergy. *Circulation* 58: 1154–63.
27. Visser CA, David GK, Kan G (1986) Two-dimensional echocardiography during percutaneous transluminal coronary angioplasty. *Am Heart J* 111: 1035–1041.
28. Clements FM, de Bruyn P (1987) Perioperative evaluation of regional wall motion by transesophageal two-dimensional echocardiography. *Anesth analg* 66: 249–261.
29. Hisanaga K, Hisanaga A, Nagata K, Yoshida S (1977) A new transesophageal real-time two dimensional echocardiographic system using a flexible tube and its clinical application. *Proc Jpn Soc Ultrason Med* 32: 43–44.
30. Hisanaga K, Hisanaga A, Nagata K, Ichie Y (1980) Transesophageal cross-sectional echocardiography. *Am Heart J* 100: 605–609.
31. Schluter M, Langenstein BA, Polster J (1982) Transesophageal cross-sectional echocardiography with phased array transducer system : Technique and initial clinical results. *Br Heart J* 48: 67–72.
32. Schluter M, Hinrichs A, Wolfgang T (1990) Transesophageal Two-dimensional Echocardiography: Comparison of ultrasonic and anatomic sections. *Am J Cardiol* 53: 1173–1178.
33. Rankin JS, McHale PA, Arentzen CE (1976) Three dimensional dynamic geometry of the left ventricle in the conscious dog. *Circ Res* 39: 304–313.
34. Cucchiara RF, Nugent M, Sewart JB (1984) Air embolism in upright neurosurgical patients: detection and localization by two-dimensional transesophageal echocardiography. *Anesthesiology* 60: 353–355.
35. Kremer P, Gahalan MK, Beaupre PN (1983) Intraoperative myocardial ischemia detected by Transesophageal Two-Dimentional Echocardiography. *Circulation* 68: 332.
36. van Daele MERM, Sutherland GR, Mitchell MM (1990) Do changes in pulmonary capillary wedge pressure adequately detect myocardial ischemia? A correlative hemodynamic, electrocardiographic and transesophageal echocardiographic study. submitted.
37. Clements FM, Hill R, Kisslo J, Orchard R (1986) How easily can we learn to recognize regional wall motion abnormalities with 2D transesophageal echocardiography? *Proc Soc Cardiovasc Anesthesiol*, 7th annual meeting, Montreal, 1986.
38. Shively BK, Schiller MB (1986) Transesophageal echocardiography in the intraoperative detection of myocardial ischemia and infarction. *Echocardiography* 3: 433–443.
39. Cahalan MK, Prakash O, Rulf EN (1987) Addition of nitrous oxide to fentanyl anesthesia does not induce myocardial ischemia in patients with ischemic heart disease. *Anesthesiology* 67–6: 925–929.
40. Schnittger I, Fitzgerald PJ, Jordan EP (1984) Computerized quantitative analysis of left ventricular wall motion by two-dimensional echocardiography. *Circulation* 70: 242–250.
41. Haendchen RV, Wyatt HL, Maurer G (1983) Quantitation of regional cardiac function by two-dimensional echocardiography. 1. Patterns of contraction in the normal left ventricle. *Circulation* 67(6): 1234–44.
42. Weyman AE, Franklin TD, Hogan RD (1984) Importance of temporal hetrogeneity in assessing the contraction abnormalities associated with acute myocardial ischemia. *Circulation* 70: 102.
43. Zieher AM, Wollschlaeger HW, Bonzel T, Kasper W, Just H (1987) Hierarchy of levels of ischemia-induced impairment in regional left ventricular systolic function in man. *Circulation* 76(4): 768–776.
44. Wyatt HL, Meerbaum S (1981) Experimental evaluation of the extent of myocardial dyssynergy and infarct size by two-dimensional echocardiography. *Circulation* 63: 607–614.
45. Braunwald E, Kloner RA (1982) The stunned myocardium: prolonged post-ischemic ventricular dysfunction. *Circulation* 66: 1146–1149.
46. Burggraf GW, Craige E (1975) Echocardiographic studies of left ventricular wall motion and dimensions after valvular heart surgery. *Am J Cardiol* 35: 473–80.

47. Ezekiel A, Areeda JS, Garcia EV, Corday SR (1987) Intelligent left ventricular contour detection results from two-dimensional echocardiograms. *Comp Cardiol* pp 603–606. Long Beach, California: IEEE Computer Society.

48. Chu CH, Delp EJ, Buda AJ (1990) Detecting left ventricular endocardial and epicardial boundaries by digital two-dimensional echocardiography. *Comp Cardiol*, pp 393–396. Long Beach, California: IEEE Computer Society.

49. Bosch JG, Reiber JHC, van Burken G (1990) Automated endocardial contour detection in short-axis 2-D echocardiograms; methodology and assessment of variability. (in press)

50. Miller JG, Perez JE, Sobel BE (1985) Ultrasonic characterization of myocardium. *Progress in Cardiovascular Diseases*, Vol 28(2): 85–110.

51. Chandraratna PAN, Jones JP, Leeman S (1988) Ultrasonic tissue characterization of the heart. *Echocardiography* 5(3): 183–198.

52. Perez JE, Miller JG, Barzilai B (1988) Progress in quantitative ultrasonic characterization of myocardium: From the laboratory to the bedside. *Journal of the American Society of Echocardiography* 1(4): 294–304.

53. Vered Z, Mohr G, Barzilai B (1989) Ultrasound integrated backscatter tissue characterization of remote myocardial infarction in human subjects. *JACC* 13(1): 84–91.

54. Berwing K, Schlepper M (1988) Echocardiographic imaging of the left ventricle by peripheral intravenous injection of echo contrast agent. *Am Heart J* 115: 399–408.

55. Feinstein FB, Heidenreich PA, Dick CD (1988) A new intravascular ultrasound contrast agent: Preliminary safety and efficacy results. *Circulation* 78 (suppl 4): II–565.

9. Silent myocardial ischemia
Clinical implications, detection and management

GIUSEPPE SPECCHIA, COLOMBA FALCONE,
CRISTINA OPASICH and MARIA TERESA LA ROVERE

Introduction

Silent myocardial ischemia can be defined as a condition of discrepancy between the supply of oxygen to the myocardium and the metabolic demand thereof to such an extent as to induce biochemical mechanical and electric alterations which are characteristic of myocardial ischemia but cause no pain. Such a situation can be transient (a silent transient ischemic attack) and end with the metabolic and functional recovery of the affected myocardial fibrous cells, or continue until it causes irreversible damage, finally leading to necrosis (silent myocardial infarction). A flow which is chronically reduced but nonetheless sufficient to keep the myocardium vital (hibernating myocardium) [1] is very often not associated with angina but with signs and symptoms of an alteration of the pump function: the term 'silent chronic ischemia', however, is questionable in view of the probable metabolic reset, which casts doubts on the definition of ischemia itself.

The silent ischemic attack is undoubtedly the most widespread form of acute myocardial ischemia not associated with pain and has been extensively studied in recent years. The following points seem to be well-established and confirmed by numerous studies:

- silent acute ischemia constitutes the vast majority of both spontaneous and induced ischemic events, regardless of the pathogenetic mechanism which induced the ischemia [2–8].
- The silent ischemic episode differs from the symptomatic one in the absence of pain. The electric, mechanical and hemodynamic alterations largely coincide [2, 6–12]. Silent episodes seem to be characterized by a shorter duration and a lower severity of the ischemia only in the case of acute transmural ischemic episodes such as those which occur in vasospastic ischemia [3, 4–13]; the value of this observation is largely undermined by extensive overlap in the data.
- The prognosis of patients with silent ischemia and with symptomatic ischemia is substantially identical [14–17].

S. Iliceto et al. (eds.), Ultrasound in Coronary Artery Disease, 83–93.
© 1991 *Kluwer Academic Publishers.*

- In the vast majority of cases, patients subject to silent ischemic attacks also suffer from episodes accompanied by angina. Though it is impossible to precisely define the prevalence of patients who are always fully asymptomatic during ischemia, the very few available studies suggest that this population is very small [18].
- The reason, or reasons, for which pain sometimes accompanies ischemia and sometimes does not are as yet unknown. It is still unclear whether the absence of pain is a specific attribute of the individual ischemic attack or a characteristic condition of the patient, who is capable of inhibiting the origin, the transmission or the subjective perception of pain in most or all of the ischemic episodes he suffers [19–23].

The frequent coexistence of silent and symptomatic ischemic episodes in the same patients and the probable rarity of patients with constantly and fully asymptomatic ischemic attacks gives a partial indication of the problems involved in identifying patients affected by silent ischemia and combines the diagnostic difficulties of silent ischemia with some which are already known for symptomatic ischemia. Among these difficulties, the greatest lies in the fact that the gold reference standard for many of the tests which are intended to explore myocardial ischemia is not myocardial ischemia itself, but angiographically encountered coronary artery obstructions.

The absence of pain which characterizes silent ischemic episodes naturally further complicates the task of recognizing a test as truly positive. The importance of this further reduction in diagnostic power varies depending on whether it is necessary to define a state of illness or rule it out in a suspected patient, or to seek the incidence of silent episodes in a patient who is known to be affected by myocardial ischemia. Since in this last case diagnostic certainty almost always arises from the fact that episodes of myocardial ischemia associated with pain have already been documented, the result is the clinical paradox that one of the parameters favoring the diagnosis of silent ischemia is the anamnestic knowledge of painful ischemia episodes in that patient.

Diagnosis of silent ischemia in always-asymptomatic patients

This population belongs to Type 1 of Cohn's classification [24] and is naturally the least well-defined; there are no clues as to its numeric extent.

Since, as mentioned, in the vast majority of cases episodes of asymptomatic ischemia are accompanied by others associated with pain in the same patient, finding always and totally asymptomatic patients may mean one of two things: either these patients are different and constitute an independent group, or for unknown reasons in these patients the ischemic attack always occurs with those characteristics which make it silent. The doubt naturally arises from our ignorance on the mechanisms which facilitate or prevent the onset of angor during ischemia.

If we consider subjects affected by coronary obstructive disease, we can envision at least two situations of always asymptomatic patients. One patient, affected by coronary artery atherosclerosis, faces in his ordinary life circumstances in which the myocardial oxygen demand exceeds the possibility of flow: ischemia occurs, but for reasons we are not aware of, it is never perceived as pain. Another patient has very similar anatomical characteristics; however, for some circumstances, such as smaller usual physical effort, lower response in heart rate and blood pressure during efforts, the development of an adequate collateral circulation, he does not reach ischemia and therefore has no symptoms.

The frequent confusion between the anatomical datum and the identification of the presence or absence of ischemia can cause confusion among the two subjects in the definition of (always) silent ischemic cardiopathy, which as a matter of fact applies only to patients who can be recognized as belonging to the first example.

If the coronary vessels are not damaged, a small percentage of the ischemic population has vasospastic angina, which in some rare cases is exclusively silent. However, in so-called healthy individuals with no coronary disease, silent acute ischemia may possibly occur with greater and totally unknown frequency. It is known that pain highly suggestive for angina may sometimes be perceived in healthy subjects as a consequence of violent central stimulations with excessive orthosympathetic responses, indicating a crisis in the oxygen demand/supply balance of the myocardium [25]. We know nothing of the likelihood with which the normal myocardium may be subject to brief periods of silent ischemia during sudden and intense metabolic stresses which are not counterbalanced by an immediate increase in coronary flow.

There are no data available to orient us as to the actual prevalence of subjects with episodes of always and totally silent acute myocardial ischemia in the general population. The numbers derived from the percentage of patients struck by sudden death or acute myocardial infarction neither preceded nor associated with angor are not very useful, since both conditions need not be preceded by episodes of transient acute ischemia [18, 26–33]. The anatomic and pathological observation of obstructive coronary lesions cannot in itself necessarily lead to the conclusion that the patient was affected by ischemic episodes [34, 35].

The only work of a certain numeric extent on the general population is the well-known study conducted by Erikssen et al. [36], who studied 2014 apparently healthy males between 40 and 59 years of age and found a positive stress test without angina and angiographically encountered obstructive coronary damage in 2.5% of them.

This datum, however, runs the risk of losing at least part of its value, since in the follow-up of these fully asymptomatic ischemic subjects 8 of the 9 deceased had painful symptoms before dying.

Therefore, even so-called always asymptomatic individuals may possibly belong to a continuous clinical spectrum in which pain is a contingent symptom which occurs constantly or often or rarely in some patients during the history of the disease and is present only in some phases in other patients, while in yet others it is completely absent perhaps because major events have prevented its occurrence by interrupting the history.

Diagnosis of silent ischemia in patients with past myocardial infarction

Patients having episodes of silent ischemia after suffering myocardial infarction belong to Cohn's Type 2 [24]. The fact that these patients have been classified in a category of their own can be justified by:

- a possible different pathogenesis of the absence of pain
- the difficulty of a diagnosis of ischemia, especially when it occurs without pain, in a patient with myocardial infarction [37].

In our experience [38, 39], on the basis of the ECG response to stress testing in patients who survived a first myocardial infarction, we observed exercise-induced ischemia in 35% of the patients; among these, 77% had ECG signs not associated with pain. The addition of a thallium test seems to confirm the ischemic significance of the ECG alterations induced by effort only in half of the patients affected by silent ischemia. On the other hand, the ergometric analysis of these patients with a recent first myocardial infarction points out an exercise-induced ischemia only in 38% of the patients having a documented disease involving two-three coronary vessels, and 86% of the positive responses are silent [40].

Post-infarction silent ischemia therefore constitutes the absolute majority of the positive responses to stress testing in these patients, but the reduced specificity of the ECG signal not associated with pain makes it very often questionable, while its reduced sensitivity leads to an important underestimation of positive cases.

The possibility that a different mechanism may have a role in determining the absence of pain during post-infarction ischemia has so far failed to find confirmation of any sort; similarly, we do not know if subjective symptoms may be modified by other events, such as for example surgery or myocardial revascularization.

Stress-induced silent ischemia in post-infarction does not seem to depend on the effort level required to reach the ischemic threshold, on the extent of the ischemic threshold in terms of double product and therefore of myocardial oxygen consumption, on the degree of ST depression, on the severity of the coronary disease, on the location of the infarction scar, while an echocardiographic score suggests a larger scar for asymptomatic patients [9, 38–40].

Another important datum is that in the vast majority of cases patients with silent post-infarction ischemia have suffered pain during the acute phase of the infarction, while there are no reliable data on the frequency of silent pre-infarction ischemia in this group of patients.

Diagnosis of silent ischemia in patients with angina

Episodes of transient acute ischemia without pain can be documented more or less frequently in all patients who also denounce symptomatic episodes, both stress-induced and at rest. In many studies [2–7, 15–17, 41], the comparison between symptomatic and asymptomatic patients was made by including the patients according to their response to an ergometric test during which the ECG signs of ischemia were associated or not with typical pain. This characteristic tends to repeat in the same patient in multiple tests performed at various time intervals, though it cannot be considered an absolute rule [42]. The two groups of patients do not differ in most of their clinical, ergometric and angiographic characteristics, but a greater tolerance [43], a higher pain threshold [20] and higher beta-endorphine blood levels [21, 44] have been indicated in the asymptomatic group.

It is still unclear which, if any, is the point of transition between patients occasionally suffering from angina, patients affected by predominantly silent episodes and always-asymptomatic patients. As we said earlier, we have the impression that there is a wide range of situations and that the two extremes are respectively constituted by patients in which only pain-associated episodes are always documented and by patients who have never complained of angina and in which always and only silent transient ischemia is found.

Despite the potentially greater danger of unperceived ischemic episodes and a possible definition of 'asymptomatic' patients as a population at higher risk, most follow-up studies agree in showing that the event frequencies of the two populations fully coincide, provided that the survival curves are corrected for the severity of the underlying coronary pathology [14–17, 45, 46].

On the other hand, prolonged episodes of silent ischemia are markers of a more severe prognosis [47–49] in patients with unstable angina, and this datum confirms that ischemia, not the presence of pain, is important in characterizing the severity of the disease.

Diagnostic flow-chart in patients with suspected silent ischemia

The tests available for diagnosing silent ischemia are naturally the same which are routinely used for diagnosing symptomatic myocardial ischemia and are therefore subject to the same limitations. Some of these tests investigate the electric or mechanical consequences of ischemia, others examine the possible metabolic alterations caused by ischemia, while still others merely document differences in perfusion among various myocardial regions, assuming that a reduced perfusion is capable of inducing ischemia. Furthermore, the sensitivity and specificity of each test have been evaluated in terms of the presence or absence of coronary disease rather than in terms of the presence or absence of ischemia, and it is widely known that these two aspects do not necessarily coincide. The predictive value of a diagnostic test also depends on the prevalence of the disease in the population being tested, as well as on its sensitivity and specificity. It is thus evident that a positive test in a population of asymptomatic individuals, in which the prevalence of coronary disease is obviously low, has a low chance of being truly positive. This entails the need to confirm the diagnosis by administering further tests, thus progressively selecting groups of patients who have the highest likelihood of being ill and increasing the predictive power of diagnostic testing [5, 8, 50, 51].

However, a systematic search for silent ischemia in a general population of asymptomatic individuals, using current investigation methods, has unacceptable cost/benefit ratio limitations. The only conceivable diagnostic scheme is therefore to act on highly selected groups of patients who despite being asymptomatic are characterized by the coexistence of multiple risk factors (sex, age, smoking, dyslipemia, hypertension) for which the prevalence of coronary disease (and therefore of assumed silent ischemia) becomes high enough to provide a good yield of the applied diagnostic tests.

In patients with a past myocardial infarction, if the disease is highly prevalent the sensitivity and specificity of the most commonly used tests, such as those employing the ECG sensor, are usually reduced by the electric alterations which are already present in basic conditions [52–54]. A positive response to stress testing in the absence of angina, especially when the ECG alterations are not very significant, suggests the need confirmation through a further test, which should be chosen among those which have a different meaning from the first test. Thus it is more advantageous to follow an ergometric test with a test giving data on mechanical or perfusion alterations [55–57].

In patients with angina, the problem to be coped with does not generally reside in finding out if the patient is ischemic, but in determining if he also has silent ischemic episodes and in evaluating the extent of this unperceived ischemia within the general scope of his disease. A first question is whether it is more useful to study stress testing response in these patients or to look out for episodes of transient ischemia during Holter monitoring. In other words, the question is whether it is more important to discover a silent ischemia induced by a maximal effort or to determine the presence of silent ischemic episodes during everyday life. These two items of information have different meanings; both can allow a better understanding of the patient. A stress test which is positive only in terms of ECG alterations and is not associated with pain in an anginous patient suggests that the patient may also incur in episodes of silent ischemia; this, as mentioned, characterizes a probably different population, though as yet it is not known to what extent this knowledge may be useful in providing better prognostic evaluation and more rational therapy.

The finding of silent ischemic episodes during Holter monitoring is probably more important in the management of the patient, provided that at least two fundamental notions are kept in mind. The specificity of the silent transitory ECG alterations during Holter monitoring is still being questioned and is much less tested for a coronary disease than ECG alterations during a classical stress test [3, 6, 58, 59]. Interpreting a Holter graph is often very difficult, and the current automatic reading systems must yet receive final validation. Some authors [4, 59–61] have suggested that silent ischemic episodes evident through Holter monitoring are characterized by a lower double product with respect to the one required to obtain ischemia during stress in the same patient. This hypothesis is questioned by other authors [62, 63]; if it is confirmed, the evidence of ischemia in Holter monitoring would become even more important. Currently, however, except for patients with ischemic cardiopathy with an obviously vasospastic pathogenesis, the search for silent ischemia in Holter monitoring is important and should be reserved most of all for patients for whom a low threshold of symptomatic or silent ischemia has been demonstrated during ergometric testing [13, 59, 64, 65].

Management of patients with silent ischemia

If silent ischemia and symptomatic ischemia have the same meaning, produce the same metabolic, mechanical and electric derangement of the myocardium and entail no substantial difference in the number of major coronary events suffered by the patient with silent ischemia with respect to the anginous patient, the indication for treatment should consequently be exactly identical.

This is true in patients in an unstable phase of the disease, when the progressive aggravation of the ischemia, whether symptomatic or silent, is associated with a high risk of death or of non-fatal infarction. The therapeutic decision must still be considered independent from the presence of the pain symptom in patients with extensive coronary disease and ischemic depression of the pump function, or in patients having anatomically severe coronary lesions, such as left main coronary artery disease; in all these cases, myocardial reperfusion has repeatedly proved to be associated with longer survival [66].

On the other hand, for many patients with chronic angina the rational indication for treatment is determined by the invalidity caused by the symptom. If the recurrence of pain resists medical therapy, PTCA or surgery are universally recommended. On the contrary, it is still to be proved that the administration of antianginous drugs or revascularization, besides eliminating pain, also reduce the risk of infarction and death in these patients. Recent data derived from clinical observation [27, 67, 68] (acute myocardial infarction is hardly ever preceded by a chronic history of angina) and from the angiographic data obtained after thrombolysis or gathered before and after acute infarction in the same patient seem to confirm that thrombosis and acute infarction are often associated with small coronary obstructive lesions which cause no ischemia or angina indeed because of their small size. All these considerations make it very difficult to decide the most appropriate course of action for patients with silent chronic ischemia when angina is missing, and other therapies (e.g. anti-aggregants) certainly have a greater rational basis than anti-ischemic treatment for preventing fatal or non-fatal thrombosis. The issue is however still hotly debated, and much discussion and investigation is still needed. It is sufficient to remember that a possible indication for the therapy of silent chronic ischemia is to prevent repeated ischemias from leading, in the course of time, to fibrosis and to chronic pump efficiency reductions, compromising survival as well as function [69, 70].

References

1. Braunwald E, Rutherford J (1986) Reversible ischemic left ventricular dysfunction: Evidence for the 'hibernating myocardium'. *J Am Coll Cardiol* 8: 1467.
2. Stern S, Gavish A, Weist G, Benhorin J, Keren A, Tzivoni D (1988) Characteristics of silent and symptomatic myocardial ischemia during daily activities. *Am J Cardiol* 61: 1223.
3. Weidinger F, Sochor H, Czerning J, Pospischil E, Glogar D (1988) Characteristics of transient ischaemic episodes in patients with silent and symptomatic exercise-induced myocardial ischaemia. *Eur Heart J* 9: 1081.
4. Cecchi A, Dovellini E, Marchi F, Pucci P, Santoro G, Fazzini F (1983) Silent myocardial ischemia during ambulatory electrocardiographic monitoring in patients with effort angina. *J Am Coll Cardiol* 3: 934.
5. Rozanski A, Berman D (1987) Silent myocardial ischemia. I. Pathophysiology, frequency of occurrence, and approaches toward detection. *Am Heart J* 114: 615.
6. Campbell S, Barry J, Rebecca G, Rocco M, Nabel E, Wayme R, Selyn A (1986) Active transient myocardial ischemia during daily life in asymptomatic patients with positive exercise tests and coronary artery disease. *Am J Cardiol* 57: 1010.
7. Cohn P, Lawson W (1987) Characteristics of silent myocardial ischemia during out-of-hospital activities in asymptomatic angiographically documented coronary artery disease. *Am J Cardiol* 59: 746.
8. Epstein S, Quyyumi A, Benow R (1988) Myocardial ischemia – Silent or symptomatic. *N Engl J Med* 318: 1038.
9. Ouyang P, Shapiro E, Chandra N, Gottlieb S, Chew P, Gottlieb SH (1987) An angiographic and functional comparison of patients with silent and symptomatic treadmill ischemia early after myocardial infarction. *Am J Cardiol* 59: 730.
10. Levy R, Shapiro L, Wright C, Mockus L, Fox K (1986) The haemodynamic significance of asymptomatic ST segment depression assessed by ambulatory pulmonary artery pressure monitoring. *Br Heart J* 56: 526.
11. Wohlgelernter B, Jaffe C, Cabin H, Yeatman L, Cleman M (1987) Silent ischemia during coronary occlusion produced by balloon inflation: Relation to regional myocardial dysfunction. *J Am Coll Cardiol* 10: 491.
12. Davies G, Bencivelli W, Fragasso G, Chierchia S, Crea F, Crow J, Crean P, Pratt T, Morgan M, Maseri A (1988) Sequence and magnitude of ventricular volume changes in painful and painless myocardial ischemia. *Circulation* 78: 310.

13. Quyyumi A, Mockus L, Wright C, Fox K (1985) Morphology of ambulatory ST segment changes in patients with varying severity of coronary artery disease: Investigation of the frequency of nocturnal ischaemia and coronary spasm. *Br Heart J* 53: 186.
14. Rozanski A, Berman D (1987) Silent myocardial ischemia. II. Prognosis and implications for the clinical assessment of patients with coronary artery disease. *Am Heart J* 114: 627.
15. Bonow R, Bacharach S, Green M, LaFreniere R, Epstein S (1987) Prognostic implications of symptomatic versus asymptomatic (silent) myocardial ischemia induced by exercise in mildly symptomatic and in asymptomatic patients with angiographically documented coronary artery disease. *Am J Cardiol* 60: 778.
16. Falcone C, De Servi S, Poma E, Campana C, Scire' A, Montemartini C, Specchia G (1987) Clinical significance of exercise – induced silent myocardial ischemia in patients with coronary artery disease. *J Am Coll Cardiol* 9: 295.
17. Weiner D, Ryan T, McCabe C, Luk S, Chaitman B, Sheffield T, Tristani F, Fisher L (1987) Significance of silent myocardial ischemia during exercise testing in patients with coronary artery disease. *Am J Cardiol* 59: 725.
18. Erikssen J, Thaulow E (1989) Follow-up of patients with asymptomatic myocardial ischemia, in: Rutishauser W, Roskamm H (eds) *Silent Myocardial Ischemia*. Berlin: Springer-Verlag.
19. Droste C, Greenlee M, Roskamm H (1986) A defective angina pectoris pain warning system: Experimental findings of ischemic and electrical pain test. *Pain* 26: 199.
20. Droste C, Roskamm H (1983) Experimental pain measurement in patients with asymptomatic myocardial ischemia. *J Am Coll Cardiol* 3: 940.
21. Falcone C, Specchia G, Rondanelli R, Guasti L, Corsico G, Codega S, Montemartini C (1988) Correlation between beta-endorphin plasma levels and anginal symptoms in patients with coronary artery disease. *J Am Coll Cardiol* 11: 719.
22. Specchia G, Falcone C, Rondanelli R, De Servi S, Opasich C, Ardissino D, Codega S, Corsico G, La Rovere MT, Tramarin R (1986) Ischemia miocardica silente. *Cardiologia* 31: 859.
23. Cohn P (1980) Silent myocardial ischemia in patients with a defective anginal warning system. *Am J Cardiol* 45: 697.
24. Cohn P (1981) Asymptomatic coronary artery disease. *Mod Concepts Cardiovasc Dis* 50: 55.
25. Cannon R (1988) Causes of chest pain in patients with normal coronary angiograms: The eye of the beholder. *Am J Cardiol* 62: 306.
26. Kreger B, Kannel W, Cupples A (1987) Electrocardiographic precursors of sudden unexpected death: The Framingham study. *Circulation* 75 (suppl II): 22.
27. Davies M, Thomas A (1985) Plaque fissuring – the cause of acute myocardial infarction, sudden ischemic death, and crescendo angina. *Br Heart J* 53: 363.
28. Meissner M, Morganroth J (1986) Silent myocardial ischemia as a mechanism of sudden cardiac death. *Cardiol Clin* 4: 593.
29. Hong R, Bhandari A, McKay C, Au P, Rahimtoola H (1987) Life-threatening ventricular tachycardia and fibrillation induced by painless myocardial ischemia during exercise testing. *JAMA* 257: 1937.
30. Sharma B, Asinger R, Francis G, Hodges M, Wyeth R (1987) Demonstration of exercise-induced painless myocardial ischemia in survivors of out-of-hospital ventricular fibrillation. *Am J Cardiol* 59: 740.
31. Kannel W, Abbott R (1984) Incidence and prognosis of unrecognized myocardial infarction: An updata on the Framingham Study. *N Engl J Med* 311: 1144.
32. Assey M, Walters G, Hendrix G, Carabello B, Usher B, Spann J (1987) Incidence of acute myocardial infarction in patients with exercise-induced silent myocardial ischemia. *Am J Cardiol* 59: 497.
33. Hohnloser S, Kasper W, Zehender M, Geibel A, Meinertz T, Just H (1980) Silent myocardial ischemia as a predisposing factor for ventricular fibrillation. *Am J Cardiol* 61: 461.

34. Warnes C, Roberts W (1984) Sudden coronary death: Relation of amount and distribution of coronary narrowing at necropsy to previous symptoms of myocardial ischemia, left ventricular scarring and heart weight. *Am J Cardiol* 54: 65.

35. Barbour D, Warnes C, Roberts W (1987) Cardiac findings associated with sudden death secondary to atherosclerotic coronary artery disease: Comparison of patients with and those without previous angina pectoris and/or healed myocardial infarction. *Circulation* 75 (suppl II): 9.

36. Erikssen J, Cohn P, Thaulous E, Nowinchel P (1987) Silent myocardial ischaemia in middle aged men: Long-term clinical course, in: von Armin T, Maseri A (eds), *Silent Ischemia Current Concepts and Management.* Darmstadt: Steinkopff Verlag and New York: Springer Verlag.

37. Gibson R, Beller G, Kaiser L (1987) Prevalence and clinical significance of painless ST segment depression during early postinfarction exercise testing. *Circulation* 75 (suppl II): 36.

38. Opasich C, Cobelli F, Assandri J, Calsamiglia G, Febo O, La Rovere MT, Pozzoli M, Tramarin R, Traversi E, Ardissino D, Specchia G (1984) Incidence and prognostic significance of symptomatic and asymptomatic exercise-induced ischemia in patients with recent myocardial infarction. *Cardiology* 71: 284.

39. Opasich C, Riccardi G, Assandri J, Calsamiglia G, Forni R, La Rovere MT, Cobelli F, De Servi S, Specchia G (1988) The effects of physical training in postmyocardial infarction patients with exercise-induced silent ischaemia. *Eur Heart J* 9 (suppl): 176–180.

40. Opasich C, Cobelli F, Farilla C, Riccardi G, Bosco L, La Rovere MT, Bramucci E, Specchia G (1988) Silent Ischaemia in post-myocardial infarction patients submitted to physical training. *Eur Heart J* 9 (suppl M): 22–27.

41. Coy K, Imperi G, Lambert C, Pepine C (1987) Silent myocardial ischemia during daily activities in asymptomatic men with positive exercise test responses. *Am J Cardiol* 59: 45.

42. Specchia G, Falcone C (1988) Exercise-induced silent myocardial ischemia in patients with coronary artery disease. *CVR and R* (suppl): 25.

43. Glazier J, Chierchia S, Brown M, Maseri A (1986) Importance of generalized defective perception of painful stimuli as a cause of silent myocardial ischemia in chronic stable angina pectoris. *Am J Cardiol* 58: 667.

44. Sheps D, Adams K, Hinderliter A, Price C, Bissette J, Orlando G, Margolis B, Koch G (1987) Endorphins are related to pain perception in coronary artery disease. *Am J Cardiol* 59: 523.

45. Cohn P, Harris P, Barry W, Rosati R, Rosenbaum P, Waternaux C (1981) Prognostic importance of anginal symptoms in angiographically defined coronary artery disease. *Am J Cardiol* 47: 233.

46. Cohn P (1986) Prognostic significance of asymptomatic coronary artery disease. *Am J Cardiol* 58: 1b.

47. Gottlieb S, Weisfeldt M, Ouyang P, Mellits D, Gerstenblith G (1987) Silent ischemia predicts infarction and death during 2 year follow-up of unstable angina. *J Am Coll Cardiol* 10: 756.

48. Nademanee K, Intarachot V, Josephson M, Rieders D, Vaghaiwalla F, Singh B (1987) Prognostic significance of silent myocardial ischemia in patients with unstable angina. *J Am Coll Cardiol* 10: 1.

49. Von Arnim T, Gerbig H, Krawietz W, Hofling B (1988) Prognostic implications of transient-predominantly silent-ischeamia in patients with unstable angina pectoris. *Eur Heart J* 9: 435.

50. Berman D, Rozanski A, Knoebel S (1987) The detection of silent ischemia: Cautions and precautions. *Circulation* 75: 101.

51. Fox K (1988) Silent ischaemia: Clinical implications in 1988. *Br Heart J* 60: 363.

52. Morris D, Rozanski A, Berman D, Diamond G, Swan H (1984) Noninvasive prediction of the angiographic extent of coronary artery disease after myocardial infarction: Comparison

of clinical, bicycle exercise electrocardiographic and ventriculographic parameters. *Circulation* 70: 192.

53. Riccardi G, Opasich C, Assandri J, Tramarin R, La Rovere MT, Calsamiglia G, Pozzoli M, Traversi E, Febo O, Cobelli F, Specchia G (1985) Correlazioni tra ventricolo-coronarografia e test da sforzo in pazienti sopravvissuti a primo infarto miocardico transmurale e senza onde Q. *Cardiologia* 30: 193.

54. Quyyumi A, Raphael M, Wright C, Bealing L, Fox K (1984) Inability of the ST segment/heart rate slope to predict accurately the severity of coronary artery disease. *Br Heart J* 51: 395.

55. Pepine C, Feldman R, Ludbrook P, Holland P, Lambert C, Conti R, McGrath P (1986) Left ventricular dyskinesia reversed by intravenous nitroglycerin: A manifestation of silent myocardial ischemia. *Am J Cardiol* 58: 38B.

56. Picano E, Masini M, Lattanzi F, Distante A, L'Abbate A (1986) Role of dipyridamole-echocardiography test in electrocardiographically silent effort myocardial ischemia. *Am J Cardiol* 58: 235.

57. Gibson R, Watson D, Craddock G, Crampton R, Kaiser D, Denny M, Beller G (1983) Prediction of cardiac events after uncomplicated myocardial infarction: A prospective study comparing predischarge exercise thallium-201 scintigraphy and coronary angiography. *Circulation* 68: 321.

58. Subramaian V (1986) Clinical and research applications of ambulatory Holter ST-segment and heart rate monitoring. *Am J Cardiol* 58: 11b.

59. Tzivoni D, Gavish A, Benhorn J, Keren A, Stern S (1986) Myocardial ischemia during daily activities and stress. *Am J Cardiol* 58: 47B.

60. Deanfield J, Ribeiro P, Oakley K, Krikler S, Selwin A (1983) Myocardial ischemia during life in patients with stable angina: Its relation to symptoms and heart rate changes. *Lancet* 1: 753.

61. Pepine C, Imperi G, Lambert C (1987) Relation of transient-silent ischemic episodes to daily activities. *Circulation* 75 (suppl II): 28.

62. Singh B, Nademanee K, Figueras J, Josephson M (1986) Hemodynamic and electrocardiographic correlates of symptomatic and silent myocardial ischemia: Pathophysiologic and therapeutic implications. *Am J Cardiol* 58: 3B.

63. Quyyumi A, Wright C, Mockus L, Fox K (1984) Mechanisms of nocturnal angina pectoris: Importance of increased myocardial oxygen demand in patients with severe coronary artery disease. *Lancet* 1: 207.

64. Quyyumi A, Crake T, Wright C, Mockus L, Fox K (1987) The role of ambulatory ST-segment monitoring in diagnosis of coronary artery disease: Comparison with exercise testing and thallium scintigraphy. *Eur Heart J* 8: 124.

65. Campbell S, Barry J, Rocco M (1980) Features of the exercise test that reflect the activity of ischemic heart disease out of hospital. *Circulation* 74: 72.

66. Weiner D, Ryan T, McCabe C, Chaitman B, Sheffield L, Grace N, Fisher L, Tristini F (1988) Comparison of coronary artery bypass surgery and medical therapy in patients with exercise-induced silent myocardial ischemia: A report from the coronary artery surgery study (CASS) registry. *J Am Coll Cardiol* 12: 595.

67. Ambrose J, Tannenbaum M, Alexopoulos D, Hjemdahl-Monsen C, Leavy J, Wels M, Borrico S, Gorlin R, Fuster V (1988) Angiographic progression of coronary artery disease and the development of myocardial infarction. *J Am Coll Cardiol* 12: 56.

68. Ellis S, Alderman E, Cain K, Fisher L, Sanders W, Bourassa M (1988) Prediction of risk of anterior myocardial infarction by lesion severity and measurement method of stenoses in the left anterior descending coronary distribution: A CASS registry study. *J Am Coll Cardiol* 11: 908.

69. Pantely G, Bristow J (1984) Ischemic cardiomyopathy. *Prog Cardiovasc Dis* 27: 95.

70. Hess O, Schneider J, Monogi H, Carroll J, Schneider K, Turina M, Krayenbuehl H (1988) Myocardial structure in patients with exercise-induced ischemia. *Circulation* 77: 967.

10. Digital cine loop technology
A new tool for the evaluation of wall motion abnormalities

VITO MARANGELLI, GAETANO D'AMBROSIO, LUIGI
CARELLA, SABINO ILICETO and PAOLO RIZZON

Introduction

Cine-loop analysis is a recent development in technology that allows the
acquisition of echocardiographic images in a digital form as a sequence of a
determined frame number, starting from a trigger signal, normally the R-wave
of QRS signal. These images can be reviewed in a cyclic manner (a 'loop') and
in a particular screen format (usually 'Quad Screen Format') aimed at comparing different loops in synchrony with the cardiac cycle. Currently the main
clinical use of cine-loop analysis consists in wall motion analysis in different
conditions. For instance it is possible to compare the same views recorded
during rest condition and post-stress condition, or at different stages of myocardial infarction. This system greatly enhances the capacity of seeing differences and changes without the disturbing interference of visual memory
pitfalls. The digital images can then be stored on floppy disks, so that the
image database can be a real tool in clinical use.

An introduction to Cine-loop technology: Hardware and software

Cine-loop systems are currently available in two forms. More commonly they
are echocardiograph independent units and normally implemented on AT-
level modified personal computers (an expanded or extended memory is
required to store and process an adequate number of images). They can be
used as normal computers or as cine-loop units. At the moment a widespread
diffusion is reached also by cine-loop systems completely integrated in echocardiographic equipment. They are more practical in use (smaller volumes),
but less flexible in the upgrading. In our Division, we have a two-year experience of both the system models.

A flow chart of a digital cine-loop system is given in Figure 1. The image
source for cine-loop analysis is usually the video signal produced by the echocardiographic machine or a video-tape-recorder (VTR). To produce a correct synchronization of acquired images between different cardiac cycles a

S. Iliceto et al. (eds.), Ultrasound in Coronary Artery Disease, 95–105.
© 1991 *Kluwer Academic Publishers.*

DIGITAL CINE LOOP TECHNOLOGY

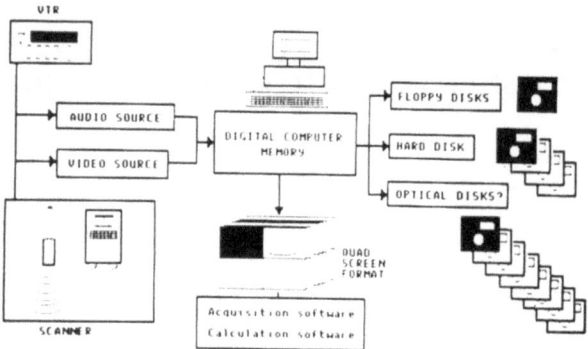

Figure 1. Flow chart showing a typical Digital Cine Loop System data flow. A VTR (video tape recorder) or the echocardiograph (Scanner) produce video and audio signals for the digital computer system, which can acquire images in particular formats such as quad screen as well as make calculations. The digitized images are then saved on various kinds of magnetic disks.

signal of physiological meaning, as a *trigger* for the acquisition start, is required: the R wave of the QRS complex is a universal marker for the beginning of ventricular systole, the echocardiograph can easily recognize the R wave and can use it for its triggering functions. The audio signal for the R wave 'beep', from the echocardiograph or the VTR, has a special input channel to the cine-loop system. It is also possible to use the video tracing of QRS signal as a trigger signal, but the quality of the signal is not as stable as required. During the examination the ECG baseline can easily be shifted up and down or affected by noise from the patient, motion of connecting cables and electrode contact problems. The image acquisition effectively starts when the user presses a pedal and the first trigger signal has been recognized. Different parameters can be set such as the trigger delay (between the triggered R wave and the first acquired image) and different modalities of triggering (video, external hardware, manual).

The core of the system is the cine-loop video-memory. Memory size is the main determinant of the maximal quantity of images stored for elaboration. Each single image represents a *frame*. More precisely a frame is the whole image information that the monitor screen can visualize. Current memories contain 32 or more frames (this number is continually changing with technological advances).

The PreVue/StressVue system produced by Nova Microsonics contains, for instance, a maximum of 32 frames. This number depends on the modality of division of the screen and on the 'image resolution' (pixel density). The screen area can be completely occupied by the source image (Single Screen mode), or it can be divided into two halves (Dual or Split Screen) or in four regions (Quad Screen). As image loops can independently be acquired in each single portion of the screen, the maximal number of stored images is

given by the maximal single frame number multiplied by the regions represented in each single screen. The acquired image is reduced so as to fit the
screen region occupied. The video-memory can also be divided into blocks:
32, 16, 12 or 8 consecutive frames. Every sequence of n consecutive frames
(n = 8, 12, 16, 32) constitutes 'a loop'. The maximum number of acquired
loops is given by the maximum frame number divided by the frame number in
each single loop. The possible numbers are: 4 loops by 8 frames, 3 loops by
12 frames, 2 loops by 16 frames, 1 loop by 32 frames. Each frame is identified by a specific progressive number (# 1–32). The technical expression for
this concept is 'dynamic video-memory'. The time interval between two consecutive frames (inter-image delay) can be selected by software. Each loop
will cover a total interval of:

$$(n - 1) * \text{inter-image delay}$$

(n = number of frames per loop). A 50 msec inter-image delay in an 8-frame
loop will cover a total of 350 msec. Since there is currently great interest in
systolic phase evaluation, this interval permits the acquisition of the whole
cardiac systole in a wide range of heart rates. The acquired series of images is
played on the computer monitor in a cyclic manner, the first frame immediately after the last one. A Play Loop Delay setting operation can speed up
or reduce the motion velocity.

The central idea in digital cine loop technology stems from the possibility
of acquiring images from the same portion of the cardiac cycle in different
conditions and simultaneous reviewing of them side by side on the screen (see
Figure 2). To make sense from a physiological point of view the two loops
must be representative of the same part of the cardiac cycle. A 'baseline'
versus a 'test' condition can then be compared, the test being a stress test or a

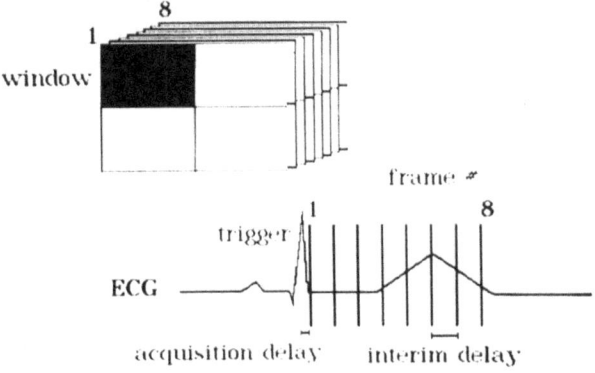

Figure 2. The Digital Cine Loop System can acquire images using the R wave of the ECG signal
as a trigger signal. It is possible to choose an acquisition and an interim (inter-image) delay
interval. At each interval, as shown, a single frame is captured and stored into the digital
memory.

drug effect study. The observer can easily and correctly evaluate changes in wall motion without 'human memory pitfalls'.

At the end the processed images can be saved on a magnetic support for permanent storage in an image database. Floppy disks or hard-disks are usually the definitive media. Stored images can easily be retrieved into the system and visualized. This procedure is quicker and more practical than traditional cassette systems. AT level personal computers can be modified, at a very low cost, to visualize images (Review Stations) without the frame grabber function. The acquisition and reviewing phases can then be split with optimization of the echo laboratory management.

An important utility of these systems is the 'mixing procedure' which can rearrange in a predefined pattern images from different loops to offer a simplification of the acquisition phase. More details will be given in the stress test procedure description.

In a digital form the image can be numerically processed and transformed. A wide range of calculations can be made on digital images, such as traditional echo doppler parameters (dimensional measurements, doppler velocities, etc.) and complex analyses (videodensitometry and endocardial or doppler velocity pattern automatic edge detection). Report utilities (wall motion evaluation and summary text reports) produce file or printed documents.

Clinical applications

At the moment the clinical use of digital cine loop technology mainly regards ventricular wall motion analysis during systole. In this chapter we will discuss what we have achieved in our own laboratory and what we know from other laboratories in Europe and the United States.

We will describe stress tests, the classic treadmill test, and new alternative stress tests analyzed in the literature of recent years and widely accepted in laboratory practice. We will briefly describe the method and for each test the practical use of our main digital cine loop system, the PreVue II system (Software release 4.035) by Nova Microsonics, Indianapolis.

Echo treadmill stress test

We routinely use a treadmill echo stress test according to a modified Bruce protocol. The recording of echo examination is performed following the two-stage protocol. The first recording is performed during the rest phase before beginning the test. Three apical views (apical four-chamber, apical two-chamber and apical long-axis) and a parasternal (the better between parasternal long-axis or short-axis) are recorded. The second recording is made immediately after interrupting exercise; the patient has been previously instructed to rapidly position himself in left lateral decubitus. This manouver can reduce the interval between stopping exercise and beginning image acquisition. The

ECHO TREADMILL STRESS TEST
CINE LOOP FORMAT

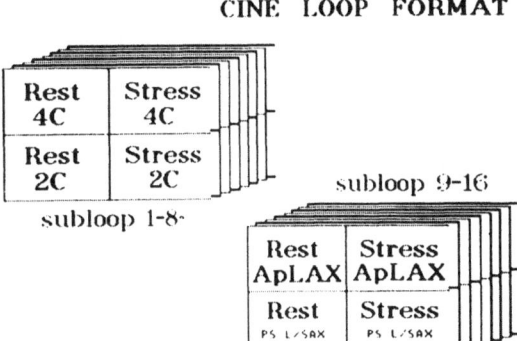

Figure 3. Cine loop acquisition format of Echo Treadmill Stress Test. Images from rest and post-exercise acquisition (Stress) are shown side by side for each view. Two subloops are needed. 4C = apical four chamber view; 2C = apical two-chamber view; AP LAX = apical long-axis view; PS L/SAX = parasternal long-axis or short axis views.

average time interval for acquiring the first view is 10–15 seconds and no more than 1.5–2 min for the last one.

The cine loop format is shown in Figure 3. A specific utility (two-stage stress protocol) can be used to obtain this format. The machine can acquire the images during the examination using an acquisition procedure which is particularly suitable for the exercise stress test. The time interval between interrupting the test and the actual beginning of image recording is particularly critical for examination usefulness. Mild wall motion abnormalities can be lost if the recording starts after an interval of even a few minutes. The software controls the acquisition of a quad screen for rest images; each of the four acquired views has a special label. The quad screen of the rest images can be saved on a floppy disk. Then the exercise images are acquired; a timer can be used to record directly on the images the exercise duration and the time interval between stopping the exercise and beginning of image acquisition; both these values can offer valuable information on the stress effectiveness and the real significance of the recorded images. Unlike the rest phase, when just a single cycle per acquisition is registered, during the post-stress study four consecutive cycles of the same view per time are captured by a single push of the pedal. The probability of acquiring a good image is then considerably increased, considering that the patient is hyperpnoic and tachypnoic and the images are impaired by the presence of lung in the explored ultrasonic window. If a good image has not been got the acquisition can immediately be repeated. Four views are consecutively acquired and automatically labelled. The user can then choose the best cycle from among those captured and an automatic combination is performed following the final format in Figure 3 (rest/post-exercise image coupling).

This format strongly facilitates the image evaluation process. Differences between rest and exercise images are enhanced on the quad screen format,

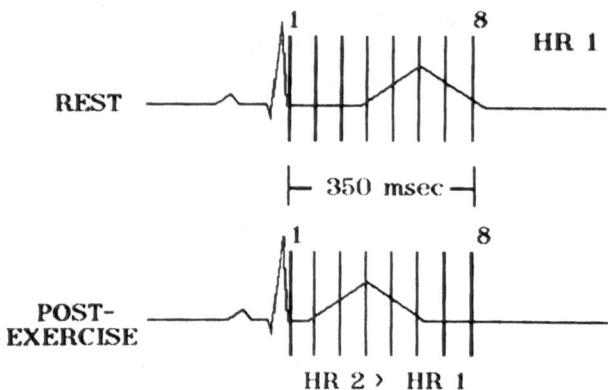

Figure 4. When the difference in heart rate between rest and post-exercise is too great, some early diastolic images during the post-exercise recording are captured. This can produce an unpleasant optical effect.

and no memory effort is required to compare images as in the traditional systems. Digital cine loop technology greatly reduces intra-observer variability in serial studies. To correctly reflect the physiological realities some technical requirements must be fulfilled and some problems be considered:

1. The ECG signal quality must be as good during post-exercise as during the baseline recording. The trigger should be taken only at the R wave. Poor signals can provoke trigger from different signals (noise, T waves). The acquired cycle begins at a different time from the early systole, thus putting rest and post-exercise images out of phase. There are no advantages in comparing a systole and a diastole.
2. Heart rate and the systole duration are different in the rest and post-exercise phases. Using the same interim delay gives the acquisition of some early diastolic images during the post-exercise recording (see Figure 4). Normally this difference is small and presents no problems in image comparison. An unpleasant optical effect is obtained when there is a great difference in heart rate between rest and post-exercise phases; the decrease in interim delay during post-exercise acquisition is then advisable.
3. As for every technical procedure, there is a 'learning curve' in optimal procedure performance. It takes no more than two weeks, if the technician is already trained in basic echocardiographic techniques, to master the multiple coordination problems due to the contemporary handling of echo probe and cine loop device. An initial effort is required to correctly manage some new imaging concepts involved in the cine loop logic. As the biological reality can be strongly affected by the complex 'technological chain' to which the image-information is subjected, the physician should pay careful attention to technical accuracy in test execution and evaluation.
4. As just one cycle is used to represent the considered condition, a sampling

defect should be avoided. Extrasystolic or post-extrasystolic cycles must be excluded to make a correct comparison possible. This is a real problem in patients affected by atrial fibrillation or stable arrhythmias.

5. The complete procedure takes 10–15 min more than the traditional ECG treadmill test. In our laboratory the stress test technician performs his traditional role during the test execution, so avoiding unacceptable double 'procedures' and increases in cost for the hospital. The echo and ergometric procedures can be perfectly well performed together since they only overlap in the initial and final stages.

6. A security power source is recommended to avoid unpleasant image failure due to power problems after the acquisition phase and before the floppy disk storage. We routinely use the video tape recording procedure in addition to the cine loop recording to avoid possible system malfunctions and to check any sampling defect in the acquired loops (see point 4).

As a conclusive remark we think that cine loop technology, if critically used, is an effective and necessary tool to improve Echo treadmill stress test evaluation. We think that a logical extension of its usefulness to bicycle stress testing can be made.

Echo dipyridamole stress test

We use the dypiridamole stress test to assess left ventricular wall motion abnormalities in patients with an indication for stress test who did not undergo this test for absolute or relative contraindications. It is one of the alternative stresses. High sensitivity and specificity values are currently reported. A videotape recording is done of three apical views (four- and two-chamber, and apical long-axis) before drug infusion and every four min after dypiridamole infusion (0.56 mg/kg b.w. in 4 min) up to 20 min. A second half-dose is administered 8 min after the first one if no modifications are seen and no disturbing collateral effects are found. Aminophylline infusion (240 mg) is administered if a premature test interruption is necessary (positive test for angina or ECG ischemia signs or new wall motion abnormalities) or if drug provoked headache persists.

In Figure 5 the cine loop format is shown. The quad screen is built following the concept of comparing the same view in four protocol stages. The 1–8 subloop takes the three apical views to examine the baseline wall motion. Each of the other three subloops takes one single view. On the upper left there is the baseline image, while on the upper right the 4-min recording, in the lower left the 12-min-one and in the lower right the 20 min image. Thirty-two frames for each test are saved on floppy disks.

The technical problems with this protocol are really minimal, unlike with the treadmill stress. The quality of images is perfectly comparable to the baseline recording, as no position problems or new conditions occur. The small chronotropic effect of dipyridamole infusion avoids the heart rate possible

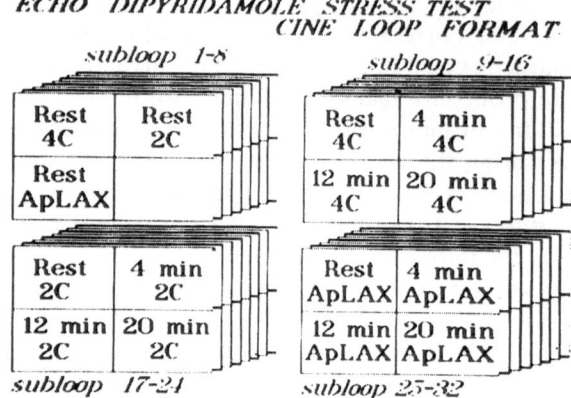

Figure 5. Cine loop acquisition format of Echo Dipyridamole Stress Test. Images from Rest Acquisition are shown in Subloop 1–8, while images from consecutive moments after the drug infusion, together with the Rest image, are shown in a single subloop for each single view. Four subloops are needed. 4C = apical four-chamber view; 2C = apical two-chamber view; AP LAX = apical long-axis view; 4 min, 12 min, 20 min = minutes after the beginning of the dipyridamole infusion.

artifacts in image comparison. The use of cine loop technology gives high quality results in this procedure.

Pharmacological tests

The technique applied in the dipyridamole protocol can easily be extended to other pharmacological tests, that aim to assess left ventricle wall motion abnormalities. The dobutamine test is in current use in this particular field and it has already been experimented using the digital cine loop technology.

Transesophageal atrial pacing 2D-Echo

This is an alternative stress test that has been used in current echo-lab practice for many years now. The protocol comprises the recording of three apical views during rest and during atrial stimulation using a transesophageal catheter at progressively increasing heart rates (110, 120, 130 beats per minute × 2 min steps and a final one at 150 beats per minute × 5 min). If there is an onset of a Wenckebach type II degree AV block, an atropine infusion (0.01 mg/kg b.w.) is administered. Interruption criteria are the onset of angina, consistent new wall motion abnormalities, intolerance to the stimulation.

There are no particular problems as regards image quality. On the other hand a real problem involves the correct triggering of the systole. The QRS is infact preceded by the stimulation artifact (usually a big spike). The echocardiograph considers the artifact as a real trigger, producing a beep for it, as for

ECHO T.A.P. STRESS TEST
CINE LOOP FORMAT

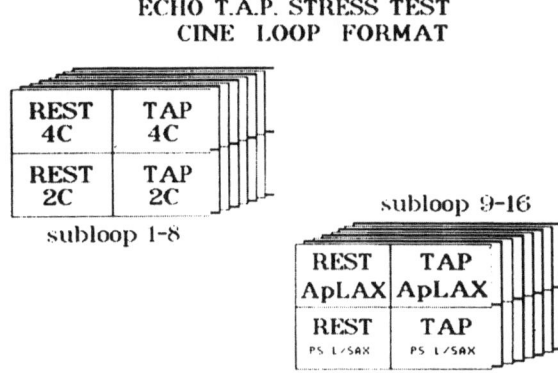

Figure 6. Cine loop acquisition format of Transesophageal Atrial Pacing (T.A.P.) Stress Test. Images from rest and pacing acquisition (Stress) are shown side by side for each view. Two subloops are needed. 4C = apical four-chamber view; 2C = apical two-chamber view; AP LAX = apical long-axis view; PS L/SAX = one of parastensl long-axis or short-axis view.

the R wave of the ECG signal. The cardiac cycle can be infact acquired from the spike. Rest and pacing images are thus not comparable. To obtain a correct acquisition of the systolic phase we acquire a loop of 32 frames and select 8 consecutive frames from the end diastolic one. Comparable images between rest and pacing are thus obtained (Figure 6).

Acute myocardial infarction follow-up

The digital cine loop technology is the ideal tool to follow the evolution of left ventricle wall motion abnormalities during the acute phase in the Coronary Care Unit and after the discharge. The images recorded over several days offer the possibility to observe the echocardiographic expression of myocardial infarction evolution (segmental wall motion changes, left ventricular function study by shortening and ejection fractions, aneurysmal evolution). We usually acquire a quad screen format showing four echocardiographic views and some images in single screen modality showing Doppler and M-mode representative tracings to assess significant aspects (valve regurgitation, velocity patterns). An image database is obtained, that permits a quick assembling of the myocardial infarction image history in each single patient.

Other applications

A wide range of echocardiographic applications are used in combination with digital cine loop technology. Regional wall motion comparisons can be made before and after a percutaneous transluminal coronary angioplasty procedure or a coronary artery bypass graft intervention. The real limitation to the pos-

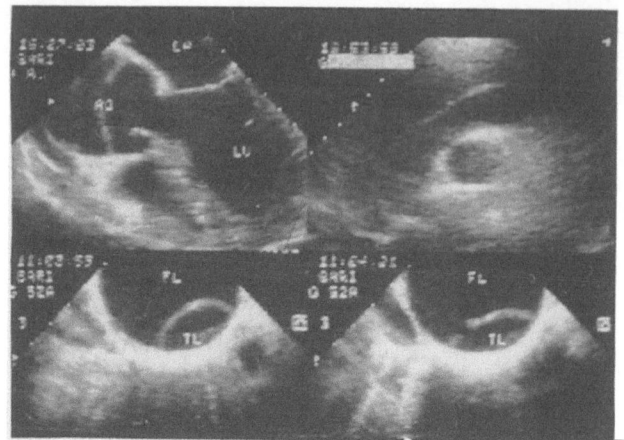

Figure 7. The capacity to visualize a complex three-dimensional structure is shown in this image: a quad screen reconstruction of a Type I Aortic Dissection has been made, showing the transesophageal recording of the dissection at the level of the ascending aorta, aortic arch and thoracic descending aorta.

sible applications of digital cine loop technology lies in the cardiologist's imagination and the specific work conditions.

Teaching applications

The cine loop quad screen format has a unique power of spatial reconstruction of a geometrical complex structure such as the heart. It can be of valuable aid in teaching for postgraduate or university courses about echocardiographic normal and pathological anatomy (Figure 7).

Laboratory management

The whole laboratory staff must be introduced to the new technology; infact digital cine loop technology requires a partial reorganization of laboratory procedures. The non-medical members need a training period to manage some features of routine procedures connected to the execution of cine-loop recordings (floppy formatting, data entering, image database management, etc.), in order to optimize procedure duration. The medical members should be introduced to the concepts and use of new devices. However the training period is not very long (about two weeks). An important managerial problem is the increase in cost per exam because of the materials involved (floppy disks). This is limited in comparison to the mean cost per echocardiographic examination and is justified for the better results in the clinical management of the patient obtained. A future new simplification of database management will be offered by optical disk technology as permanent memory. Their memory capacity is much higher than that of current floppies and they will probably make it possible to store on a single optical disk the whole year's routine activity of an average size echo laboratory.

References

1. West SR, Feigenbaum H, Armstrong WF, Green D, Dillon JC (1984) Split screen simultaneous digital imaging of rest and stress echocardiogram – A new method for evaluation of exercise induced wall motion abnormalities. *J Am Coll Cardiol* 3: 563 (abstract).
2. Robertson WS, Feigenbaum H, Armstrong WF, Dillon JC, O'Donnell J (1983) Exercise echocardiography: A clinically practical addition in the evaluation of coronary artery disease. *J Am Coll Cardiol* 2: 1085.
3. Limacher MC, Qinones MA, Polner LR, Nelson JG, Winters WL Jr, Waggoner AD (1983) Detection of coronary artery disease with exercise two-dimensional echocardiography. *Circulation* 67: 1211.
4. Berberich SN, Zager JRS, Plotnick GD, Fisher ML (1983) A practical approach to exercise echocardiography: Immediate postexercise echocardiography. *J Am Coll Cardiol* 1: 1002.
5. Feigenbaum H (1986) *Echocardiography*, 4th edition, pp 471–475. Philadelphia: Lea & Febiger.
6. Picano E, Distante A, Masini M, Morales AM, Lattanzi F, L'Abbate A (1985) Dipyridamole-echocardiography test in effort angina pectoris. *Am J Cardiol* 56: 452–456.
7. Picano E, Lattanzi F, Masini M, Distante A, L'Abbate A (1986) High dose dipyridamole-echocardiography test in effort angina pectoris. *Am J Cardiol* 8: 848–854.
8. Iliceto S, Sorino M, D'Ambrosio G, Papa A, Favale S, Biasco G, Rizzon P (1985) Detection of coronary artery disease by two-dimensional echocardiography and transesophageal atrial pacing. *J Am Coll Cardiol* 5: 1188–97.

PART TWO

Evaluation of myocardial infarction

11. Two-dimensional echocardiography in the early management of acute myocardial infarction

LUCIANO AGATI, MARIA PENCO, CARMINE D. VIZZA, MARCO RENZI and ARMANDO DAGIANTI

Introduction

In the past, emphasis has been placed on the accurate diagnosis, monitoring and antiarrhythmic therapy of acute myocardial infarction. This approach could have been appropriate in an era when therapy was primarily directed on the prevention of complications. In patients with acute myocardial infarction (AMI), therapy is now directed toward the early use of thrombolytic agents in order to achieve coronary reperfusion. Several clinical studies have demonstrated that a sustained reperfusion of a coronary artery can preserve left ventricular function reducing the infarct size [1–7]. Thus, imaging techniques able to accurately visualize the size and the extent of myocardial damage could play a predominant role in the emergency room [8]. The advantages of performing an echocardiographic study in the earliest stages of acute myocardial infarction are many.

Early diagnosis of acute myocardial infarction

Wall motion and thickening cease whithin seconds after coronary artery occlusion and are often replaced by paradoxic motion and thinning due to passive bulging of the ischemic segment. Such regional wall motion abnormalities can be detected in patients with AMI with approximately 90% sensitivity by echocardiography [8]. The correlation between the extent of wall motion abnormalities detected by two-dimensional echocardiography and the location and extent of the myocardial infarction as determined by electrocardiographic criteria, left ventricular angiography, radionuclide thallium imaging and autopsies studies has been excellent [9–12]. Moreover, the contractile thickening and thinning properties of the myocardium may be directly visualized by two-dimensional echocardiography, whereas angiographic or radionuclide methods indicate only endocardial motion. Thus, two-dimensional echocardiography is the imaging technique of choice for evaluating patients in the earliest stages of AMI. The diagnosis of acute myocardial

S. Iliceto et al. (eds.), Ultrasound in Coronary Artery Disease, 107–119.
© 1991 Kluwer Academic Publishers.

infarction, based on prolonged chest pain and typical ST segment elevation, is usually easily made. An early evaluation by two-dimensional echocardiography has little to offer in this clinical setting.

On the contrary, in a population of patients presenting with a chest pain syndrome without diagnostic ECG findings of AMI, two-dimensional echocardiography provides a rapid, sensitive and specific noninvasive tool to aid in the establishment of the correct diagnosis [13, 14]. In our series of 48 patients with AMI undergoing echocardiographic study within 5 hours following onset of chest pain (mean time 3.1 ± 1.3 h) it was possible to observe persistent wall motion abnormalities in 91% of patients presenting with ST segment elevation and in 70% of patients presenting with ST segment depression.

We must stress the importance of this finding; as a matter of fact it has been demonstrated that patients with acute myocardial infarction presenting with ST segment depression had a very unfavourable coronary anatomy with a high prevalence of multivessel disease and high prognostic risk [15–17]. Thus an early correct diagnosis of acute myocardial infarction in this subgroup of patients has important clinical implications suggesting a more aggressive management.

Evaluation of infarct size and left ventricular function

In clinical assessment of patients with AMI frequently global left ventricular function (i.e. ejection fraction) has been measured [18]. There are some disadvantages of utilizing exclusively indexes of global left ventricular performance to evaluate patients with AMI.

(a) Global left ventricular performance may be preserved even in the setting of profound myocardial ischemia. In fact, normal non-ischemic myocardium may be hyperkinetic, thus mantain global left ventricular function in the normal range.

(b) The ejection fraction changes may either underestimate recovery of regional function in the infarct site after reperfusion or overestimate recovery if reperfusion benefits function in both the infarct and non-infarct regions [5, 18–20]. Although the severity of left ventricular disfunction correlates with infarct size, the relationship between these two parameters is not linear; it is not close enough to allow an accurate assessment of the amount of the infarcted myocardium.

(c) Depressed systolic function, impaired diastolic relaxation and mechanical expansion of the infarcted segment are the causes of a volume overload in acute myocardial infarction [21]. This disproportionate infarct dilation (LV remodeling) is an acute phenomenon present within 1 hour of transmural myocardial infarction [22–23] and seems to be beneficial because the myocardium calls on the Frank Starling mechanism as an acute compensatory response of the damaged myocardium [24]. The systolic disadvantage determined by a compliant dyskinetic region [22] resulting in a wasted work [23] is subsequently reduced by increased infarct stiffness [25]. These changes would enable to maintain the ejection fraction within normal ranges.

(d) Finally, the quantitative assessment of ejection fraction by two-dimensional echocardiography could not be accurate in all patients, it is tedious, time consuming and requires a skilled operator. For all these reasons regional wall motion analysis was included in the clinical evaluation of patients admitted in coronary care unit. For this purpose left ventricular walls were subdivided into 9, 11 or 14 segments. A numerical score corresponding to the wall motion analysis (normal, hyperkinetic, hypokinetic, akinetic or dyskinetic) was assigned to each segment.

There is universal consensus that such analysis of wall motion abnormalities overpredict anatomic infarct size [26–28]. Wyatt et al. [29] suggested that infarcted muscle fibers may act as a parallel mechanical resistor and impede contraction in adjacent, normally perfused segments. Ischemia at distance [30–31], may also contribute to overestimate the infarct size. Experimental studies have demonstrated [32] that in the peripheral infarct region the circumferential extent of hypokinesia increased between 30 min and 48 h after permanent coronary occlusion, suggesting that an early worsening in wall motion occurred in the peripheral infarct region. This early deterioration in function of the peripheral infarct region may be due to a withdrawal of endogenous cathecolamine activity, to which the decline in hyperkinesia of the noninfarct region has been attributed [1]. This phenomenon could also be a consequence of an infarct expansion or extension [33]. Thus, echocardiographic wall motion analysis more than a measure of the anatomic infarct size is a reflex of the 'functional infarct size' adding important information on a residual myocardial jeopardy.

Indication to emergency interventions

Heyndrickx et al. [34] have experimentally demonstrated that reperfusion even after brief coronary occlusion is not immediately followed by recovery of left ventricular function in the central infarct region. During this delay the 'stunned' myocardium repairs damaged metabolic processes [35–36]. In the peripheral infarct region left ventricular function begins to recover within these early hours [1, 37–38].

Sheehan et al. [1] observed that reperfusion accelerates functional recovery in the central infarct region and enhances contractility in the peripheral noninfarcted region resulting in a significant early benefit to global left ventricular function. This functional recovery starts three days after reperfusion is achieved. Therefore echocardiographic studies performed within three days after a successful reperfusion should not show any significant changes either in global or in regional left ventricular function. The early improvement of left ventricular function seems to be the major determinant of the enhancement of survival observed after thrombolytic therapy [1–7, 39–40]. This improvement is strictly dependent on the delay between the onset of symptoms and the beginning of a sustained reperfusion. Experimental and clinical studies [37–40] have shown that salvage of myocardium is possible if reperfusion takes place within 2 to 3 hours after coronary occlusion.

In our series of 76 patients [41] with AMI who underwent thrombolytic therapy within 6 hours after the onset of symptoms we found no significant difference for changes of infarct size and ejection fraction, between admission and predischarge echocardiograms, as compared to controls. When time from onset of symptoms to treatment is considered thrombolysis group can be subdivided in two subgroups: early treatment (< 3 h 30 min: 41 patients) and late treatment (> 3 h 30 min: 33 patients). In the first group a significant infarct size decrease was observed between admission and predischarge echocardiograms. It has been demonstrated that the greatest improvement in ejection fraction after a successful reperfusion occurs in those patients who had a depressed ejection fraction (< 45%) in the acute phase [20, 42]. Changes in wall motion after reperfusion correlate significantly with the acute severity of regional disfunction such that the greatest improvement occurs among patients who had akinesia or dyskinesia acutely [18]. Thus, patients showing severely depressed ventricular function and large infarct size in the acute phase potentially receive more benefits if reperfusion is achieved at an early stage.

On the contrary, Huey et al. [43] reported that many patients with small admission infarct size and non-Q wave myocardial infarction have spontaneous reperfusion and high grade residual stenosis subtending viable but jeopardized myocardium. In these patients mechanical revascularization and calcium channel blockers rather than thrombolytic therapy might be indicated. Patients whose acute myocardial infarction is followed by infarct extension have a 2.5 time greater in-hospital mortality rate and a 30% decrease in 1 year survival when compared with those who do not experience this complication [44].

Two-dimensional echocardiography allows immediate identification of infarct extension at the time the study is performed and does not require the lag time needed for ECG evolution or serum creatinine kinase elevation [44]. The assessment of the functional infarct size by two-dimensional echocardiography, during the first hours after the symptom onset, may identify a subgroup of patients high extension risk, can easily separate large from small infarctions [45] and thus aid in the choice between conventional therapy and immediate interventions such as emergency coronary angioplasty or thrombolytic therapy.

Recently, Kaul et al. [46] have experimentally demonstrated that a direct estimation of the area at risk, by means of myocardial contrast echocardiography, may be performed. If these results are reproduced safely in humans, in the future it might be possible to determine the presence or absence of areas at risk and its size at bedside, in emergency room, and therefore to formulate rational therapeutic decisions.

Prognostic implications of the early echocardiographic study

The most powerful predictor of prognosis in patients with AMI is the degree of left ventricular disfunction [47–48]. Two-dimensional echocardiography is an ideal noninvasive method for the determination of both regional and global function, therefore it should be routinely used for the risk stratification of patients with acute myocardial infarction. Many investigators have shown an important relationship between the two-dimensional echocardiographic extent of acute dysfunction and serious in-hospital AMI complications (death, cardiogenic shock, heart failure and arrhythmias) [9, 49–51]. When functional impairment exceeds 20% of the left ventricle or involves multiple noncontiguous regions, in-hospital complications rise substantially.

Nishimura et al. [51] demonstrated that the initial wall motion score index allows to predict hemodynamic deterioration in patients whose poor left ventricular function is initially compensated and therefore unsuspected on the basis of clinical data. Moreover some studies (12, 52, 53) did demonstrate that a higher predischarge wall motion score can accurately predict the occurrence of congestive heart failure and angina in a mean follow-up period.

In our series of 156 patients (L. Agati et al., unpublished data), survived an acute myocardial infarction, a wall motion score was calculated by two-dimensional echocardiography within 12 hours after admission to the coronary care unit and at predischarge (11 segments; normal wall motion = 0, hypokinetic = 1, akinetic = 2, dyskinetic = 3). All patients were followed perspectively for a mean of 10 months (range 3–15 months). Throughout follow-up, the presence of congestive heart failure (NYHA III or IV), the presence of angina, major coronary events (recurrence of myocardial infarction, coronary artery bypass grafting) and death were considered.

Both admission and predischarge two-dimensional echocardiograms were useful in identifying a subset of patients at increased risk of complications after acute myocardial infarction. Patients with extensive left ventricular impairment are more likely to experience serious cardiac complications during follow-up. (Figures 1, 2) Moreover patients with normal wall motion or with mild hypokinesia in the early phases of acute myocardial infarction are most of all likely to experience major coronary events in the follow-up period. (Figure 1) While changes in the wall motion score index during the acute infarction period did not have predictive value for the determination of in-hospital complications [51], both a score increase or decrease did have a high

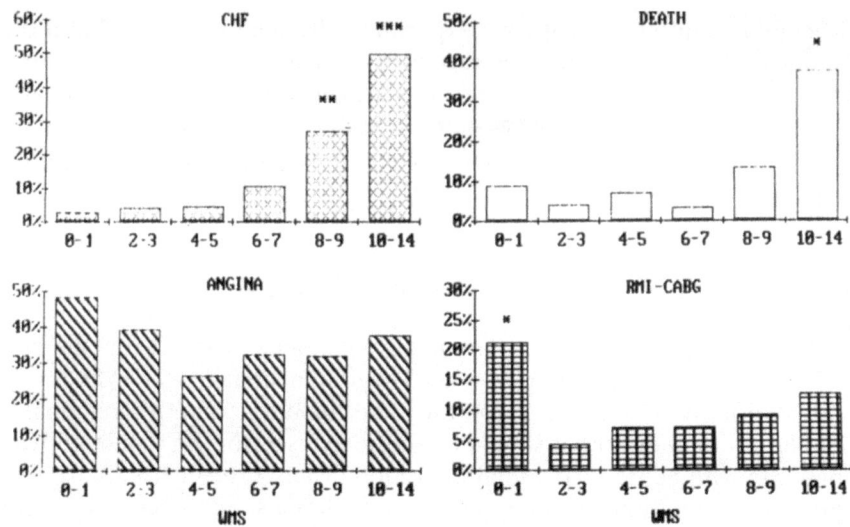

Figure 1. Analysis of admission wall motion score (WMS) and complications during follow-up study.

CHF = Congestive Heart Failure (Class III, IV).
*** $p < 0.001$ compared with 0–1, 2–3, 4–5, 6–7.
** $p < 0.01$ compared with 0–1, 2–3, 4–5, 6–7.
DEATH
* $p < 0.05$ compared with each subset.
RMI-CABG = Recurrent Myocardial Infarction-Coronary Artery Bypass Grafting
* $p < 0.05$ compared with 2–3, 4–5, 6–7, 8–9.

predictive value for the determination of complications during follow-up.

In our study, 75% of patients with changes in the wall motion score from the initial to the final echo study experienced complications during follow-up, whereas only 30% of patients with unchanged wall motion score had complications during this period ($p < 0.001$). Particularly, in the first group 61% of patients had new coronary events compared to 21% in the second group ($p < 0.001$). On the contrary, patients whose infarct size is small to moderate and does not change during the acute period, are more likely to have a free-complications outcome. The high incidence in this study population of patients undergoing thrombolytic therapy (53%) and the presence of 30% of patients with subendocardial infarction might explain the results. Many investigators have observed that the combination of coronary narrowing with retained wall motion in the area of infarction may contribute to the increased frequency of new coronary events (unstable angina and reinfarction) during follow-up [43, 54–61].

Wilson et al. (58) have shown that also among patients with uncomplicated infarction and single vessel disease, the presence of residual ischemia within the infarct zone predicted a higher recurrent ischemic event rate than that of patients without infarct zone ischemia. Patients with non-Q wave myocardial

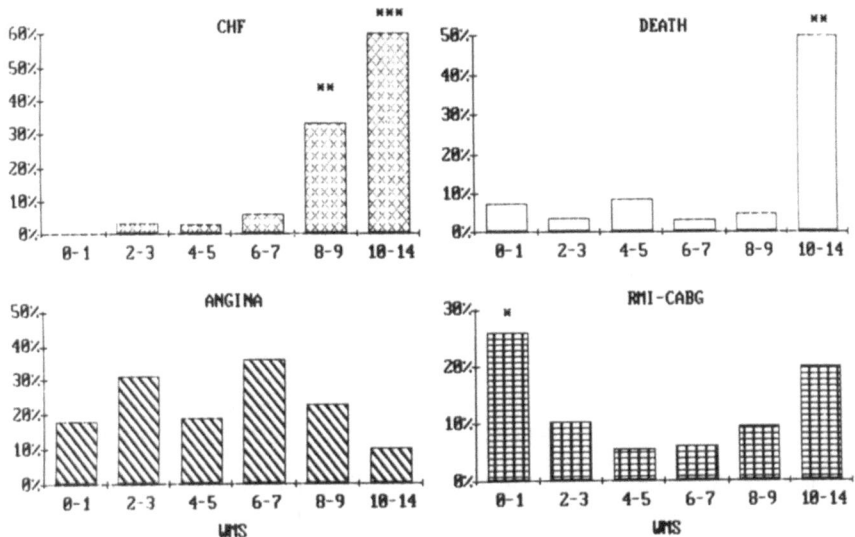

Figure 2. Analysis of predischarge wall motion score (WMS) and complications during follow-up study.

CHF = Congestive Heart Failure (Class III, IV).

*** $p < 0.001$ compared with 0–1, 2–3, 4–5, 6–7.

** $p < 0.01$ compared with 0–1, 2–3, 4–5, 6–7.

DEATH

** $p < 0.01$ compared with each subset.

RMI-CABG = Recurrent Myocardial Infarction-Coronary Artery Bypass Grafting

* $p < 0.05$ compared with 2–3, 4–5, 6–7, 8–9.

infarction frequently complain of post-infarction angina; these patients are at particularly high risk for recurrent infarction and have a marked increase in mortality in the late follow-up period (2-3 years). A residual jeopardized viable myocardium is frequent observed in this subgroup of patients [43, 54–60].

This anatomical substratum was also frequently observed after thrombolytic therapy was performed as a consequence of a significant residual stenosis in the infarct area. The survival in patients with partial reperfusion is nearly as poor as that of patients without reperfusion [18]. Furthermore Gissi study [40] showed that although early thrombolysis enhances short and long term survival, patients undergoing systemic fibrinolytic therapy are more likely to have major coronary events during follow-up than controls.

Recent comparative trials between thrombolytic therapy and combined therapy with percutaneous angioplasty have demonstrated the importance of reducing the residual stenosis by mechanical interventions to salvage more myocardium and to reduce post-infarction angina and recurrent myocardial infarction [62, 63]. Thus, regardless of myocardial infarction type (site, Q or non-Q wave, single or multivessel disease) the presence of a normal wall motion or a mild hypokinesia in the infarct zone and the observation of changes in wall motion score during the acute phase of myocardial infarction could identify a viable but jeopardized myocardium suggesting more aggressive interventions.

References

1. Sheehan FH, Doerr R, Schmidt WG, Bolson EL, Uebis R, von Essen R, Effert S, Dodge HT (1988) Early recovery of left ventricular function after thrombolytic therapy for acute myocardial infarction: An important determinant of survival. *J AM Coll Cardiol* 12: 289–300.
2. Kennedy JW, Ritchie JL, Davis KB, Fritz JK (1983) Western Washington randomized trial of intracoronary streptokinase in acute myocardial infarction. *N Engl J Med* 309: 1477–82.
3. Kennedy JW, Martin GV, Davis KB, Maynard C, Stadius M, Sheenan F, Ritchie JL (1988) The Western Washington intravenous streptokinase in acute myocardial infarction randomized trial. *Circulation* 77: 345–52.
4. The ISAM Study Group (1986) A prospective trial of intravenous streptokinase in acute myocardial infarction (ISAM): Mortality, morbidity and infarct size at 21 days. *N Engl J Med* 314: 1465–71.
5. Serruys PW, Simmons ML, Suryapranata H, Vermeer F, Wijus W, Van den Brand M, Bar F, Zwaan C, Krauss XmM, Remme WJ, Res J, Verhengt FW, Van Domburg R, Lubsen J, Hugenholtz PG (1986) Preservation of global and regional left ventricular function after early thrombolysis in acute myocardial infarction. *J Am Coll Cardiol* 7: 729–42.
6. White HD, Norris RM, Brown MA, Takayama H, Maslowsky A, Bass NM, Otrmiston JA, Whitlock T (1987) Effect of intravenous spreptokinase on left ventricular function and early survival after acute myocardial infarction. *N Engl J Med* 317: 850–5.
7. Kennedy JW, Atkins JM, Goldstein S, Jaffe AS, Lambrew CT, McIntyre KM, Mueller HS, Paraskos JA, Weaver WD (1988) Recent changes in management of acute myocardial infarction: Implications for emergency care physicians. *J Am Coll Cardiol* 11: 446–9.
8. Kloner RA, Parisi AF (1987) Acute myocardial infarction: Diagnostic and prognostic applications of two-dimensional echocardiography. *Circulation* 75: 521–24.
9. Heger JJ, Weyman AE, Wann LS, Dillon JC, Feigenbaum H (1977) Cross-sectional echocardiography in acute myocardial infarction: Detection and localization of regional left ventricular asynergy. *Circulation* 60: 531–8.
10. Kisslo JA, Robertson D, Gilbert BW, Bon Kamm O, Bhar VS (1977) A comparison of real-time two-dimensional echocardiography and cine-angiography in detecting left ventricular asinergy. *Circulation* 55: 134–41.
11. Nixon JV, Narahara KA, Smitherman TC (1980) Estimation of myocardial involvement in patients with acute myocardial infarction by two-dimensional echocardiography. *Circulation* 62: 1248–55.
12. Agati L, Penco M, Pastore LR, Fedele F, Di Renzi L, Dagianti A (1981) Studio settoriale della cinesi ventricolare sinistra mediante ecocardiografia 2D. Utilita' per la diagnosi e la prognosi dell'infarto acuto del miocardio. *Giorn It Cardiol* 11: 201–7.
13. Loh IK, Charuzi Y, Beeder C, Marshall LA, Ginsburg JH (1982) Early diagnosis of nontransmural myocardial infarction by two-dimensional echocardiography. *Am Heart J* 104: 963–67.
14. Quinones MA, Roberts RR (1985) Role of two-dimensional echocardiography in acute myocardial infarction. *Echocardiography* 3: 213–16.
15. Gei P, Cuccia C, Bonaldi E, Pagnoni N, Volpini M, Berra P, Ettori F, Niccoli L, Riva S (1988) Studio coronarografico nei pazienti con infarto miocardico non-Q: correlazioni con l'aspetto elettrocardiografico iniziale e prognosi. *Giorn It Cardiol* 18: 90–96.

16. Gibson RS (1987) Clinical, functional and angiographic distinctions between Q wave and non-Q wave myocardial infarction: Evidence of spontaneous reperfusion and implications for interventions trials. *Circulation* 75 (suppl V): 128.

17. Willich S, Stone P, Muller J, Toffler GH, Crowder J, Parker C, Rutherford JD, Turi ZG, Robertson T, Passamani E, Braunwald E and MILIS Study Group (1987) High-risk subgroups of patients with non-Q wave myocardial infarction based on direction and severity of ST segment deviation. *Am Heart J* 114: 1110.

18. Sheehan FH (1987) Determinants of improved left ventricular function after thrombolytic therapy in acute myocardial infarction. *J Am Coll Cardiol* 9: 937–44.

19. Sheehan FH, Szente A, Mathey DG, Dodge HT (1985) Assessment of left ventricular function in acute myocardial infarction: The relationship between global ejection fraction and regional wall motion. *Eur Heart J* 6(suppl E): 117–25.

20. Raizner AE, Tortoledo FA, Verani MS, Vanreet RE, Young JB, Rickman FD, Cashion WR, Samuels DA, Pratt CM, Attar M, Rubin HS, Lewis JM, Klein MS, Roberts R (1985) Intracoronary thrombolytic therapy in acute myocardial infarction: A prospective, randomized, controlled trial. *Am J Cardiol* 55: 301–8.

21. Warren SE, Royal HD, Markis JE, Grossman W, McKay R (1988) Time course of left ventricular dilation after myocardial infarction influence of infarct-related artery and success of coronary thrombolysis. *J Am Coll Cardiol* 11: 12–9.

22. Kass DA, Maughan WL, Ciuffo A, Graves W. Healy B, Weisfeldt ML (1988) Disproportionate epicardial dilation after transmural infarction of the canine left ventricle: acute and chronic differences. *J Am Coll Cardiol* 11: 177–85.

23. Mc Kay RG, Pfeffer MA, Pasternak RC, Markis JE, Come PC, Shoichiro N, Alderman JD, Ferguson JJ, Safian RD, Grossman W (1986) Left ventricular remodeling after myocardial infarction: A corollary to infarct expansion. *Circulation* 74: 693–702.

24. Russel RO (1988) Disproportionate dilation after transmural infarction-reflections on its meaning. *J Am Coll Cardiol* (1980) 11: 186.

25. Bogen DK, Raibnowitz SA, Needleman A, Mc Mahon TA, Abelman WH (1980) An analysis of the mechanical disadvantage of myocardial infarction in the canine left ventricle. *Circ Res* 47: 728–41.

26. Lieberman AN, Weirs JL, Jugdutt BI, Becker L, Bulkley BH, Garrison JG, Hutchins GM, Kallman CA, Weisfeldt ML (1981) Two-dimensional echocardiography and infarct size: relationship of regional wall motion and thickening to extent of myocardial infarction in the dog. *Circulation* 63: 739–44.

27. Niemminen M, Parisi AF, O'Boyle JE, Folland ED, Khuri S, Kloner RA (1982) Serial evaluation of myocardial thickening and thinning in acute experimental infarction: identification and quantification using two-dimensional echocardiography. *Circulation* 66: 174–80.

28. Weiss JL, Bulkley BH, Hutchins GM, Mason SJ (1981) Two-dimensional echocardiographic recognition of myocardial injury in man: Comparison with postmortem studies. *Circulation* 63: 401–9.

29. Wyatt HL, Forrester JS, da Luz PL, Diamond GA, Chagrasulis R, Swann HJC (1976) Functional abnormalities in nonoccluded regions of myocardium after experimental coronary occlusion. *Am J Cardiol* 37: 366–72.

30. Schuster EH, Bulkley BH (1980) Ischemia at distance after acute myocardial infarction: a cause of early postinfarction angina. *Circulation* 62: 509–15.

31. Stamm RB, Gibson RS, Bishop HL, Carabello BA, Beller GA, Martin RP (1983) Echocardiographic detection of infarct-localized asynergy and remote asynergy during acute myocardial infarction: Correlation with the extent of angiographic coronary disease. *Circulation* 67: 233–45.

32. Gibbson EF, Hogan RD, Franklin TD, Nolting M, Weyman AE (1985) The natural history of regional dysfunction in a canine preparation of chronic infarction. *Circulation* 71: 394–402.

33. Hutchins GM, Bulkey BH (1978) Infarct expansion versus extension: two different complications of acute myocardial infarction. *Am J Cardiol* 41: 1127–32.
34. Heyndrickx GR, Millard RW, McRitchie RJ, Maroko PR, Vatner SF (1975) Regional myocardial functional and electrophysiological alterations after brief coronary artery occlusion in conscious dogs. *J Clin Invest* 56: 978–85.
35. Braunwald E, Kloner RA (1982) The stunned myocardium: prolonged, postischemic ventricular disfunction. *Circulation* 66: 1146–9.
36. Jennings RB, Steenbergen JR (1985) Nucleotide metabolism and cellular damage in myocardial ischemia. *Ann Rev Physiol* 47: 727–49.
37. Ellis SG, Henschke CL, Sandor T, Wynne J, Braunwald E, Kloner RA (1983) Time course of functional and biochemical recovery of myocardium salvaged by reperfusion. *J Am Coll Cardiol* 1: 1047–55.
38. Lavallee M, Cox D, Patrick TA, Vatner SF (1983) Salvage of myocardial function by coronary artery reperfusion 1, 2, and 3 hours after occlusion in conscious dogs. *Circ Res* 53: 235–47.
39. GISSI Trial (1986) Effectiveness of intravenous thrombolytic treatment in acute myocardial infarction. *Lancet* 1: 397–401.
40. GISSI Trial (1987) Long-term effects of intravenous thrombolysis in acute myocardial infarction: final report of GISSI study. *Lancet* 2: 871–4.
41. Penco M, Fedele F, Agati L, Pastore RL, Modena MG, Mattioli G, Dagianti A (1988) Effects of thrombolytic treatment on recovery of left ventricular function in acute myocardial infarction, in: *Echocardiography 1988*, pp 113–21. Amsterdam: Elsevier Science Publisher.
42. Smalling RW, Fuentes F, Freud GC, Reduto LA, Wanta-Matthews M, Gaeta JM, Walker W, Sterling R, Gould KL (1982) Beneficial effects of intracoronary thrombolysis up to eighteen hours after onset of pain in evolving myocardial infarction. *Am Heart J* 104: 912–20.
43. Huey BL, Gheorghiade M, Crampton RS, Beller G, Kaiser DL, Watson DD, Nygaard TW, Craddock GB, Sayre SL, Gibson RS (1987) Acute non-Q wave myocardial infarction associated with early ST segment elevation: Evidence for spontaneous coronary reperfusion and implications for thrombolytic trials. *J Am Coll Cardiol* 9: 18–25.
44. Isaacsohn JL, Earle MG, Kemper AJ, Parisi AF (1988) Postmyocardial infarction pain and infarct extension in the coronary care unit: Role of two-dimensional echocardiography. *J Am Coll Cardiol* 11: 246–51.
45. Pandian NG, Skorton DJ, Colins SM, Koyanagi S, Kieso R, Marcus ML, Kerber RE (1985) Myocardial infarct size threshold for two-dimensional echocardiographic detection: Sensitivity of systolic wall thickening and endocardial wall motion abnormalities in small versus large infarcts. *Am J Cardiol* 55: 551–8.
46. Kaul S, Glasheen W, Ruddy TD, Pandian NG, Weyman AE, Okada RO (1987) The importance of defining left ventricular area at risk in vivo during acute myocardial infarction: an experimental evaluation with myocardial contrast two-dimensional echocardiography. *Circulation* 75: 1249–60.
47. Sanz G, Castaner A, Betriu A, Magrina J, Roig E, Coll S, Pare' JC, Navarro Lopez F (1982) Determinants of prognosis in survivors of myocardial infarction: A prospective clinical angiographic study. *N Engl J Med* 306: 1065–70.
48. Taylor GJ, Humphries JO, Mellits ED, Pitt B, Schulze RA, Griffith LSC, Achuff S (1980) Predictors of clinical course, coronary anatomy, and left ventricular function after recovery from acute myocardial infarction. *Circulation* 62: 960–70.
49. Gibson RS, Bishop HL, Stamm RB, Crampton RS, Beller GA, Martin RP (1982) Value of early two-dimensional echocardiography in patients with acute myocardial infarction. *Am J Cardiol* 49: 1110–12.
50. Horowitz RS, Morganroth J (1982) Immediate detection of early high-risk patients with acute myocardial infarction using two-dimensional echocardiographic evaluation of left ventricular regional wall motion abnormalities. *Am Heart J* 103: 814–22.

51. Nishimura RA, Tajik AJ, Shub C, Miller FA, Ilstrup DM, Harrison C (1984) Role of two-dimensional echocardiography in the prediction of in-hospital complications after acute myocardial infarction. *J Am Coll Cardiol* 4: 1080–7.

52. Nishimura RA, Reeder GS, Miller FA, Ilstrup DM, Shub C, Seward JB, Tajik AJ (1984) Prognostic value of predischarge 2-dimensional echocardiogram after acute myocardial infarction. *Am J Cardiol* 53: 429–32.

53. Dagianti A, Agati L, Di Renzi L, Fedele F, Pastore LR, Penco M (1985) Il cardiologo moderno tra tecnologia e clinica nella valutazione della cardiopatia ischemica. *Cardiologia* 30: 759.

54. Marmor A, Geltman EM, Schechtman K, Sobel BE, Roberts R (1982) Recurrent myocardial infarction: clinical predictors and prognostic implications. *Circulation* 66: 415–21.

55. Marmor A, Sobel BE, Roberts R (1981) Factors presaging early recurrent myocardial infarction ('Extension'). *Am J Cardiol* 48: 603–10.

56. Krone RJ, Friedman E, Thanavaro S, Miller JP, Kleiger RE, Oliver GC (1983) Long-term prognosis after first Q-wave (transmural) or non Q-wave (nontransmural) myocardial infarction: analysis of 539 patients. *Am J Cardiol* 52: 234–9.

57. Mahias-Narvarte H, Adams KF, Willis PW (1987) Evolution of regional left ventricular wall motion abnormalities in acute Q and non-Q wave myocardial infarction. *Am Heart J* 113: 1369–75.

58. Wilson WW, Gibson RS, Nygaard TW, Craddock GB, Watson DD, Crampton RS, Beller GA (1988) Acute myocardial infarction associated with single vessel coronary artery disease: An analysis of clinical outcome and the prognostic importance of vessel patency and residual ischemic myocardium. *J Am Coll Cardiol* 11: 223–34.

59. Ferlinz J (1988) Clinical options in patients with single vessel coronary artery disease and acute myocardial infarction. *J Am Coll Cardiol* 11: 235–6.

60. Bissett JK, Matts J, Sharma B (1987) Program On Surgical Control For Hyper lipidemia-Study Group (POSCH). Residual myocardial jeopardy in patients with Q-wave and non-Q wave infarctions. *Br Heart J* 58: 460–4.

61. Brown KA, Weiss RM, Clements JP, Wackers FJ (1987) Usefulness of residual ischemic myocardium within prior infarct zone for identifying patients at high risk late after acute myocardial infarction. *Am J Cadiol* 60: 15–9.

62. Topol EJ, O'Neill WW, Langburd AB, Walton J Jr, Bourdillon PDV, Bates ER, Grines CL, Schork MA, Kline E, Pitt B (1987) A randomized placebo-controlled trial of intravenous recombinant tissue-type plasminogen activator and emergency coronary angioplasty in patients with acute myocardial infarction. *Circulation* 75: 420.

63. Topol EJ, Califf RM, George BS, Kereiakas DJ, Abbotsmith CW, Candela RJ, Lee KL, Pitt B, Stack RS, O'Neill WW (1987) and the Thrombolysis and Angioplasty in Myocardial Infarction Study Group. A randomized trial of immediate versus delayed elective angioplasty after intravenous tissue plasminogen activator in acute myocardial infarction. *N Engl J Med* 317: 581.

12. Left ventricular shape changes and modelling during acute myocardial infarction

PAOLO MARINO, GIORGIO GOLIA and PIERO ZARDINI

Introduction

During acute transmural ischemia the ipoxic myocardium, unable to develop adequate pressure, undergoes a process of passive stretching secondary to the contraction of the nonischemic muscle [1]. Concomitantly, the opposing non-ischemic myocardium demonstrates an increase in wall thickening or shortening [2–3]. The combined effect of these different regional and global deformations would be to alter the shape of the left ventricle (Figure 1).

Ventricular shape analysis

The examination of ventricular shape has generally relied on eccentricity indices or on the perimeter/area ratio of a ventricular silhouette to that of a circle [4–5]; furthermore, it has been mainly limited to two-dimensional information derived from cineventriculographic images, an ideal technique for the assessment of deformations in the long axis of the ventricle. In the normal heart the systolic contraction is always associated with a progressive elongation of the left ventricular cavity. This ventricular shape change has a clear functional significance: as the perimeter/area ratio for any planar contour is smallest for a perfect circle, the absence for the ventricle of any elongation in its long axis during systole would determine, for a given amount of reduction in the perimeter of the cavity, a smaller change in area, which, if extrapolated to volume, would lead to a significant reduction of volume ejected [4]. It has been shown, in fact, that the larger the ventricular chamber volume the rounder the shape is, and that when stroke volume is reduced dynamic shape change is similarly decreased [4, 6–7].

Shape changes during acute ischemia

These methodological approaches (eccentricity, perimeter/area ratio), how-

S. Iliceto et al. (eds.), Ultrasound in Coronary Artery Disease, 121–131.
© 1991 Kluwer Academic Publishers.

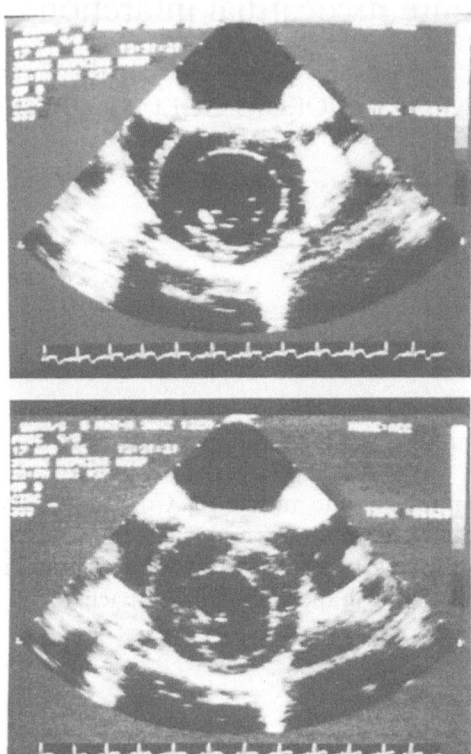

Figure 1. Left ventricular cross-sectional view, at the level of the papillary muscles, during acute ischemia in an open chest animal model. There is a net endocardial shape deformation (elongation) from diastole *(top)* tos systole *(bottom)*.

ever, do not characterize the precise nature of shape deviation from the model geometry for a given contour. In addition, they are relatively insensitive to shape changes, particularly when applied to cross-sectional views [8]. Because of the relative insensitivity of these traditional measurements, only few studies have addressed the problem of shape quantification in the 'true' short axis of the ventricle, comparing antero-posterior vs. septal-lateral dimensions using sonomicrometer cristals or two-dimensional echocardiography [9–11]. One of these studies reported increased cross-sectional elongation of the canine left ventricle at end-systole during occlusion of the circumflex coronary artery, as indexed by eccentricity [9]. In that work, during transmural ischemia, the systolic cross-sectional shape of the left ventricle, imaged in a short axis view at the level of the papillary muscles, changed from its normal circular configuration to a flattened one, the dysfunctioning posterolateral wall of the ventricle serving as a flattened side of an elliptical shaped contour. This elongated ventricular cavity configuration, which likely reflects radial inhomogeneity of wall stress and strain, has been invoked as responsible for the functional impairment of the nonischemic muscle bordering the risk region during acute ischemia in the experimental animal [9]. Shape changes, in fact, could alter loading conditions on adjacent nonischemic myocardium and be responsible for overstress imposed on particular segments of the ventricular wall through local changes in the radius of curvature.

Differences between anterior vs. posterior ischemia

We have recently confirmed these prior observations on shape changes during acute ischemia in the territory of the circumflex artery using the more sensitive Fourier shape analysis technique, and we have further demonstrated that the occlusion of the left anterior descending coronary artery produces

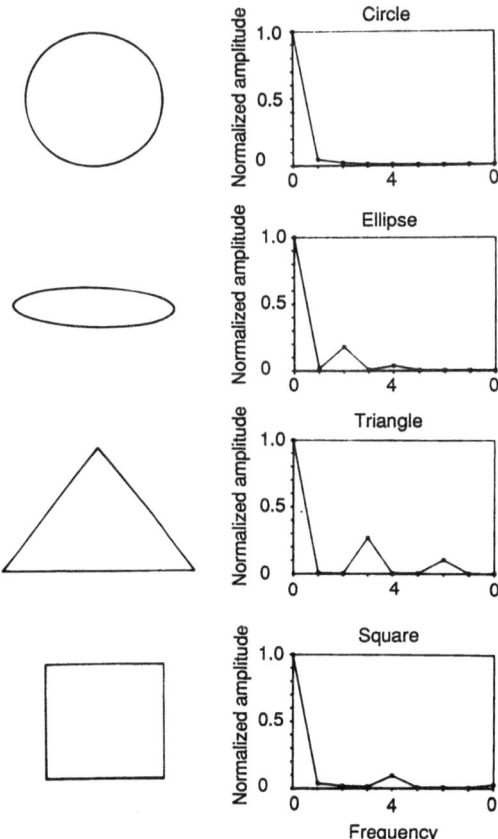

Figure 2. Fourier shape analysis. Each term of the series corresponds to a primary shape. From top: zero order term (circle); 2nd order term (ellipse); 3rd order term (triangle); 4th order term (square). Increases or decreases in the amplitude of any particular component would indicate more or less of a contribution of the associated shape in the overall geometry of the ventricular silhouette.

124   P. Marino

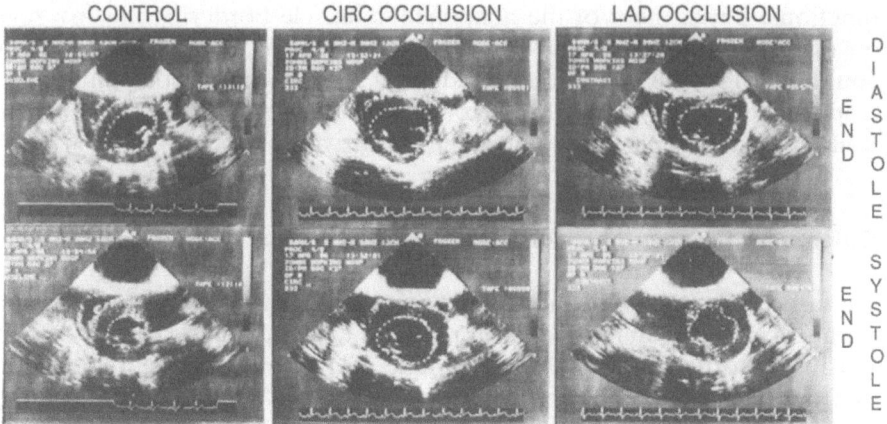

Figure 3. Diastolic (top) and systolic *(bottom)* short axis echocardiograms during control, and ischemia in the territory of the circumflex (CIRC) and left anterior descending (LAD) coronary artery. Specific cavity shape changes for each condition are grossly detectable (from Marino P et al. (1988) *Am J Physiol* 254: H547–557).

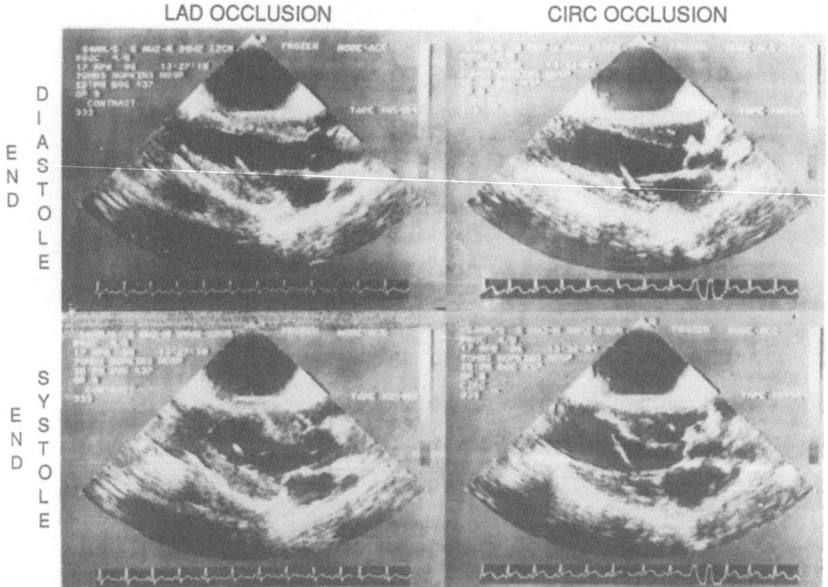

Figure 4. Diastolic *(top)* and systolic *(bottom)* long axis echocardiograms during occlusions of the left anterior descending (LAD) and circumflex (CIRC) coronary artery. With LAD occlusion there is a clear systolic bulging of the anteroseptal wall distal to the first centimeter from the base of the heart. No such bulging is detectable in the inferoposterior wall during CIRC ischemia (from Marino P et al. (1988) *Am J Physiol* 254: H547–557).

and end-systolic deformation change that is different from both control con-dition and circumflex ischemia [12]. In that study the ventricular geometry was imaged in a short axis view and characterized by a methodological approach which provided a complete architectural description of cavity shape, allowing to relate each individual component of the Fourier shape spectrum to specific aspects of shape deformation [8, 13] (Figure 2).

The results demonstrated that there are different and characteristic shape deformations in the short axis endocardial left ventricular contour, that are dependent on the site of the ischemic injury, and that cannot be attributed to different extents of the risk region in the two territories. While control condi-tion is characterized by a more circular shape at end-systole, compared to end-diastole (Figure 3), reflecting the tendency, for the normal heart, to even-ly distribute stress around the cavity at high intraventricular pressure, during circumflex occlusion the endocardial configuration becomes elongated, making the shape of the ventricle to appear, in the short axis plane, more elliptical at end-systole compared to end-diastole (Figure 3). This change in shape reflects radial inhomogeneity of wall stress and strain during acute ischemia, and differs from shape deformations induced by occlusions in the territory of the anterior descending coronary artery. During ischemia in this territory the ventricle assumes a triangular shape (Figure 3), due to the bulg-ing of the portion of the circumference at risk (anteroseptal wall, Figure 4), the abrupt step-like discontinuity involving the wall at a level which is a func-tion of the extent of the proximity of the stenosis and the variability of the coronary distribution for each given animal.

Mechanisms of shape differences

While several potential mechanisms may contribute to the disparity in shape deformation and regional systolic thickening of nonischemic myocardium [14] between ischemia in the territory of the circumflex vs. the anterior de-scending coronary artery, differences in regional muscle wall architecture deserve special comments. The left anterior descending artery perfuses the anterior wall, which has a smaller radius of curvature and is thinner than the posterolateral basilar region perfused by the circumflex artery. The thinner wall, smaller radius of curvature, and more concentric geometry of the distal anteroapical region may make it more susceptible to bulging during ischemia than the thicker and less curved posterolateral myocardium. This disparity, which is partly responsible for the different shape changes deformations de-tected in the short axis view during ischemia in the two vessels, has also been proposed as an explanation for the greater incidence of dilation (expansion) following infarction of the anterior, as opposed to posterolateral, wall [15].

Functional shape alterations resulting from acute transmural ischemia have, in fact, been suggested as the first step in the process of infarct expan-sion. Experimental studies have shown that reversible early shape changes induced by acute coronary occlusion later become irreversible as necrotic softening occurs [16]. This observation may explain discrepancies between studies in living patients which demonstrate infarct expansion during the first 72 h after infarction [17–18] and post mortem studies in which expansion is much less apparent in that early period [19]. It has been shown, in fact, that systolic stretching of ischemic zone segments during ischemia results in sarcomere stretching, with myofiber thinning and segment lengthening [20]. The subsequent normalization of the length of the infarct zone seen at early autopsy may be caused by elastic retraction; the disrupted sarcomeres, however, remain lengthened and the myofibers must buckle producing wavy fiber changes easily detectable at light microscopy [20].

Effect of reperfusion on ventricular volume and shape changes after myocardial infarction

Among the factors affecting the process of expansion after myocardial infarction, early reperfusion seems to play a major role. It has been demonstrated that necrosis spreads over time from the endocardium to the epicardium [21]; thus, if reperfusion would save jeopardized myocardium, the salvage would most likely occur in the epicardial region. This small rim of epicardial myocardium might be sufficient to prevent or lessen infarct expansion [22], as shown in a recent study where perfusion of the infarct-related artery during the healing phase of myocardial infarction prevented continuing infarct expansion and subsequent left ventricular dilation [23].

We were able to confirm the beneficial effect that thrombolytic treatment exerts on the process of infarct expansion from the analysis of two-dimensional echocardiographic examinations of a cohort of 331 patients enrolled in the GISSI trial [24–25]. Patients assigned to thrombolytic treatment exhibited, at predischarge echocardiography, significantly smaller end-diastolic and end-systolic volumes ($p = 0.01$ and $p = 0.04$ respectively) compared with patients assigned to standard care. No difference was detectable for ejection fraction ($p = 0.64$). For both groups there was a significant relationship between end-systolic volume and a qualitatively assessed regional wall motion score (Infarct Size Index), which was assumed as an estimate of infarct size. For large and comparable extents of infarct size, the end-systolic volume was smaller in patients assigned to thrombolysis than in patients assigned to standard care. This finding, which was peculiar of patients with anterior infarction (Figure 5), further supports the experimental and clinical data suggesting that reperfusion of the infarct-related artery should limit expansion, independently of myocardial salvage [22, 26–28].

The effect of reperfusion on *early* left ventricular volume and *shape changes* after myocardial infarction has been preliminary addressed in a consecutive series of infarcted patients, who underwent echocardiography serial-

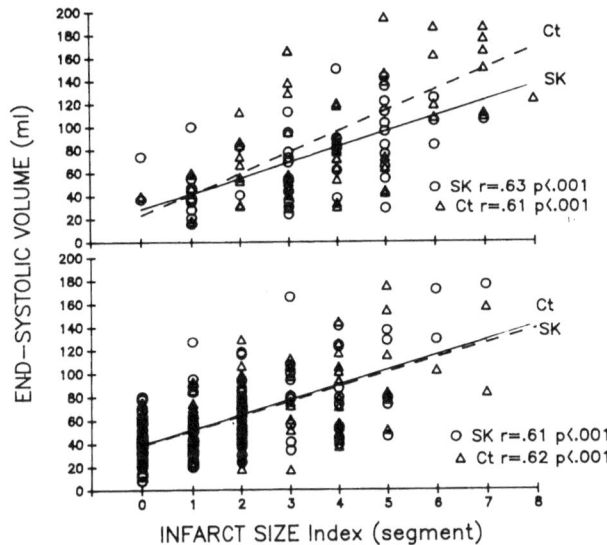

Figure 5. End-systolic volume plotted against a qualitative estimated regional wall motion score (Infarct Size Index) in patients who did (SK: n = 161) or did not (Ct: n = 170) receive thrombolytic treatment. For large and comparable extents of infarct size, end-systolic volume is smaller for SK than for Ct in patients with anterior myocardial infarction *(top)*. With infarction in an alternative location (inferior, lateral, multiple, S-T depression) *(bottom)*, no difference in end-systolic volume can be detected between patients assigned to thrombolytic or conventional treatment.

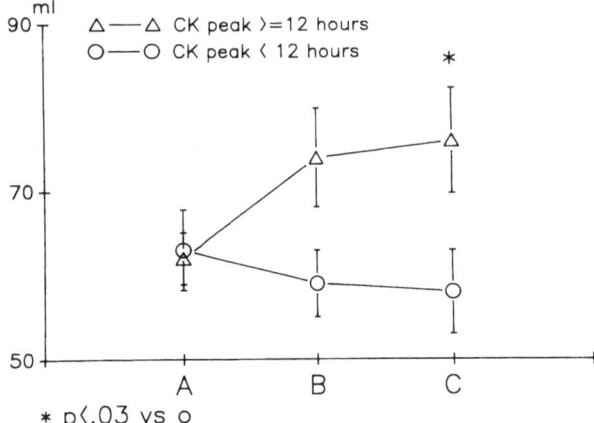

Figure 6. Serial changes (mean ± SE) of end-systolic volume during the first two weeks after acute myocardial infarction in patients with early and late CK time to peak. End-systolic volume averages the same between the two groups at the first examination *(A)*, performed within 24 h from the onset of symptoms. At predischarge echocardiogram *(C)*, however, end-systolic volume is significantly larger in patients with late than in patients with early CK peaking.

ly in the two weeks after the acute episode [29]. The study population was divided into two groups according to the CK time to peak (< 12 h; $> = 12$ h), which was considered as a marker of spontaneous or induced reperfusion. Although the baseline characteristics were comparable between the two groups (only the delay in thrombolytic treatment was significantly greater in patients with late compared with those with early peak), patients with late CK peaking showed a progressive left ventricular dilatation, which became significant by two weeks (Figure 6). Patients with early peak did not show any change in ventricular volume throughout the study.

Shape changes paralled changes in volume. A shape descriptor, which would increase if left ventricular shape changed from the normal (elliptical) toward the spherical configuration, was very comparable, at 24 h from the onset of symptoms, between patients with early and late CK peak (3.6 ± 0.5 vs 3.7 ± 0.9, p = 0.32). At the predischarge examination, however, when differences in volume between the two groups were grossly evident, the shape index was significantly increased in patients with late CK peak (3.9 ± 0.6 vs 3.5 ± 0.7, p = 0.03), reflecting increased ventricular roundness with increasing volume [P. Marino, unpublished].

Effect of unloading on shape changes and ventricular dilation after myocardial infarction

While functional shape alterations and increased ventricular volume with ischemia may take as long as 24 hours to develop in fixed morphologic changes [18], experimental evidence suggests that such early changes may be reversed by ventricular unloading [16].

The prevention of expansion by unloading has been investigated clinically in two randomized trials where a vasodilating drug (nifedipine or nitroglycerin) or placebo was given to acutely infarcted patients who underwent serial two-dimensional echocardiographic examinations in the first two weeks after the acute event [30, 31]. In both studies it was shown that vasodilating therapy limits the extent of infarct expansion, postulating that this favourable effect is afterload mediated. Furthermore, chronic vasodilator therapy should prevent left ventricular sphericity, which has been shown to be linked to the level of exercise capacity and be predictor of subsequent clinical course in patients after acute myocardial infarction [32].

These favourable clinical results of left ventricular unloading on myocardial function and geometry confirm the experimental findings showing that chronic vasodilator therapy with a converting enzyme inhibitor drug attenuates left ventricular dilation and functional deterioration after myocardial infarction in rats [33].

Conclusion

The relatively recent and extensive use of two-dimensional echocardiography in the setting of acute ischemia and myocardial infarction has definitely confirmed the major role of this technique in the noninvasive and serial assessment of the evolutionary changes in shape and geometry which characterize the left ventricle during the acute stage of the illness [34]. At present, further experience is needed to assess the effects of interventions (unloading, reperfusion) directed to restore the original cardiac topography and to define their impact on the natural hystory of the disease. Finally, future investigations have to be conceived focusing on the role of hypertrophy of remote noninfarcted myocardium in the maintenance of an acceptable left ventricular cavity-to-wall thickness relationship, and observing the effects of hypertrophy on the ventricular function and their possible prognostic significance for morbidity and mortality [35].

References

1. Akaishi M, Weintraub WS, Schneider RM, Klein LK, Agarwal JB, Helfant RH (1986) Analysis of systolic bulging. Mechanical characteristics of acutely ischemic myocardium in the conscious dog. *Circ Res* 58: 209–217.
2. Kerber RE, Marcus ML, Wilson R, Ehrhardt J, Abboud FM (1976) Effects of acute coronary occlusion on the motion and perfusion of the normal and ischemic interventricular septum. An experimental echocardiographic study. *Circulation* 54: 928–935.
3. Theroux P, Ross J Jr, Franklin D, Kemper WS, Sasayama S (1976) Regional myocardial function in the conscious dog during acute coronary occlusion and responses to morphine, propanolol, nitroglycerin, and lidocaine. *Circulation* 53: 302–314.
4. Gibson DG, Brown DJ (1975) Continuous assessment of left ventricular shape in man. *Br Heart J* 37: 904–910.
5. Fischl SJ, Gorlin R, Herman MV (1977) Cardiac shape and function in aortic valve disease: physiologic and clinical implications. *Am J Cardiol* 39: 170–176.
6. Vokonas PS, Gorlin R, Cohn PF, Herman MV, Sonnenblick EH (1973) Dynamic geometry of the left ventricle in mitral regurgitation. *Circulation* 48: 786–796.
7. Lewis RP, Sandler H (1971) Relationship between changes in left ventricular dimensions and the ejection fraction in man. *Circulation* 44: 548–557.
8. Kass DA, Traill TA, Keating M, Altieri PI, Maughan WL (1988) Abnormalities of dynamic ventricular shape change in patients with aortic and mitral valvular regurgitation: assessment by Fourier shape analysis and global geometric indexes. *Circ Res* 62: 127–138.
9. Lima JAC, Becker LC, Melin JA, Lima S, Kallman CA, Weisfeldt ML, Weiss JL (1985) Impaired thickening of nonischemic myocardium during acute regional ischemia in the dog. *Circulation* 71: 1048–1059.
10. Goto Y, Yamamoto J, Saito M, Haze K, Sumiyoshi T, Fukami K, Hiramori K (1985) Effects of right ventricular ischemia on left ventricular geometry and the end-diastolic pressure-volume relationship in the dog. *Circulation* 72: 1104–1114.
11. Akaishi M, Schneider RM, Mercier RJ, Naccarella FF, Agarwal JB, Helfant RH, Weintraub WS (1985) Relation between left ventricular global and regional function and extent of myocardial ischemia in the canine heart. *J Am Coll Cardiol* 6: 104–112.
12. Marino P, Kass D, Lima J, Maughan WL, Graves W, Weiss JL (1988) Influence of site of regional ischemia on LV cavity shape change in dogs. *Am J Physiol* 254: H547–557.

13. Ehrlich R, Weinberg B (1970) An exact method for characterization of grain shape. *J Sediment Petrol* 40: 205–212.
14. Marino PN, Becker LC, Lima JAC, Weiss JL (1987) Greater dysfunction of non-ischemic myocardium during acute anterior vs. inferior transmural ischemia (abstr). *J Am Coll Cardiol* 9: 92A.
15. Pirolo JS, Hutchins GM, Moore GW (1986) Infarct expansion: Pathologic analysis of 204 patients with a single myocardial infarct. *J Am Coll Cardiol* 7: 349–354.
16. Nicklas JM, Becker LC, Bulkley BH (1982) Ultrasonic detection of regional shape changes after acute transmural myocardial infarction: time course in the dog model (abstr). *Am J Cardiol* 49: 1038.
17. Eaton LW, Weiss JL, Bulkley BH, Garrison GB, Weisfeldt ML (1979) Regional cardiac dilatation after acute myocardial infarction. *N Engl J Med* 300: 57–62.
18. Erlebacher JA, Weiss JL, Weisfeldt ML, Bulkley BH (1984) Early dilation of the infarcted segment in acute transmural myocardial enlargement. *J Am Coll Cardiol* 4: 201–208.
19. Hutchins GM, Bulkley BH (1978) Infarct expansion versus extension: Two different complications of acute myocardial infarction. *Am J Cardiol* 41: 1127–1140.
20. Erlebacher JA, Richter RC, Alonso DR, Devereux RB, Gay WA Jr (1985) Early infarct expansion: structural or functional? *J Am Coll Cardiol* 6: 839–844.
21. Reimer KA, Lowe JE, Rasmussen MM, Jennings RB (1977) The wavefront phenomenon of ischemic cell death. 1. Myocardial infarct size vs duration of coronary occlusion in dogs. *Circulation* 56: 786–794.
22. Weisman HF, Healy B (1987) Myocardial infarct expansion, infarct extension, and reinfarction: Pathophysiologic concepts. *Prog Cardiovasc Dis* 30: 73–110.
23. Jeremy RW, Hackworthy RA, Bautovich G, Hutton BF, Harris PJ (1987) Infarct artery perfusion and changes in left ventricular volume in the month after acute myocardial infarction. *J Am Coll Cardiol* 9: 989–995.
24. GISSI (1986) Effectiveness of intravenous thrombolytic treatment in acute myocardial infarction. *Lancet i*: 397–402.
25. Marino P, Zanolla L, Golia G, Zardini P (1988) Effects of intravenous streptokinase on left ventricular modelling after myocardial infarction: the GISSI trial (abstr). *Circulation* 78: II–275.
26. Hochman JS, Choo H (1985) Coronary reperfusion inhibits infarct expansion independent of myocardial salvage (abstr). *Circulation* 72: III–67.
27. Shatkin BJ, Swinford RD, Honig SC, Brown EJ, Cohn PF (1987) Dissociation between infarct reduction and myocardial expansion with reperfusion (abstr). *J Am Coll Cardiol* 9: 93A.
28. Slepian MJ, Schipke JD, Segiura S, Kass DA, Maughan WL (1988) Reperfusion of ischemic canine hearts prevents pressure mediated left ventricular dilatation (abstr). *J Am Coll Cardiol* 11: 253A.
29. Marino P, Golia G, Scazzina L, Prioli MA, Zanolla L, Zardini P (1990) Effect of reperfusion on left ventricular remodelling after myocardial infarction, in: Proceedings 6th International Contress on Echocardiography, Rome 1988. Amsterdam: Elsevier Science Publishers. (in press)
30. Jugdutt BI, Warnica JW (1988) Intravenous nitroglycerin therapy to limit myocardial infarct size, expansion, and complications. Effect of timing, dosage, and infarct location. *Circulation* 78: 906–919.
31. Gottlieb SO, Gerstenblith G, Shapiro EP, Chandra N, Healy B, Weisfeldt NL, Weiss JL (1985) Nifedipine reduces early infarct expansion: Results of a double-blind, randomized trial (abstr). *Circulation* 72: III–274.
32. Lamas GA, Vaughan DE, Parisi AF, Pfeffer MA (1988) LV shape predicts exercise capacity following anterior MI: Effects of captopril (abstr). *Circulation* 78: II–470.
33. Pfeffer JM, Pfeffer MA, Braunwald E (1985) Influence of chronic captopril therapy on the infarcted left ventricle of the rat. *Circ Res* 57: 84–95.

34. Marino PN, Weiss JL (1987) Use of the echocardiogram for identifying infarct expansion, in: Califf RM, Wagner GS (eds), *Acute Coronary Care:* 265–279, Boston: Martinus Nijhoff Publisher.
35. Rubin SA, Fishbein MC, Swan HJC (1983) Compensatory hypertrophy in the heart after myocardial infarction in the rat. *J Am Coll Cardiol* 1: 1435–1441.

13. Two-dimensional echocardiographic quantification of myocardial infarct size

NATESA G. PANDIAN and BRENDA S. KUSAY

Introduction

Echocardiography has become the most commonly used imaging technique in the evaluation of patients with acute myocardial infarction [1, 2]. Two-dimensional echocardiography provides excellent morphologic and functional information. Conventional and color Doppler modalities reveal alterations in blood flow dynamics. The result is a comprehensive examination of the infarcted heart. Among the various pathophysiologic abnormalities associated with an infarction, infarct size has remained the crucial factor influencing the patient's clinical course. Recently, due to the progress of thrombolysis and other interventional approaches, the knowledge of infarct size has gained major therapeutic importance as well.

For many decades, clinicians carefully examined the electrocardiographic abnormalities and enzymatic changes to get an understanding of the size of an infarct. Although these techniques provide important information, their pitfalls in estimating infarct size are well-known. Echocardiography can aid in the diagnostic, prognostic and therapeutic evaluation of a patient with myocardial infarction by furnishing information on the presence, location and size of infarction and associated complications. In this chapter we will review the strengths and limitations of two-dimensional echocardiography when estimating the size of a myocardial infarction.

Recognition of myocardial ischemia and infarction

Ischemia and infarction cause rapid changes in myocardial function, often within a few beats. Generally, if ischemia is transient, normal function is regained. On the other hand, prolonged myocardial ischemia usually results in cellular necrosis within about an hour. Resultant myocardial dysfunction then becomes persistent. Regional myocardial dyssynergy caused by ischemia or infarction affects both diastolic and systolic performance. Although diastolic dysfunction often precedes and persists longer than systolic dysfunction,

S. Iliceto et al. (eds.), Ultrasound in Coronary Artery Disease, 133–141.
© 1991 *Kluwer Academic Publishers.*

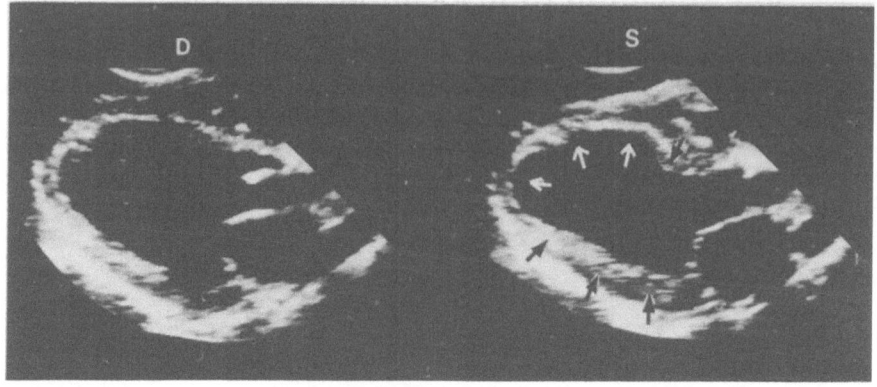

Figure 1. Two-dimensional echocardiographic long-axis image (*left*, diastole; *right*, systole) from a canine experiment showing regional myocardial dyssynergy associated with acute myocardial infarction resulting from left anterior descending coronary artery occlusion. The left ventricular cavity is enlarged. The middle and distal portions of the septum and the apex exhibit systolic thinning and bulging (white arrows).

diastolic properties are relatively more difficult to evaluate. Hence, systolic wall thickening and endocardial motion have been studied in more detail. Depending on the extent and magnitude of ischemia, abnormalities in systolic wall thickening can manifest as decreased thickening, lack of thickening or systolic thinning. Similarly, endocardial motion abnormalities can be categorized as hypokinetic, akinetic, or dyskinetic.

In the past, sonomicrometry was the technique most widely used to study contractile abnormalities in vivo. Comparison of two-dimensional echocardiography to sonomicrometry in animal models of ischemia has demonstrated similar values for sensitivity and specificity [3]. When echocardiography was compared to force-gauge mapping, another experimental technique used in detecting myocardial dyskinesis, similar results were obtained [4]. Anatomic-echocardiographic correlative studies in animals and humans have confirmed that morphologic evidence of infarction is almost always associated with regional contraction abnormalities noted on two-dimensional echocardiography [5–7] (Figure 1). Accordingly, this technique has proven to be highly valuable in the detection of ischemia and infarction.

Localization of myocardial infarction

The ability of two-dimensional echocardiography to localize myocardial ischemia and infarction has been confirmed by a large body of experimental and clinical investigations [7–11]. In canine studies, the site of wall thickening or wall motion abnormalities always corresponds to the perfusion territory of the obstructed coronary artery. Occlusion of the left anterior descending coronary artery causes contractile dysfunction in the anterior wall, anterior portion of the interventricular septum and the apex. Occlusion of the circumflex coronary artery, which supplies the inferoposterior wall in dogs, leads to reginal dysfunction in this area.

The relationship between wall motion abnormalities and post-mortem site of infarction has been well corroborated in humans as well. In anterior infarction caused by occlusion of the left anterior coronary artery, asynergy occurs in the anterior wall, the anterior interventricular septum and the apex (Figure 2). The anterolateral wall exhibits abnormal contractions when lesions of the diagonal branches from the left anterior coronary artery are the culprits. In inferior myocardial infarctions resulting from right coronary artery disease, the left ventricular inferoposterior wall becomes dysfunctional (Figure 2). Occlusion of the circumflex coronary artery impairs function of the lateral and posterolateral walls and, to a variable extent, the posterior wall.

Clinical investigations have established a good correlation between echocardiography and electrocardiography in determining the location of myocardial infarction. In detecting left ventricular asynergy, substantial agreement between echocardiography and contrast cineangiography has been noted as well [11]. In addition, it has been confirmed that wall motion abnormalities on two-dimensional echocardiograms parallel the site of coronary disease on

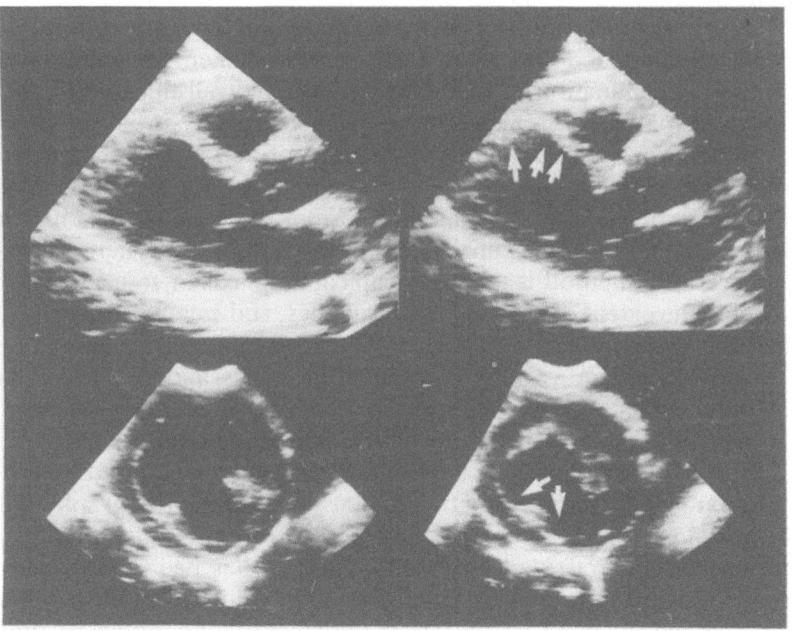

Figure 2. Two-dimensional echocardiographic images from two patients with acute myocardial infarction (*left*, diastole; *right*, systole). Top panel shows long-axis images from a patient with acute anterior myocardial infarction. The interventricular septum and apex manifest dyssynergy. The bottom panel shows short-axis images from a patient with acute inferior myocardial infarction; the inferoposterior wall and the posterior portion of the septum exhibit contraction abnormalities.

selective coronary arteriograms. Thus, echocardiography is also useful in identifying the coronary artery involved.

Estimation of infarct size

The diagnostic ability of two-dimensional echocardiography to identify and localize myocardial infarction, provided the impetus to use this modality in quantifying infarct size. A number of workers focused on devising two-dimensional echocardiographic methods to quantitate infarct size in experimental and clinical investigations. In animal investigations, it is possible to obtain high quality images of the left ventricle with excellent border definition in both long-axis and short-axis planes. The use of detailed quantitative approaches is therefore possible in canine investigations. The approach most commonly used is imaging the ventricle in the short-axis orientation from base to apex [4–7]. The endocardial and epicardial borders of the ventricle are either traced manually or digitized using a computer program. The center of the chamber is identified and multiple radii are advanced to intersect the endocardial and epicardial borders. The number of radii can be as small as 8 or as large as 120 or more. Using this approach, the end-diastolic and end-systolic frames, or all frames from end-diastole to end-systole, are analyzed.

Measurements of wall thickness, the length of the radius from the center to the endocardium, and the area of each sector are taken. Measuring wall thickness allows examination of alterations in systolic wall thickening; measuring endocardial radii or the cavity sector area allows analysis of endocardial motion. In addition, the circumferential extent of abnormal wall thickening or endocardial motion in the short-axis orientation is estimated and expressed as a percentage of the total circumference. From these values, taken at multiple short-axis planes, overall spatial extent of myocardial dyssynergy can be computed. Another method is to employ apical long-axis or four-chamber views, determine the extent of regional abnormalities, and calculate the total amount of dysfunctional myocardium [12]. By obtaining long-axis images along multiple orthogonal planes, or by combining long-axis and short-axis data, the three-dimensional extent of myocardial dyssynergy can be appreciated [13].

Information derived from the above mentioned approaches in canine models of myocardial ischemia and infarction has documented that the functional infarct size estimated by two-dimensional echocardiography correlates well with morphologic infarct size [4–7]. While a certain degree of over-estimation of the infarct size by echocardiography has been observed in some investigations, precise quantitation of infarct size was found in others. The differences may be due to variations in the types of quantitative methods used and/or modifications in the definition of abnormal function. Over-estimation by two-dimensional echocardiography has also been explained by the presence of abnormal contraction in segments adjacent to infarcted myocardium resulting from either a mechanical tethering effect, ischemia, or myocardial stunning.

Despite some differences noted among various studies, one fact has been well validated. The extent of regional dysfunction has a definite correlation with infarct size – except when the infarct size is very small, or small and sub-endocardial. If less than one third of the transmural myocardial thickness or less than one third of the short-axis ventricular circumference is infarcted, regional dysfunction may not be present [5, 7]. In various animal studies, an excellent relationship between infarct size and myocardial area at risk following coronary occlusion has been demonstrated [6, 14]. In these studies, the risk area was measured by contrast myocardial echocardiography or post-mortem coronary arteriography. Contrast myocardial echocardiography is considered to be a superior technique because of its ability to define the risk area in vivo [14]. In humans, morphologic infarct size, measured post-mortem, corresponds well to the functional infarct size defined by ante-mortem two-dimensional echocardiography. While a small sub-endocardial infarct is not associated with myocardial asynergy, the absence of wall motion abnormalities excludes a transmural infarction. This was observed in animal investigations as well. Also, in a setting of a single, fresh infarcted region unaffected by reperfusion, the morphologic infarct size is never bigger than that demonstrated by echocardiography.

Sophisticated, quantitative analysis has been used in some human studies to echocardiographically determine the magnitude of regional dyssynergy and the functional infarct size. However, detailed computerized methods may not be employable in all patients due to difficulties in obtaining clear border definition in all of the necessary images. On the other hand, visual analysis of wall motion abnormaties during real-time two-dimensional imaging is possible in most patients. Visual examination easily integrates wall movement throughout systole and has proven to be reproducible; therefore, this approach is frequently used in human studies [10, 11]. During the review of a two-dimensional echocardiogram, the ventricle is visually divided into a number of segments in different views and a wall motion score is assigned to each segment. The number of segments may vary from 9 to 20. Based on the degree of motion of each segment, it is assigned a value. In one scheme, the value of 1 is assigned to the segment if it has normal motion, 2 for hypokinesis, 3 for akinesis, 4 for dyskinesis, and 5 for aneurysmal bulging. From these values, a comprehensive wall motion score is derived.

A large number of clinical investigations have examined the reliability of two-dimensional echocardiography in estimating the functional infarct size compared to other imaging modalities such as contrast cineangiography, radionuclide ventriculography, and thallium scanning [1, 8–11]. In general, there is a good correlation between echocardiography and the other techniques. A good relationship has also been noted between echocardiographic functional infarct size and enzymatic size of infarction. The significance of assessing functional infarct size is further illustrated by studies which indicate that knowing the extent of regional dyssynergy provides information about immediate and long-term prognosis [10].

Ultrasonic tissue characterization of myocardial infarction

Acoustic properties of the myocardium are altered in the setting of ischemia and infarction. A number of investigators are examining the potential use of acoustic signal analysis to provide information about structural changes associated with ischemia, infarction, and reperfusion. In one approach, raw radio-frequency data is analyzed and measurements of attenuation and backscatter are recorded. In another approach, echocardiographic gray level data is processed and quantitative statistical analysis of average regional amplitude and spatial distribution of amplitudes is performed. Initial investigations demonstrated that these approaches are capable of detecting ischemia and infarction, but their value in quantitating infarct size requires further study.

Assessment of infarct size in right ventricular infarction

Right ventricular myocardial infarction occurs frequently in patients with acute inferior myocardial infarction. When compared to the amount of information available about left ventricular infarction, information about right ventricular infarct size, its area at risk, and the extent of right ventricular dyssynergy is scant. Two-dimensional echocardiography is capable of detecting right ventricular infarction with excellent sensitivity (92%) [15]. In one canine study, only 2 out of 26 myocardial slices with right ventricular infarct did not demonstrate right ventricular dyssynergy. In these two, the infarct size was very small, less than 6% of the right ventricle. Recent animal investigations, using two-dimensional and contrast myocardial echocardiography, have indicated a definite correspondence between right ventricular risk area and infarct size. A close correlation was documented – not only after the infarct had been well established (r = 0.93), but also when the risk area was measured immediately after coronary occlusion (r = 0.92). Correlation between infarct size and the extent of right ventricular dyssynergy has also been noted to be close (r = 0.92).

Effect of reperfusion and stunned myocardium on quantitation of infarct size

When ischemic episodes are multiple but brief, or when an ischemic episode is protracted but not long enough to cause an infarction, prolonged myocardial dysfunction may occur even after resolution of ischemia. Such prolonged post-ischemic dysfunction is termed stunned myocardium. This phenomenon can be encountered when reperfusion follows coronary occlusion. Abnormal energy transduction, altered calcium flux, production of free radicals, abnormal deposition and behavior of white blood cells, disruption of sympathetic neural responsiveness, and heterogenous improvement in perfusion have all been purported, either as a lone influence or in combination, to be responsible for stunning of the myocardium.

Myocardial regions within the risk territory or adjacent to an infarction may demonstrate persistent regional dysfunction even though the muscle in that region is not infarcted. Consequently, the extent of myocardial dyssynergy may not correlate with the amount of necrosed muscle. In animal studies, a poor correspondence has been noted between infarct size and the extent of myocardial contraction abnormalities following reperfusion. In patients, prolonged post-ischemic dysfunction, reverting back to normalcy much later, is frequently encountered following reperfusion achieved by thrombolytic therapy or angioplasty. Studies have shown that dysfunctional myocardium that has not been permanently damaged has the ability to respond to stress with augmented contractility. When inotropic drugs such as epinephrine, isoproterenol or dopamine, and unloading agents such as hydralazine are used, the stunned myocardium is able to exhibit better contraction, indicating a functional reserve in these regions [16]. Because of the prognostic and therapeutic significance, it is important to be able to discriminate whether myocardial dysfunction in a given region is due to ischemia and infarction or due to stunned myocardium. Recovery of function in serial imaging studies would indicate the presence of earlier stunning, but recovery may take variable periods of time and thus would not be useful in immediate management.

The stunned myocardial state has important clinical implications. Evaluation of ventricular function immediately after reperfusion therapy may not indicate the success of such therapy. Depressed cardiac performance after interventional therapy or surgery should not be associated with a negative prognostic connotation. On the other hand, it is conceivable and indeed postulated that recurrent stunning episodes may lead to permanent myocardial dysfunction. If such a long-term consequence is a possibility, attempts should be made to avoid or reduce ischemia during diagnostic and interventional procedures since multiple mild ischemic episodes can lead to recurrent myocardial stunning. Understanding the causes, mechanisms, clinical correlates, and prognostic and therapeutic implications of stunned myocardium needs further research.

Prognostic value of echocardiographic estimation of functional infarct size

Assessment of the extent of myocardial wall motion abnormalities by two-dimensional echocardiography can indicate the likely in-hospital course of a patient with acute myocardial infarction [10]. The incidence of complications such as death, shock, heart failure and arrhythmias is higher when the functional infarct size exceeds 20% of the ventricle or when multiple non-contiguous regions are dysfunctional [1]. The incidence of complications is markedly lower in the setting of a small functional infarct. Generally, the extent of wall motion abnormality does not vary significantly within the first few days. Therefore, in acute myocardial infarction, an early assessment of wall motion abnormality can be used as a guide when implementing in-hospital management. Functional infarct size influences long-term prognosis as well. Many studies have shown that a larger functional infarct and a higher wall motion score index are associated with greater long-term mortality. A change in the shape of the ventricle, due to infarct expansion or ventricular aneurysm formation, is another factor which has a bearing on prognosis. These patients are likely to have a higher short-term and long-term incidence of complications and death.

The myocardial area at risk and infarct size influence global left ventricular function. Global left ventricular function is an important determinant of morbidity and mortality following myocardial infarction. Left ventricular ejection fraction, estimated by two-dimensional echocardiography, provides a valuable prognostic index [17]. Thus, early evaluation of functional infarct size, ventricular shape, and global left ventricular function provides valuable information on the likely course of a patient with acute myocardial infarction.

Conclusion

Two-dimensional and Doppler echocardiographic techniques have a proven role in the assessment of complications of myocardial infarction. A large body of evidence has clearly demonstrated that two-dimensional echocardiographic assessment of the left ventricle can yield reliable estimates of the size of a myocardial infarction. The importance of such echocardiographic quantitation has been substantiated by clinical studies which have pointed out the diagnostic and prognostic value of determining functional infarct size. The ability of two-dimensional echocardiography and contrast myocardial echocardiography to provide risk-infarct ratio is of use in assessing the efficacy of interventional therapy. With further work in the study of right ventricular infarction, stunned myocardium, and ultrasonic tissue characterization, echocardiography is likely to play an even bigger role in patients with complicated and uncomplicated myocardial infarction.

References

1. Kloner RA, Parisi AF (1987) Acute myocardial infarction: diagnostic and prognostic applications of two-dimensional echocardiography. *Circulation* 75: 521.
2. Pandian NG, Skorton DJ, Kerber RE (1984) Role of echocardiography in myocardial ischemia and infarction. *Modern Conc of Cardiovas Dis* 53: 19.
3. Pandian NG, Kerber RE (1982) Two-dimensional echocardiography in coronary stenosis I. Sensitivity and specificity in the detection of transient myocardial dyskinesis. *Circulation* 66: 597.
4. Wyatt HL, Meerbaum S, Heng MK, Rit J, Gueret P, Corday E (1981) Experimental evaluation of the extent of myocardial dyssynergy and infarct size by two-dimensional echocardiography. *Circulation* 63: 739.
5. Lieberman AN, Weiss JL, Jugdutt BI, Becker LC, Bulkley BH, Garrison JG, Hutchins GM, Weisfeldt ML (1981) Two-dimensional echocardiography and infarct size: Relationship of

regional wall motion and thickening to the extent of myocardial infarction in the dog. *Circulation* 63: 739.

6. Pandian NG, Koyanagi S, Skorton DJ, Collins SM, Eastham CL, Kieso RA, Marcus ML, Kerber RE (1983) Relations between two-dimensional echocardiographic wall thickening abnormalities, myocardial infarct size and coronary risk area in normal and hypertrophied myocardium in dogs. *Am J Cardiol* 52: 1318.

7. Pandian NG, Skorton DJ, Collins SM, Koyanagi S, Kieso R, Marcus ML, Kerber RE (1985) Myocardial infarct size threshold for two-dimensional echocardiographic detection: sensitivity of systolic wall thickening and endocardial motion abnormalities in small versus large infarcts. *Am J Cardiol* 55: 551.

8. Visser CA, Lie K, Kan G, Meltzer R, Durrer D (1981) Detection and quantification of acute, isolated myocardial infarction by two-dimensional echocardiography. *Am J Cardiol* 47: 1020.

9. Horowitz RS, Morganroth J, Parrotta C, Chen CC, Soffer J, Pauletto FJ (1982) Immediate diagnosis of acute myocardial infarction by two-dimensional echocardiography. *Circulation* 65: 323.

10. Heger JJ, Weyman AE, Wann S, Rogers EW, Dillon JC, Feigenbaum H (1980) Cross-sectional echocardiographic analysis of extent of left ventricular asynergy in acute myocardial infarction. *Circulation* 61: 1113.

11. Kisslo JA, Robertson D, Gilvert BW, Von Ramm O, Behar VS (1977) A comparison of real-time, two-dimensional echocardiography and cineangiography in detecting left ventricular asynergy. *Circulation* 55: 134.

12. Parisi AF, Moynihan P, Folland ED (1981) Quantitative detection of regional left ventricular contraction abnormalities by two-dimensional echocardiography. II. Accuracy in coronary artery disease. *Circulation* 63: 761.

13. Guyer DE, Foale RA, Gillam LD, Wilkins GT, Guerrero L, Weyman AE (1986) An echocardiographic technique for quantifying and displaying the extent of regional left ventricular dyssynergy. *J Am Coll Cardiol* 8: 830.

14. Kaul S, Glasheen W, Ruddy T, Pandian NG, Weyman A, Okada R (1987) The importance of defining left ventricular area at risk in vivo during acute myocardial infarction: An experimental evaluation utilizing myocardial contrast two-dimensional echocardiography. *Circulation* 75: 1249.

15. Pandian NG, Wang SS, Brockway B, Chuttani K (1988) Sensitivity of regional right ventricular myocardial dyssynergy in the detection of right ventricular infarction, and its quantitative value in estimating infarct size (abstracts). *Circulation* 78: II–418.

16. Becker LC, Levine JH, DiPaula AF, Guarnierin T, Aversano T (1986) Reversal of dysfunction in postischemic stunned myocardium by epinephrine and postextrasystolic potentiation *J Am Coll Cardiol* 7: 580.

17. Kan G, Visser CA, Lie KI, Durrer D (1984) Early two-dimensional echocardiographic measurement of left ventricular ejection fraction in acute myocardial infarction. *Eur Heat J* 5: 210.

14. Detection and evaluation of left ventricular thrombosis in myocardial infarction
Role of echocardiography

ANTONIO F. AMICO, SABINO ILICETO, CATALDO MEMMOLA, GIOVANNI PICCINNI, CARLO CAIATI, CESARE PELLEGRINI and PAOLO RIZZON

Introduction

Intraventricular thrombosis is a complication met with relatively frequently during acute anterior myocardial infarction [1], especially if there is also an aneurysmatic dilatation. In this clinical situation, before the advent of echocardiography, diagnosis was retrospective and based on the appearance of a systemic embolism. After the acute phase of myocardial infarction, the only available diagnostic method was contrast ventriculography: this method has the drawback of being neither very sensitive (it cannot visualize laminated thrombi) nor specific (it may show up false filling defects in large ventricles). Moreover, its poor repeatability means it is not very suitable for following up the behaviour of thrombi.

Apart from echocardiography, a variety of noninvasive methods have been suggested for diagnosing intracardiac thrombi. Among these, 131–I fibrinogen scanning [2] and radiolabeled antibodies to fibrinogen [3] are the most sophisticated but least clinically useful as they cannot define the site of the thrombus even though they do identify its presence. Though relatively noninvasive, radionuclide ventriculography [4] has the same sensitivity limitations as contrast ventriculography.

Computed tomography [5] and indium 111 platelet scintigraphy [6] are the two methods most commonly proposed as an alternative to echocardiography when this proves technically inadequate. Their diagnostic accuracy is comparable to that of echocardiography and indium 111 platelet scintigraphy also gives additional information on the active incorporation of fibrinogen and platelets into the thrombus.

Diagnostic power of echocardiography in intraventricular thrombosis

Even though M-mode echocardiography has occasionally enabled diagnosis of intraventricular thrombi [7], it has not been very useful from a practical point of view as it is not able to visualize the cardiac apex where most thrombi

S. Iliceto et al. (eds.), Ultrasound in Coronary Artery Disease, 143–149.
© 1991 *Kluwer Academic Publishers.*

are found. In earlier experiences of using two-dimensional echocardiography [8] it emerged that, for technical reasons, echocardiography runs the risk of giving false postives. An initial study comparing echocardiographic with angiographic, surgical and autoptic findings defined the characteristic morphological aspects to be sought in the event of intraventricular thrombi [9]. The series included 21 patients selected from 2,657 consecutive echocardiograms. This study concluded that:

– left ventricular thrombi are always associated with wall motion abnormalities;
– the thrombi are, as a rule, apical and this is probably because of the blood stasis which is made worse by the reduced wall motion;
– to clearly distinguish the surface of the endocardium from that of the thrombus, different gain and reject adjustments need to be tried, as well as a reduced depth so as to reduce the near field artifact;
– the thickness of the ventricular wall is an important element which needs to be considered in the case of a ventricular aneurysm. Given the thin walls of the latter, if an aneurysmatic wall of normal thickness is found, one would suspect an associated wall thrombus (Figure 1);
– the presence of scars on the walls may produce anomalous echoes which, in order to establish whether they are artefacts or not, need to be investigated using multiple tomographic planes;
– the echodensity of the thrombus varies according to whether it is protruding or laminated; moreover probably the age of the thrombus also has an effect, as those of older age are generally more echo dense than the more recent ones (Figure 2).

In order to reduce the possibility of false positive diagnoses one must bear in mind the possibility of technical artefacts, such as how near the apex is to the ultrasound source and the presence of strongly echo-reflecting structures with reverberations. In general, the margin of a thrombus should have a constant

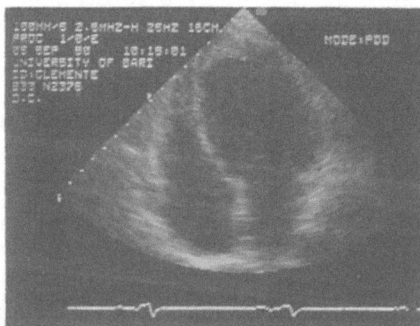

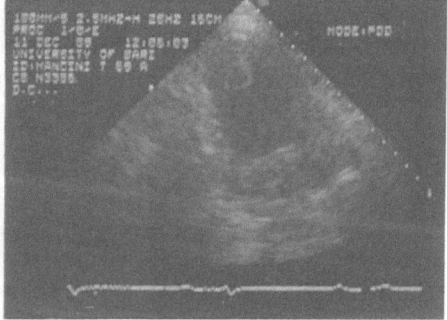

Figure 1. Apical four-chamber view: when there is a aneurysmal dilation of the left ventricle a localized thrombus is observed at the apex.

Figure 2. Apical two-chamber view: apical thrombus the superficial layers of which appear to be strongly echo-reflecting.

and reproducible position in different planes, which is not generally the case with artefacts. Finally, one should consider that there may be a series of normal or pathological structures which can mimic the presence of a thrombus such as the papillary muscles, abnormal trabeculae and muscular bridges and tendon structures.

Stratton et al. [10] have defined the sensitivity and specificity of two-dimensional echocardiography in the diagnosis of thrombi in a series of 78 patients. True positive diagnosis was made in 95% of cases and the possibility of a thrombus was correctly excluded in 86% of cases. The predictive value of a negative study was 98%. They found that in the echocardiograms defined as equivocal the probability of false positive diagnoses was higher, indicating that cases where the presence of a thrombus is not clear should be considered negative. Furthermore, false positive diagnoses occurred more often for thrombi with a diameter of less than one centimetre.

The above data, from retrospective studies, on the diagnostic accuracy of echocardiography have been confirmed by a prospective study of 67 patients in whom diagnosis was confirmed or excluded during aneurysmectomy or autopsy [11]. Sensitivity was 92% while specificity was 88%. In order to reduce the incidence of false positives, quantitative image analysis techniques have been proposed, based on the analysis of phase and amplitude relations of the echoes reflected by the thrombi [12].

Echocardiography in the follow-up of ventricular thrombosis

Systemic embolisms are a complication of acute myocardial infarction [13]; the incidence of embolisms is, on the whole, small in the population of patients with infarction, reports of it being between 1.3% [14] and 3.4% [15]. Consequently it would not be advisable to propose a preventive therapy for this complication across the board to all patients with infarctions. Echocardiography could be used to select a group of patients with intracardiac thrombosis in whom the presence of a greater risk factor would justify the use of particular therapies which affect coagulation. Various studies have shown that in patients in whom ventricular thrombosis during acute myocardial infarction is echocardiographically ascertained, there is a greater incidence of systemic embolisms [16–18]. Embolic potential seems to be greater during the first few days after infarction, probably because of the structural instability of the thrombotic mass: an echocardiographic exam, done between 3 and 12 weeks after the acute phase on 200 patients following a rehabilitation programme, diagnosed the presence of intraventricular thrombi in 40, none of whom had had embolisms [19]. It is likely that a variety of factors all play a part in the embolising process which starts from intracardiac thrombi: the age of the thrombus may well be an important parameter since as in more recent thrombi spontaneous lysis and stratification are more active; if this is so, it might explain the echocardiographically documented spontaneous changes in the shape and mobility of thrombi in the early phase of infarction [20].

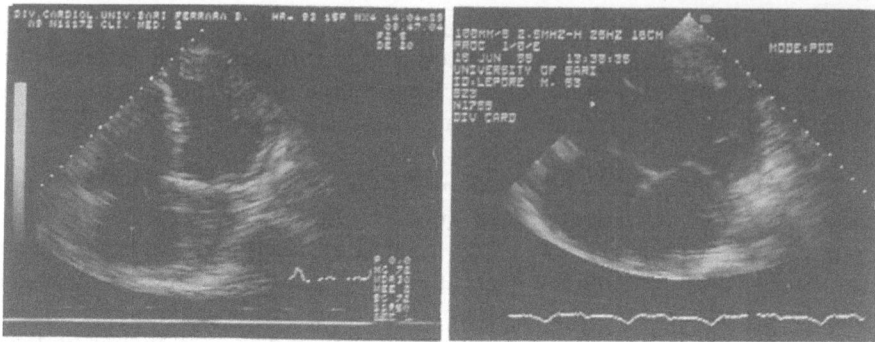

Figure 3. Apical left ventricular thrombosis: the left Figure shows a thrombus with greater risk of embolism than the one shown on the *right* (see text).

A relationship between morphological aspect and embolic potential of the thrombus has been suggested in several studies [17, 18, 21]. Thrombi which protrude into the left ventricular chamber, with a surface whose thrombus-blood interface is opposite in sign to the curvature of the adjacent left ventricular wall, and those which move independently of the adjacent wall, should be considered 'at risk' (Figure 3). The important problem of the therapeutic approach to be adopted in these situations has not yet been resolved despite the important information supplied by echocardiography. Anticoagulant treatment does not seem able to prevent the formation of thrombi [22], nor has it been proved that this treatment does actually reduce the incidence of embolisms in patients with apparently 'at risk' thrombi: this is because the low incidence of the phenomenon means that one would need an extremely large-scale study of the sort which can only be had in large multi-centre studies. A study of this kind, recently carried out in Italy [23], evaluated the efficiency of a *non* anticoagulating treatment (Ca-heparin at moderate dosages) in preventing left endoventricular thrombi from forming in patients with acute anterior myocardial infarction: of 167 patients with no signs of thrombi at the first echocardiogram taken within 24 h of the infarct symptoms, 87 underwent Ca-heparin 12500 U treatment every 12 h while the other 80 received no treatment whatsoever. Only five of the patients in the first group developed thrombi (5.7%) as opposed to 21 (26.2%) in the second group (p = 0.0002). This result is particularly important considering how safe this therapeutic approach is: out of 360 treated patients, the incidence of bleeding was only 4.4%

It has been claimed that anticoagulation treatment helps to solve or at least reduce the size of the thrombus [24], even though this does sometimes happen spontaneously [25]. Thrombolytic therapy promises to be the most efficient for doing this and it has, indeed, proven to be able to dissolve recently-formed thrombi [26]. It seems more than likely that the adoption of thrombolysis as a part of routine treatment of acute infarction has led to a reduction in the incidence of intraventricular thromboses since, in large trials, fewer peripheral embolisms have been documented than in the data found in literature in the pre-thrombolysis era [27–29].

Echocardiography and endocardiac thrombosis: future perspectives

The above clearly shows how great a contribution echocardiography has made to the study of this specific chapter of ischemic heart disease. It also justifies frequent echocardiographic controls in the early phases of anterior myocardial infarction so as to monitor the development of thrombi and guide the physician when deciding on anticoagulant therapy. However, ultrasounds can probably play an important part in studying the pathogenetic mechanisms of the thrombotic phenomenon. Furthermore, improvements in image processing techniques could lead to a more in-depth analysis of the thrombotic formation itself, thus perhaps supplying more detailed information on its composition, age, etc.

In the past, there have been reports of an association, detected unexpectedly by echocardiography, between spontaneous echocontrast and the formation of intraventricular thrombi [30]. This phenomenon has also been found in patients with mitral stenosis, enlarged left atrium and atrial fibrillation [31]. Apart from finding that it was associated with thrombi, it has also been noticed that it is not affected by anticoagulating therapy. However, it has been suggested that this finding is an expression of different 'thrombophylic' situations. In a classification we proposed [32], the spontaneous echocontrast secondary to blood stasis was defined as type I and two more aspects have since been distinguished: type IA, characterized by the presence of a cloud of minute echoes that move in a whirling smokelike manner within a single area with poorly defined outlines and in which thrombi can be sometimes observed; and type IB, which seems more homogeneous than type IA. Its outlines fluctuate and are extremely mobile, though relatively well defined with a better echoreflectivity than that of blood. This type of spontaneous contrast echo is also often found near thrombi. Type IA could be formed by extremely mobile masses of red cells that form in conditions of stasis while type IB could correspond to masses of red cells caught in fibrin nets, which are less mobile and acoustically denser than the previous type. In our observations type IA was detected in several settings of slow blood flow (dilated cardiomyopathies, left ventricular aneurysm, enlarged left atrium etc.) while type IB was fairly rare, occuring in large ventricular aneurysms and in the pericardial sac in one case with a pericardiocentesis induced hemopericardium.

Connected to these observations, the literature reports experimental studies which have investigated the acoustic properties of thrombi [33] and the possibility, by means of analysis of the grey scale and other variables which can be derived from the echocardiographic image, of predicting the embolic potential of the thrombotic formation [34].

Conclusions

Thromboses are complex phenomena which have aroused the interest of researchers, especially because of the introduction of powerful thrombolytic drugs which have radically changed the therapeutic approach to the problem. Echocardiography has gained a prominent place not only in the diagnosis of intracardiac thromboses but, in the future too, ultrasounds are likely to be applicable in monitoring the evolution of the biological process itself.

References

1. Asinger RW, Mikell FL, Elsperger J, Hodges M (1981) Incidence of left ventricular thrombosis after acute transmural myocardial infarction. Serial evaluation by two-dimensional echocardiography. *N Engl J Med* 305: 297–302.
2. Frisbie JH, Tow DE, Sasahara AA, Barsamian EM, Parisi AF (1976) Non invasive detection of intracardiac thrombosis. 131–I fibrinogen cardiac survey. *Circulation* 6: 989–991.
3. Kramer RS, Ashburn WL, Vasko JS (1967) Detection of intracardiac thrombi using radioiodinated antifibrinogen (RIAF) and precordial scanning: Experimental and clinical studies. *Ann. Surg* 166: 173–177.
4. Stratton JR, Ritchie JL, Hammermeister KE, Kennedy JW, Hamilton GW (1981) Detection of left ventricular thrombi with radionuclide angiography. *Am J Cardiol* 48: 565–72.
5. Tomoda H, Hoshiai M, Furuya H, Kuribayashi S, Ootaki M, Matsuyama S, Koide S, Kawada S, Shotsu A (1983) Evaluation of intracardiac thrombus with computed tomography. *Am J Cardiol* 51: 843–52.
6. Ezekowitz MD, Wilson DA, Smith EO, Burow RD, Harrison LH, Parker DE, Elkins RC, Peyton M, Taylor FB (1982) Comparison of indium 111 platelet scintigraphy and two-dimensional echocardiography in the diagnosis of left ventricular thrombi. *New Engl J Med* 306: 1509–13.
7. Horgan JH, O'M Shiel F, Goodman AC (1976) Demonstration of left ventricular thrombus by conventional echocardiography. *J Clin Ultrasound* 4: 287–8.
8. Meltzer RS, Guthaner D, Rakowski H, Popp RL, Martin RP (1979) Diagnosis of left ventricular thrombi by two-dimensional echocardiography. *Br Heart J* 42: 651–5.
9. Asinger RW, Mikell FL, Sharma B, Hodge M (1981) Observations on detecting left ventricular thrombus with two-dimensional echocardiography: Emphasis on avoidance of false positive diagnoses. *Am J Cardiol* 47: 145–56.
10. Stratton JR, Lighty GW, Pearlman AS, Ritchie JL (1982) Detection of left ventricular thrombus by two-dimensional echocardiography: Sensitivity, specificity and causes of uncertainty. *Circulation* 66: 156–66.
11. Visser CA, Kan G, David GK, Lie KI, Durrer D (1983) Two-dimensional echocardiography in the diagnosis of left ventricular thrombus: A prospective study of 67 patients with anatomic validation. *Chest* 83: 228–32.
12. Green SE, Joynt LE, Fitzgerald PJ, Rubenson DS, Popp RL (1983) In vivo ultrasonic tissue characterization of human intracardiac masses. *Am J Cardiol* 51: 231–6.
13. Hellerstein HK, Martin JW (1946) Incidence of thromboembolic lesions accompanying myocardial infarction. *Am Heart J* 32: 443–52.
14. Working party on anticoagulant therapy in coronary thrombosis: Assessment of short-term anticoagulant administration after cardiac infarction. *Brit Med J* (1969) 1: 335–42.
15. Veterans Administration Cooperative Clinical Trial Group (1973) Anticoagulants in acute myocardial infarction. Results of a cooperative clinical trial. *JAMA* 225: 724–29.

16. Keating AC, Gross SA, Schlamowitz RA, Glassman JG, Mazur JH, Pitt WA, Miller D (1983) Mural thrombi in myocardial infarctions. Prospective evaluation by two-dimensional echocardiography. *Am J Med* 74: 989–95.
17. Haugland JM, Asnger RW, Mikell FL, Elsperger J, Hodges M (1984) Embolic potential of left ventricular thrombus detected by two-dimensional echocardiography. *Circulation* 70: 588–98.
18. Visser CA, Kan G, Meltzer RS, Dunning A, Roelandt J (1985) Embolic potential of the ventricular thrombi after myocardial infarction: A two-dimensional echocardiographic study of 119 patients. *J Am Coll Cardiol* 5: 1276–80.
19. Tramarin R, Pozzoli M, Vecchio C (1982) Trombosi ventricolare nell'infarto miocardico recente. Studio ecocardiografico. *G. Ital Cardiol* 12: 397–404.
20. Domenicucci S, Bellotti P, Chiarella F, Lupi G, Vecchio C (1987) Spontaneous morphologic changes in left ventricular thrombi: A prospective two-dimensional echocardiographic study. *Circulation* 75: 737–43.
21. Stratton JR, Resnick AD (1987) Increased embolic risk in patients with left ventricular thrombi. *Circulation* 75: 1004–11.
22. Friedmand MJ, Carlson K, Marcus FI, Woolfenden JM (1982) Clinical correlations in patients with acute myocardial infarction and left ventricular thrombus detected by two-dimensional echocardiography. *Am J Med* 72: 894–8.
23. The SCATI Group (1989) Randomized Controlled Trial of Subcutaneous Calcium-heparin in acute myocardial infarction. *Lancet* (July 22): 182–186.
24. Tramarin R, Pozzoli M, Febo O, Opasich C, Colombo E, Cobelli F, Specchia (1986) Two-dimensional echocardiographic assessment of anticoagulant therapy in left ventricular thrombosis early after acute myocardial infarction. *Eur Heart J* 7: 482–492.
25. Spirito P, Bellotti P, Chiarella F, Domenicucci S, Sementa A, Vecchio C (1985) Prognostic significance and natural history of left ventricular thrombi in patients with acute anterior myocardial infarction: A two-dimensional echocardiographic study. *Circulation* 72: 774–80.
26. Kremer P, Fiebig R, Tilsner V, Bleifeld W, Mathey DG (1985) Lysis of left ventricular thrombi with urokinase. *Circulation* 72: 112–8.
27. Gruppo Italiano per lo Studio della Streptochinasi nell'Infarto Miocardico (GISSI) (1985) Effectiveness of intravenous thrombolytic treatment in acute myocardial infarction. *Lancet* 1: 397–422.
28. Wilcox RG, Von Der Lippe G, Olsson CG, Jensen G, Skene AM, Hampton JR for the ASSET Study Group (1988) Trial of tissue plasminogen activator for mortality reduction in acute myocardial infarction. Anglo-Scandinavian Study of Early Thrombolysis (ASSET). *Lancet* 2: 525–30.
29. The ISAM Study Group (1986) A prospective trial of intravenous streptokinase in acute myocardial infarction (ISAM): Mortality, morbidity and infarct size at 21 days. *N Engl J Med* 314: 1465–71.
30. Mikell FL, Asinger RW, Elsperger KJ, Anderson RW, Hodges M (1982) Regional stasis of blood in the dysfunctional left ventricle echocardiographic detection and differentiation from early thrombosis. *Circulation* 66: 755–63.
31. Iliceto S, Antonelli G, Sorino M, Biasco G, Rizzon P (1985) Dynamic intracavitary left atrial echoes in mitral stenosis. *Am J Cardiol* 55: 603–6.
32. Iliceto S, Papa A, Antonelli G, Sorino M, Amico A (1985) Spontaneous contrast echocardiography. *Echocardiography* 5: 455–65.
33. Mikell FL, Asinger RW, Elsperger KJ, Anderson RW, Hodges (1982) Tissue acoustic properties of fresh left ventricular thrombi and visualization by two dimensional echocardiography: Experimental observations. *Am J Cardiol* 49: 1157–65.
34. Lloret RL, Cortada X, Bradford J, Metz MN, Kinney EL (1985) Classification of left ventricular thrombi by their history of systemic embolization using pattern recognition of two-dimensional echocardiograms. *Am Heart J* 110: 761–5.

15. Two dimensional echocardiography and Doppler findings in right ventricular infarction

M.A. GARCÍA-FERNANDEZ, J. LÓPEZ-SENDÓN
and M. MORENO YANGÜELA

Introduction

Two dimensional and Doppler echocardiography constitutes a safe, non-invasive, easily repeatable diagnostic examination that provide reliable and valuable information about the structure and function of the heart. In this chapter we will discuss the usefulness of two dimensional echocardiography and Doppler to evaluate right ventricular function in ischemic heart disease and to diagnose right ventricular infarction and associated complications.

Two dimensional echocardiographic terminology and image display of the right ventricle

The right ventricle may be visualized in the long axis, short axis and four chamber views from several positions of the transducer, the parasternal, apical and subcostal areas [1–3] (Figure 1). All these tomographic planes provide information about different areas of the right ventricle and a variety of methods have been developed to divide the right ventricular wall in several segments.

Parasternal area

The parasternal long axis view of the left ventricle demonstrates the left atrium, aortic root, left ventricle and a portion of the right ventricular outflow tract. By rotating the transducer, two additional long axis views may be obtained. The parasternal long axis view of the right ventricle is rotating the transducer counterclockwise and orienting the sector beam through the right atrium, tricuspid valve and inflow tract of the right ventricle. In this view, the anterior and posterior leaflets of the tricuspid valve as well as the anterior and inferior right ventricular walls are imaged. From this position, orienting slightly the transducer to the right, the modified long axis view of the right ventricle is

S. Iliceto et al. (eds.), Ultrasound in Coronary Artery Disease, 151–181.
© 1991 *Kluwer Academic Publishers.*

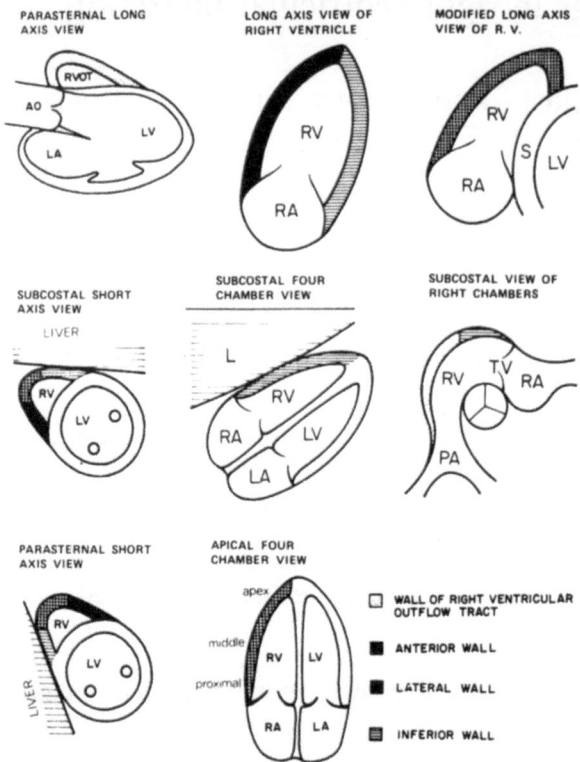

Figure 1. Schematic representation of different echocardiographic views of the right ventricle. AO: aorta; LA: left atrium; LV: left ventricle; RA: right atrium; RV: right ventricle; RVOT: right ventricular outflow tract.

obtained, in which the lateral and septal right ventricular walls, right atrium and the anterior and septal tricuspid leaflets are visualized.

Parasternal short axis view. The right ventricle is visualized in the left upper portion of the image and its wall may be divided into three segments: anterior, lateral and posterior. The interventricular septum and the left ventricle are also identified in this view. The short axis view allows the identification of three segments of the right ventricular wall; however, from the parasternal area it is difficult to obtain good quality images of the right ventricle.

Apical area

The apical four chamber view is optimal to study the movement of the interventricular septum and the right ventricular diameters. The right ventricle is transected in its long axis, from the inflow tract to the apex. The lateral right ventricular wall is longitudinally transected.

Subcostal area

Subcostal four chamber view. Equivalent to the apical four chamber view, identifies both ventricles and atria as well as the interventricular septum. The segment of the right ventricular wall visualized in this plane corresponds to a longitudinal section of the inferior or lateral right ventricular wall.

Subcostal short axis view. This view is similar to the parasternal short axis view with an inverted spatial orientation, and can also be obtained at different levels from apex to base. The right ventricle is better visualized employing this transducer position. In a group of 70 patients with acute myocardial infarction, good quality images of the subcostal transversal plane were obtained in 62 patients while adequate imaging of the parasternal plane could only be achieved in 42 cases [5].

Subcostal right chamber view. Equivalent to the anteroposterior angiocardiographic imaging of the right heart, allows the visualization of the inferior vena cava, right atrium, right ventricular inflow and outflow tracts and pulmonary artery. Other echocardiographic planes may be obtained such as the left ventricular short axis with right ventricular outflow tract and pulmonary valve [4], but the aforementioned views are the most commonly employed for the study of the right ventricle.

Right ventricular function in right ventricular infarction

A – *Right ventricular contraction abnormalities*

A strong correlation between segmental left ventricular contraction abnormalities and myocardial ischemia or necrosis has been demonstrated by several techniques including cineangiography [6], radioisotopic ventriculography [7] and two dimensional echocardiography [8, 9]. For this reason, regional abnormalities of left ventricular wall motion have become a hallmark of both acute and chronic coronary artery disease. Asynergy of the right ventricular free wall has been demonstrated in patients with acute myocardial infarction or ischemia using radionuclide [7, 10, 11] and angiographic [12] techniques, and echocardiography has proved to be a feasible method to determine such abnormalities of right ventricular contraction [4, 5, 13–28].

After acute right ventricular infarction, asynergy may be identified in all segments of the right ventricular wall, including the outflow tract, ventricular apex and the anterior wall, but in general it is specifically located in the posterior right ventricular wall [5, 14–18, 21, 22, 24–27] (Figure 2). Contraction abnormalities in this segment are best identified in simultaneous M mode tracings. Abnormal segmental wall motion without posterior wall involvements is not frequently found [5].

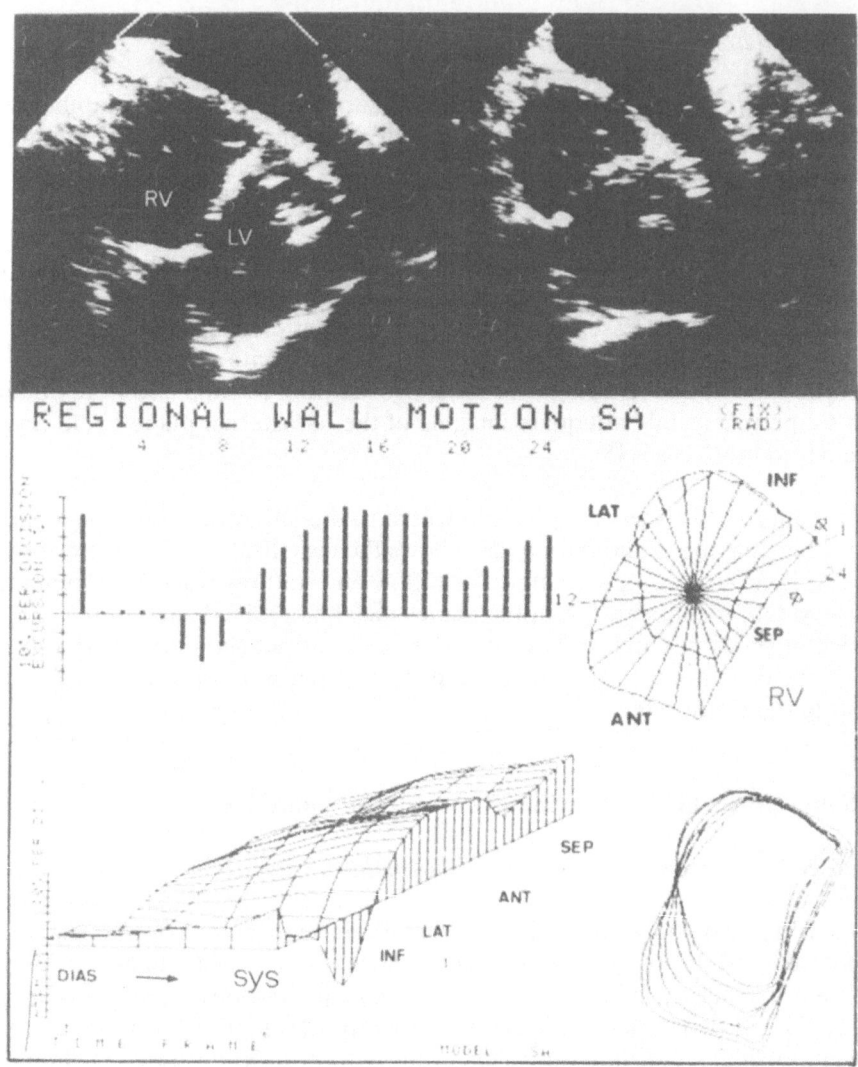

Figure 2. Subcostal short axis view in a patient with acute right ventricular infarction. Akinesia of the inferior right ventricular wall is evident in the computerized bar histogram, were diskinesia of the lateral wall can also be identified. Analysis of segmental right ventricular contraction through systole (inferior panel) demonstrates that the contraction abnormality begins in early systole and is maximal at end diastole. Dias: end diastole; Sys: end systole; Ant, inf, lat: anterior, inferior and lateral wall of the right ventricle (RV); LV: left ventricle; Sep: interventricular septum.

In our experience, over 60% of patients with right ventricular infarction present abnormalities of contraction confined to the posterior segments of the right ventricular wall; in 20% there is also abnormal contraction of the lateral wall and only 10% of the patients present asyneresys both in the anterior, lateral and porterior segments of the right ventricular wall. Moreover, anatomopathologic studies indicate that, in many cases, right ventricular infarction is confined to its posterior wall [29]. For this reason, the best single echocardiographic view to investigate segmental right ventricular function after acute myocardial infarction is the short axis view. To this respect, an adequate image of the right ventricular wall is best obtained from the subcostal position [5, 27]. The greater frequency of wall motion abnormalities in the long axis and four chamber planes reported in other studies in patients with inferior myocardial infarction and right ventricular involvement [13, 14], can be attributed to a more rigid criteria of patient selection, inclusion being restricted to patients with strong clinical evidence of right ventricular infarction. Although infarction involving only the right ventricular anterior wall is relatively frequent after occlusion of the anterior descending coronary artery [29], no prospective echocardiographic studies have been made to investigate the possible segmental contraction abnormalities in such cases.

Segmental right ventricular contraction and right ventricular necrosis
Recent echocardiographic isotopic and anatomic studies [8, 9, 30] have demonstrated that necrotic segments of the left ventricle almost always present motion abnormalities, but the latter far less frequent imply myocardial infarction, and a number of nonnecrotic myocardial segments show segmental wall motion abnormalities. In absence of transmural necrosis, asynergy has been attributed to local ischemia [8, 9], small inlands of infarcted tissue [9] and myocardial dysfunction due to mechanical tethering in zones adjacent to the necrosis [31].

These findings indicate that wall motion abnormalities found in two dimensional echocardiography are very sensitive but not very specific for myocardial infarction. On the basis of these previous studies performed in the left ventricle, one can hypothesize that regional abnormalities of right ventricular contraction are sensitive for detection of right ventricular infarction, but may also be present in patients with right ventricular ischemia without necrosis. Parodi et al. [32] have reported transient right ventricular dilatation and hypokinesis of the right ventricular inferior wall in two patients with coronary spasm involving the middle portion of the right coronary artery, and transient right ventricular dysfunction may be also demonstrated during exercise in patients with significant lesions in the right coronary artery without infarction. Nevertheless, Panidis et al. [19] studied the right ventricular function in coronary artery disease and found that regional wall motion abnormalities of the right ventricular inferior wall were frequent after acute right ventricular infarction, but no ventricular segmental wall motion abnormalities were found in a group of 17 patients with greater than 75% obstruction of the right coronary artery and absence of infarction. This observation shows that segmental right ventricular wall motion is usually normal in patients with significant disease of the right coronary artery unless ischemic damage of the right ventricle due to infarction has occurred.

Correlation between hemodynamics and wall motion abnormalities

Abnormal wall motion and abnormal hemodynamics. In a previous study, we found a strong relation between hemodynamic alterations indicative of ischemic right ventricular dysfunction after acute myocardial infarction and the presence and extent of abnormalities in regional wall motion demonstrated by two dimensional echocardiography [5]. All patients studied by us presented some contraction abnormalities and those patients with the most severe right ventricular dysfunction (right atrial pressure equal to or higher than pulmonary capillary pressure) presented a higher number of right ventricular wall segments with abnormal motion [5]. The same results were reported by Yung-Dae et al. [13], D'Arcy et al. [14], Vanucci et al. [15], and others [15–17, 20, 21, 23]. Furthermore, abnormalities in right ventricular wall motion may still be present after normalization of the hemodynamic variables of ischemic right ventricular dysfunction. That was the case in 8 of 13 patients studied by us, 5 of 13 patients reported by Yung-Dae et al. [13] and several patients studied by De'll Italia et al. [21]. These findings may be of interest when considering ischemic right ventricular involvement in subacute or chronic heart disease [33, 34]. Although further studies are needed to evaluate the long term evolution of right ventricular wall dynamics after acute myocardial infarction. Bellamy et al. [27] studied a group of 22 patients with acute right ventricular infarction. In 18 survivors right ventricular wall motion abnormalities persisted after one week of evolution and during a follow-up during 13–30 weeks resolved completely in 12 of them and all but 2 had at least some improvement in segmental wall motion.

Normal wall motion and abnormal hemodynamics. From another point of view, some patients with mild and transient right ventricular dysfunction may present normal right ventricular wall motion [5]. When one considers that the hemodynamic alterations of ischemic right ventricular dysfunction after acute myocardial infarction are highly specific for right ventricular necrosis [29], this finding may be explained by several mechanisms:

– Although asynergy usually persists for several days or weeks after acute myocardial infarction [5, 20, 33–35], some segmental wall motion abnormalities can be transient, even in the presence of transmural myocardial infarction [7], if some islands of normal tissue are preserved, and may be manifested only under stress conditions such as exercise [33].
– Small defects can be occult to the echocardiographic examination if several transverse planes are not obtained [8]. To this respect, equilibrium gated blood pool studies may be more sensitive than echocardiography [27].
– Simple observations of endocardial excursion from end diastole to end systole may fail to detect important wall motion abnormalities and, in some cases, may miss dyskinetic segments completely [36, 37]. Two dimensional echocardiographic studies have shown that maximal myocardial expansion

within ischemic segments may occur early in the systolic contraction period rather than at end systole [37, 38]. Figure 3 illustrates one of such cases in which a clear dyskinetic movement can be only appreciated during mid systole. Also, hypokinesis and small abnormalities in ventricular motion are very difficult to evaluate after right ventricular infarction mainly because of the technical difficulties and the lack of definition of normal contracting patterns. Further methodologic refinement and the application of computer aided technology will allow a more precise evaluation and quantification of regional wall motion and endocardial thickening, the lat-

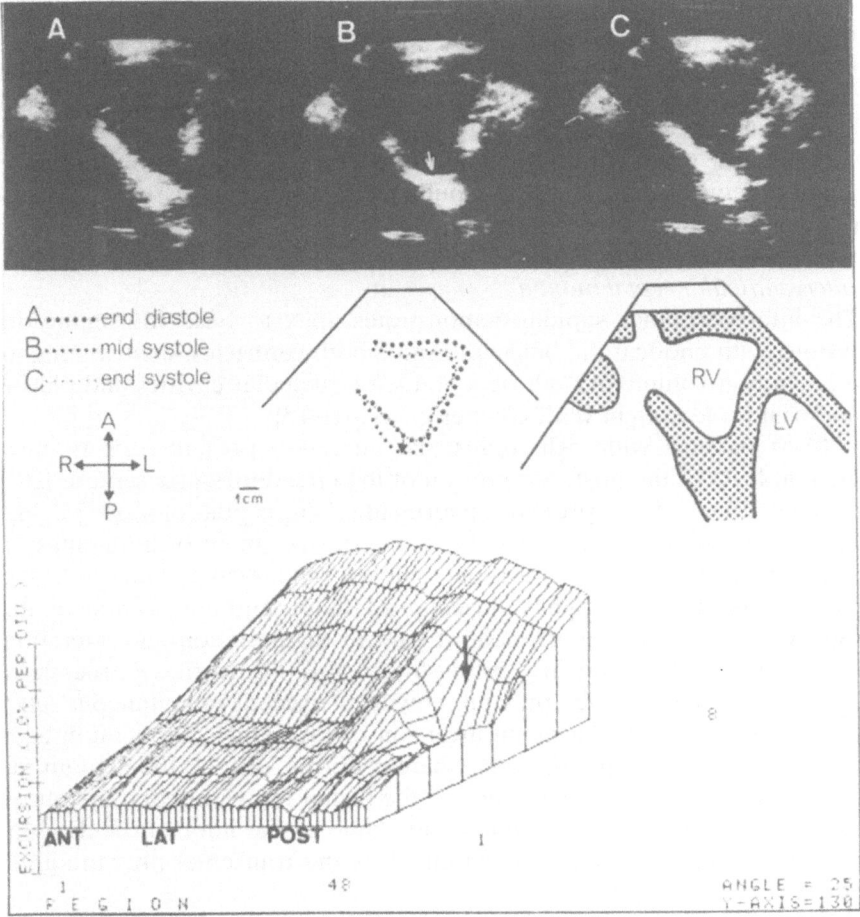

Figure 3. Parasternal short axis view in a patient with acute right ventricular infarction. Analysis of right ventricular silhouettes at end diastole (A) and end systole (C) shows normal contraction of the right ventricular wall. However, asyneresys of the posterior right wall (arrow) is evident when several silhouettes are imaged through systole. Ant, Inf. Post: anterior, inferior and posterior segments of the right ventricular wall. LV: left ventricle; RV: right ventricle.

ter being a sensitive and specific variable of ventricular function in acute myocardial infarction [9].
- There is always the possibility that the transient and borderline hemodynamic changes right ventricular function after acute myocardial infarction may be due to ischemia rather than necrosis [32, 34].

Abnormal wall motion and normal hemodynamics. Also interesting is the observation that some patients without right ventricular disfunction during the acute phase of myocardial infarction may present abnormal right ventricular wall motion [5, 23]. It can be the result of transient ischemia rather than infarction [35–38], but those patients with right ventricular asynergy without any hemodynamic alterations at all presented electrocardiographic criteria of right ventricular necrosis (ST segment elevation in leads V_{3R} and V_{4R}), a finding highly indicative of acute right ventricular infarction [39, 40]. This finding strongly suggests that wall motion abnormalities can be more sensitive than hemodynamics in detecting acute right ventricular infarction. This may be specially true when left ventricular dysfunction is impaired, preventing a close relation between right atrial and pulmonary capillary pressure suggestive of right ventricular involvement [5, 29].

Interventricular septal motion
The interventricular septum demonstrates apex to base shortening during systole, with endocardial bulging towards both ventricles, contributing to the reduction in volume of both right and left ventricular cavities and playing an important role in right ventricular ejection [41–43].
Most patients with right ventricular infarction present necrotic involvement at least of the posterior portion of the interventricular septum [29] and probably near 50% present abnormalities of septal motion [5, 44, 46]. Paradoxical septal motion, defined as the displacement of both sides of the interventricular septum towards the right ventricular cavity during systole, is a common finding after right ventricular infarction and has been attributed to right ventricular volume overload, tricuspid regurgitation and alterations in right ventricular compliance [5, 12–44, 26, 44–47]. In these circumstances, right ventricular diastolic pressure equals or exceeds simultaneous left ventricular pressure, producing an inversion of the ventricular septum towards the left ventricle during diastole whereas during systole, the septum moves towards the right ventricle because of the higher left ventricular systolic pressure. In other words, the position and shape of the interventricular septum through the cardiac cycle is determined by the transeptal pressure gradient [46, 48].
The role of the interventricular septum abnormalities in right and left ventricular function remains conjectural. The discrepancy between the lack of conspicuous deterioration of right ventricular function after destruction of the right ventricular free wall in some experimental studies and the more profound hemodynamic deterioration in the typical clinical syndrome of right

ventricular infarction has been attributed to ischemic abnormalities of the interventricular septum, only present in the clinical setting. In the most severe forms of dysfunction, there is a striking paradoxical septal motion and change in shape becoming convex towards the left ventricle in diastole and towards the right ventricle in systole [5, 45, 46]. Probably, in these circumstances the septal behaviour distorts the left ventricular geometry impairing the left ventricular function [45] rather than right ventricular dynamics. Nevertheless, in experimental studies right ventricular ischemia causes a leftward shift of the interventricular septum in end diastole and an alteration of the left ventricular end diastolic pressure volume relationship is enhanced by the intact pericardium, but without changing left ventricular myocardial performance [49]. Furthermore, this abnormal septal movement perhaps could even be considered as a compensatory mechanism of severe free wall motion abnormalities and right ventricular volume overload. The same pattern of contraction and geometry distortion has been described in pulmonary hypertension and right ventricular volume overload [50–52].

Quantitative assessment of segmental right ventricular wall contraction
The precise identification of regional contraction abnormalities depends on the use of a method which could separate normal from abnormal wall motion more reliably than the subjective interpretation of a qualitative assessment. Attempts to define the normal contractile patterns of the right ventricle have been made in angiographic and isotopic studies [7], but there is an almost complete lack of information regarding the normal contraction of the right ventricle imaged by two dimensional echocardiography [53].

Several problems have to be faced when trying to define the normal contracting pattern of the right ventricle. Its particular shape, the cardiac movement of rotation and translation of the heart through the cardiac cycle, the possible existence of different directions of contraction in different segments and the election of the most representative and reproducible echocardiographic plane are among the most obvious if not the most significant problems to approach before any attempt to study the normal segmental right ventricular contraction.

Kaul et al. [34, 53], using simple quantitative methods, measured the area between the mid right ventricular diameter and the lateral right ventricular wall in the apical four chamber view. The *systolic change in area* was considered to represent right ventricular free wall motion, and its value in ten normal individuals was calculated as $40 \pm 3\%$. Besides, the *percentual shortening of the right ventricular end diastolic mid chordae length* was also calculated resulting in a normal value limit of 22% in the apical four chamber plane. These simple methods were useful to demonstrate abnormalities of contraction in patients with myocardial infarction, but can only be considered as an initial approach to a complex problem.

The same authors [53] found a close correlation between right ventricular ejection fraction measured by radionuclide angiography and the *tricuspid annular plane systolic excursion* calculated from two dimensional echocardio-graphic images in the apical four chamber view. In normal subjects, the values of this parameter were always above 15 mm while in patients with right ven-tricular infarction and reduced right ventricular ejection fraction (< 35%) was always inferior to 12 mm, and when there was a marked depression of right ventricular ejection fraction (< 25%) the tricuspid annular plane systolic excursion was less than 8 mm. This parameter may be useful in a clinical setting, not only for its simplicity but also because its good correlation with right ventricular ejection fraction probably explained by the fact that in the right ventricle the apex to base shortening is more pronounced than the trans-versal shortening [53, 54].

Also as an initial approach to the study of normal segmental right ventricu-lar contraction we made a study in 20 normal individuals [55]. Images from the apical four chamber and subcostal short axis views were selected for com-puterized measurements of segment shortening (Figures 4, 5).

In correcting for changes in ventricular position due to heart movements, several forms of image superimposition at end systole and end diastole were made. In the four chamber plane the following were considered (Figures 4, 6):

– superimposition of both long axis of the ventricular silhouette and its mid points;
– superimposition of the center of gravity and
– simple superimposition without any attempt to correct passive movements.

In the short axis view two methods were analized (Figures 5, 7): superimposi-tion of centers of gravity, and simple superimposition without any correction.

In each case, a system of radial coordinates dividing the silhouette in 12 segments was defined and the change in segment areas was calculated. In the subcostal short axis view the inferior right ventricular wall was defined by 2 areas, the lateral wall by 3 and the interventricular septum was divided in 2 segments, anterior and posterior, each including 2 areas (Figure 4). In the

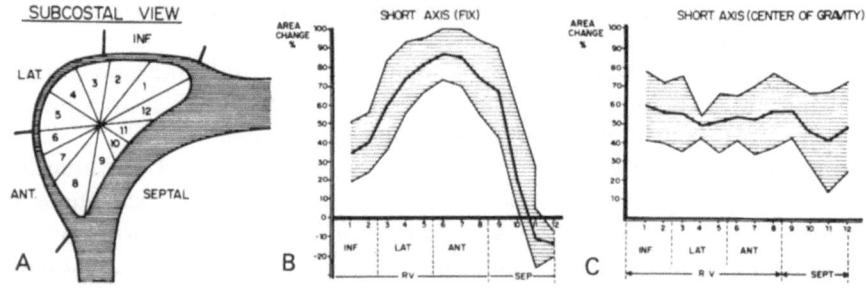

Figure 4. Normal segmental right ventricular wall contraction in the subcostal short axis view. Values obtained in 20 normal volunteers. A: areas studied. B: percentual area change (× ± 1.96s), measured after simple superposition of end diastolic and end systolic images. C: percentual area change after superimposition of the centers of gravity of the end diastolic and end systolic images.

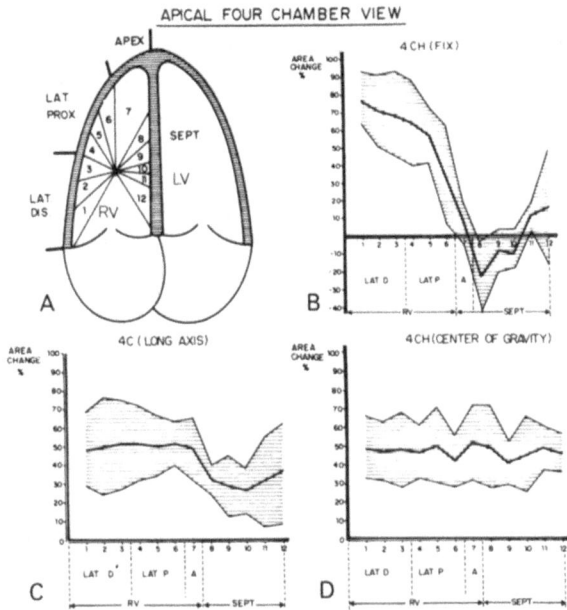

Figure 5. Normal segmental right ventricular wall contraction studied in the apical four chamber view. Values obtained in 20 normal volunteers. A: areas studied, B, C and D: percentual area change (×±1.96s) observed employing three different methods of superimposition of end diastolic and end systolic right ventricular silhouettes. B: simple superimposition; C: superimposition of long axis and D: superimposition of centers of gravity.

apical four chamber view, the proximal segment of the lateral wall included 3 areas, the distal segmento of the lateral wall 3, the right ventricular apex 1 and the septum included 5 areas (Figure 5).

The results are presented as histograms in Figures 4 and 5 which show the percentual change in area for each segment. Figure 8 shows the normal pattern of contraction in the subcostal short axis view and Figures 2 and 9 illustrate different abnormalities of contraction.

Data corresponding to measurements in the short axis view, once correction for movements of the heart was made, show that the right ventricle presents a homogeneous wall contraction of approximately 50% through systole. Differences observed between the corrected and uncorrected methods are probably secondary to the movements of the heart itself. This movement is basically a temporary rotation shift of the ventricular wall towards the inferior wall. This means that there is a swinging movement between the anterior and posterior portions of the interventricular septum. This theory is based in the fact that in the uncorrected study the anterior septum seems to contract while the posterior septum presents a pseudodyskinetic movement (Figure 4). When the correction techniques are applied, it becomes clear that the interventricular septum contributes to right ventricular emptying. The active participation of the septum to right ventricular contrac-

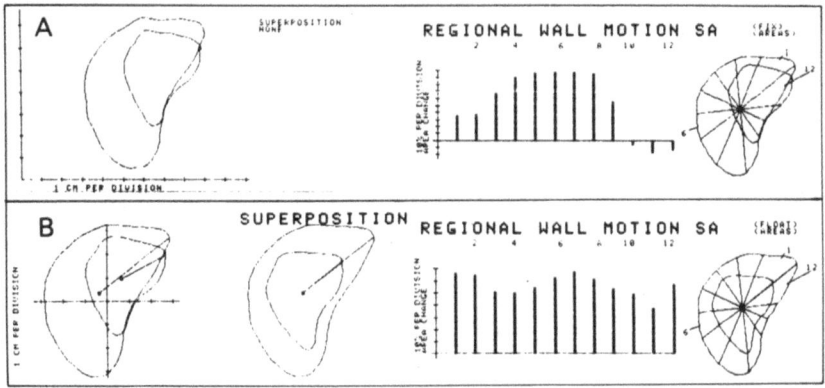

Figure 6. Normal segmental right ventricular wall contraction measured in the subcostal short axis view. A: simple superimposition of end systolic and end diastolic silhouettes. B: superimposition of centers of gravity.

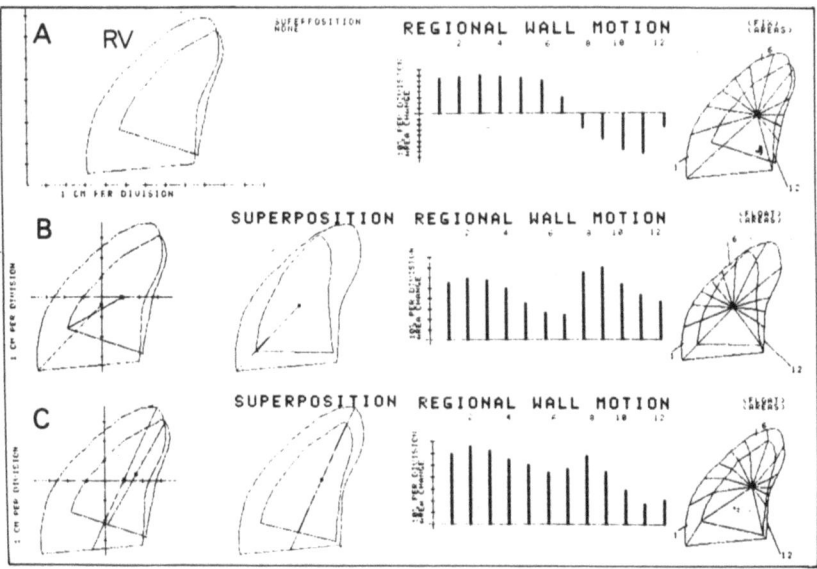

Figure 7. Normal segmental right ventricular wall contraction measured in the apical four chamber view. A: simple superimposition of end systolic and end diastolic silhouettes. B: superimposition of centers of gravity. C: superimposition of long axis.

tion is confirmed when septal shortening is studied in its whole length, as in the apical four chamber plane, with the correction techniques being applied. With the uncorrected method the septum appears to rotate around segments 10 and 11. Thus, segments 8, 9 and 10 shift towards the left ventricular cavity while segments 11 and 12 shift towards the right ventricular cavity. When correction techniques are employed it is clear that the interventricular septum presents an uniform shortening towards the right ventricular cavity. These

results are in accordance with those of angiographic [41] and isotopic [7] studies, and demonstrate the active contribution of the interventricular septal contraction to right ventricular emptying.

B – *Right ventricular dilatation*

Dilatation of the thin walled right ventricle occurs early in many pathologic conditions involving the right heart, including acute and old right ventricular infarction [13–15, 20, 25, 34, 44, 46, 56].

Gomes et al. [56 bis] found an increased right ventricular diastolic dimension in 6 of 9 patients with inferior myocardial infarction, and attributed this

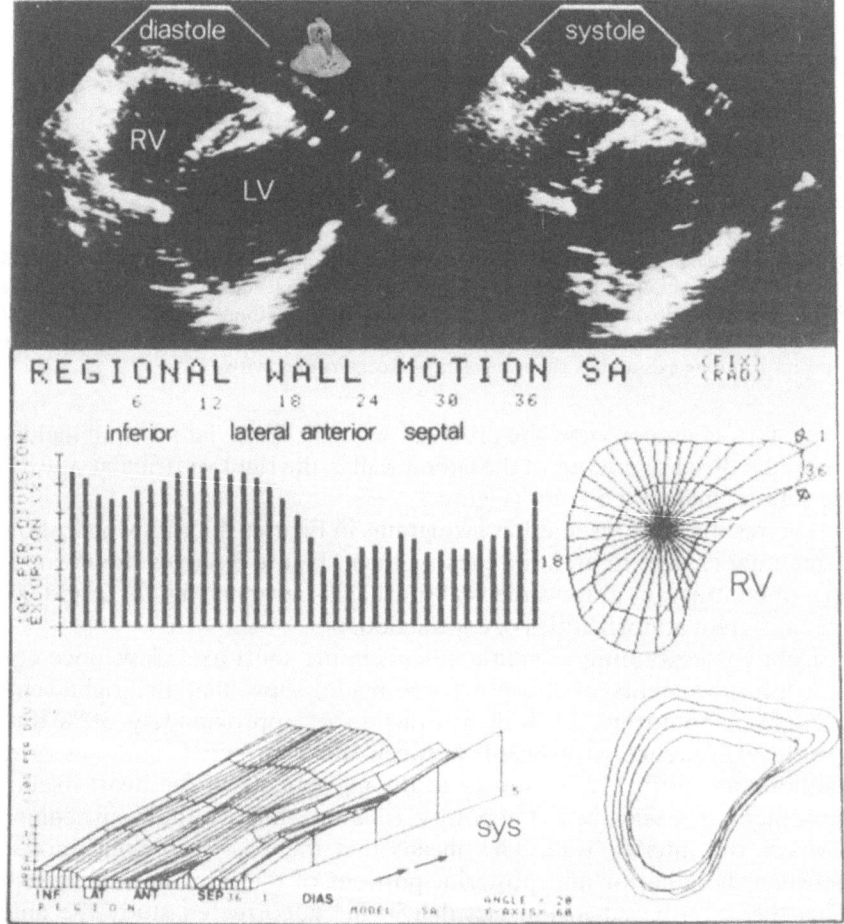

Figure 8. Subcostal short axis view. Normal pattern of contraction (superimposition of centers of gravity. All segments of the right ventricular wall, including the interventricular septum, contribute to shortening of the right ventricular dimensions. Dias: end diastole; LV: left ventricle; RV: right ventricle; Sys: end systole.

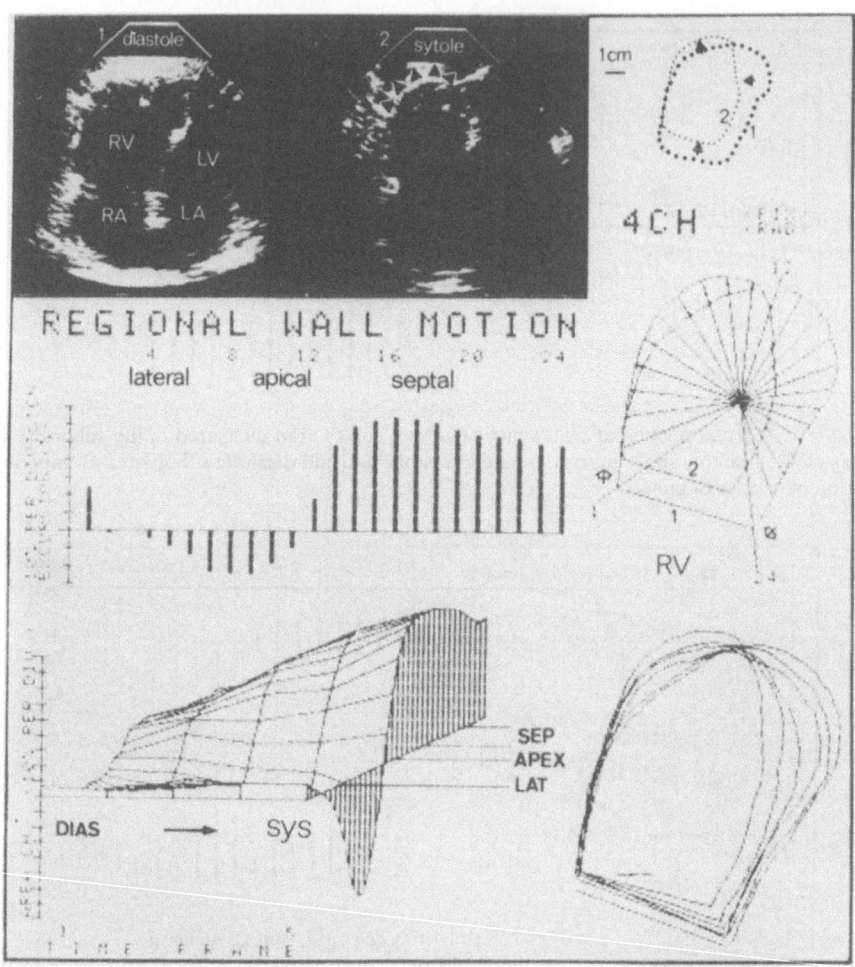

Figure 9. Apical four chamber view in a patient with acute right ventricular infarction. Analysis of segmental right ventricular contraction demonstrates the diskinesia of the lateral wall and apex. Dias: end diastole. Sys: end systole. Sep: septal. Rv: Right ventricle.

finding to right ventricular infarction. Sharphe et al. [56] demonstrated a high incidence of right ventricular dilatation (82%) in those patients with anomalous uptake of technetium pirophosphate in the right ventricular free wall. We were able to demonstrate [46] that a right ventricular diastolic dimension greater than 18 mm/m^2 is highly indicative of ischemic right ventricular disfunction provided that other causes of right ventricular dilatation such as pulmonary or valvular heart disease are excluded. The same is true for a RVDD/LVDD ratio greater than 0.63. Similar findings have been reported by Sharpe [56]. Unfortunately the sensitivity of this findings is low as nearly half of the patients with isquemic right ventricular infarction present a normal ventricular diastolic dimension.

The calculation of right ventricular volume is conceptually more difficult than that of the left ventricle. Attempts to determine right ventricular volume by echocardiography are scarce and, to date, limited practical results have been obtained with single and biplane techniques [57–63]. With the use of one area and one length from each of two intersecting echocardiographic views the right ventricular volume can be accurately assessed [57]. Furthermore, a three dimensional reconstruction of the right ventricle may ultimately be possible [64, 65], but it will require the imaging of multiple planes and complex calculations. Besides, one of the main technical problems to study the echocardiographic characteristics of the right ventricular cavity, the definition of the endocardial surfaces, may be partially solved employing digital substraction processing of contrast echocardiograms [66].

Few two dimensional echocardiographic studies offer measurements of the right ventricular cavity as ventricular diameters or silhouette areas [20, 26]. The upper normal limit of the maximal short axis in the apical four chamber view was calculated as 30 to 45 mm [4, 48]. The right ventricular diastolic area in a group of normal individuals was calculated as 10 cm^2 in the apical four chamber view and 6 cm^2 in the subcostal four chamber view [53]. Jugdutt et al. [20] calculated the right ventricular volume and ejection fraction in 17 patients with right ventricular infarction using a complex formula and found that these parameters were abnormal in those patients who died as the consequence of right ventricular dysfunction, but their results and methods for estimating right ventricular volume have to be validated in future studies.

C – *Indirect echocardiographic findings of right ventricular disfunction*

There are a number of indirect findings that may support the non invasive diagnosis of right ventricular dysfunction:

Analysis of tricuspid valve movements
The study of the echocardiographic characteristics of tricuspid valve motion could provide a noninvasive tool for assessing right ventricular function. Although not pathonomonic of ischemic right ventricular disfunction a B plateau can be found in those patients with right ventricular failure and right atrial pressure above 10 mmhg [68]. The A wave may be increased reflecting a powerful atrial contraction, or may be absent in cases of atrial infarction or supraventricular arrhythmias. Other parameters such as AC or PR-AC intervals are of little value as they do not correlate well with right atrial or right ventricular diastolic pressure [68].

Analysis of pulmonary valve motion
The A wave of the pulmonic valve may be increased in patients with right ventricular infarction [69]. This finding is more evident during inspiration and reflects the importance of right atrial contraction in some of these patients.

Opening of the pulmonary valve before atrial contraction has been report-

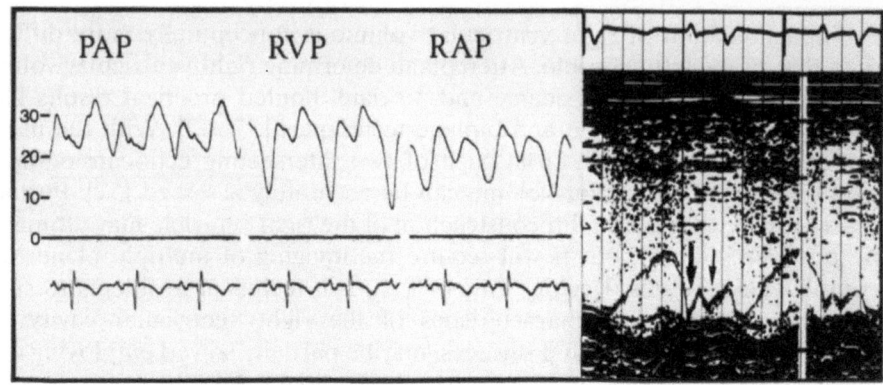

Figure 10. Premature pulmonic valve opening before atrial contraction in a patient with right ventricular infarction (first arrow). A second opening movement follows atrial contraction (second arrow), and again the valve reaches the full opening position during ventricular contraction (second arrow). Right atrial (RAP) and right ventricular (RVP) pressures are higher than pulmonary artery pressure (PAP) during diastole and a prominent A wave can be observed in both RAP and RVP. In the PAP a diastolic wave can be appreciated.

ed in several diseases including right ventricular infarction [7] (Figure 10) and in every case a common hemodynamic finding can be observed: A significant elevation of right ventricular diastolic pressure which equals or exceeds simultaneous pulmonary artery pressure during diastole. This hemodynamic alteration can be the consequence of right ventricular volume overload, decreased right ventricular compliance or both [70, 71]. In patients with isquemic right ventricular disfunction, premature pulmonic valve opening can be observed continuously or only during inspiration, depending on the presence of a continuous or intermittent right ventricular diastolic pressure above simultaneous pulmonary artery pressure.

The premature pulmonic valve opening reflects a profound alteration in phasic right ventricular flow, and supports the validity of one of Cohn's theories about the physiopathology of right ventricular infarction; pulmonary flow is passively transmitted from right to left atrium through a low resistance pulmonary vascular bed due to a mere pressure gradient between both chambers [71 bis].

Analysis of inferior vena cava
Mintz et al. [31] demonstrated a good correlation between different parameters of inferior vena cava dimensions or motion and right ventricular function. There is some degree of correlation between end-diastolic inferior vena cava dimension and right atrial pressure. Although the correlation is not so close as to permit an exact quantification of right heart pressures, an inferior vena cava dimension greater than 10 mm/mm^2 is indicative of an increased right atrial pressure above 10 mmHg. However, some patients with increased right atrial pressure may show a normal vena cava dimension.

An A wave superior to 125% of the end diastolic vena cava dimension is indicative of an increased right ventricular diastolic pressure above 10 mmHg in 100% of patients, but its sensitivity is low, and sometimes the A wave can not be properly identified.

Finally, in normal conditions the inferior vena cava dimension decreases by more than 50% during inspiration while in patients with right ventricular failure there is not inspiratory decreased and even an increase in inferior vena cava dimension can be observed. An important finding is that the increase in flow from inferior vena cava is preserved in cardiac tamponade. This feature may be helpful to differentiate isquemic right ventricular disfunction from cardiac tamponde secundary to cardiac rupture [132].

Abnormal shape of the interatrial septum
Inversion of the normal convexity of the interatrial septum can be demonstrated in patients with right ventricular disfunction. This abnormal shape is caused by an increased of right atrial pressure above pulmonary capillary values. In a previous echocardiographic study in patients with acute myocardial infarction [133] inverted interauricular septum had been identified only when right atrial pressure was equal to or higher than pulmonary capillary pressure, a condition almost exclusive of right ventricular infarction or cardiac tamponade after acute myocardial infarction (Figure 11).

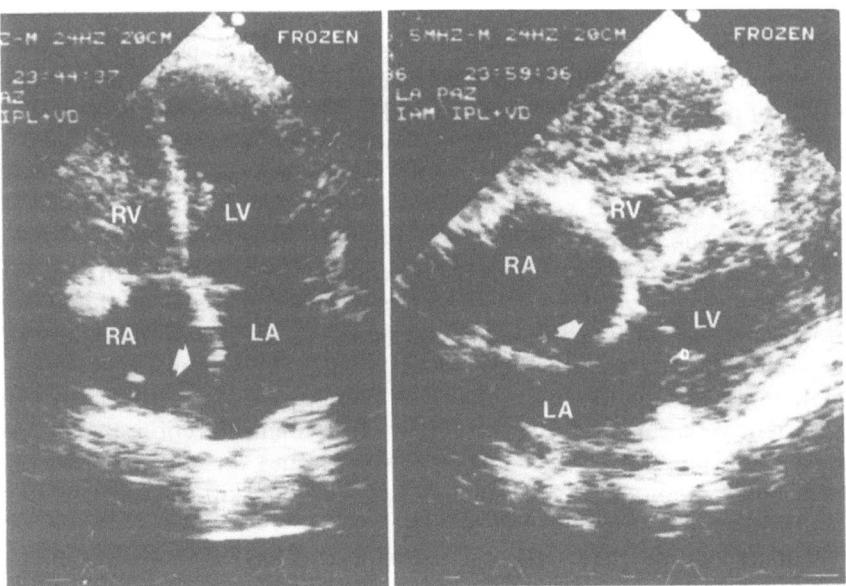

Figure 11. Apical and subcostal four chamber view in a patient with right ventricular infarctium. We can detected and abnormal inversion of the normal convexity of the interatrial septum (arrows). RA: right atrium. LA: left atrium. LV: left ventricle. RV: right ventricle.

Complications of right ventricular infarction

Right ventricular aneurysms

Ventricular aneurysms may be defined as localized protusions of a ventricular wall. Cabin and Roberts [67] classified the ventricular aneurysms in three different types: An *anatomic aneurysm* is a localized protusion of the ventricular wall both during ventricular systole and diastole, whereas a *functional aneurysm* is a protusion of a segment of the ventricular wall only evident during systole. This distinction is useful because the wall of a functional aneurysm may consist of ischemic, and potentially reversible, tissue whereas the wall of an anatomic aneurysm consist of either necrotic or fibrous tissue or both and neither is reversible. An anatomic aneurysm may be either true of false. A *true anatomic aneurysm* has a mouth that is as wide than the maximal diameter of the aneurysm; its wall was formely the wall of the ventricle. A *false anatomic aneurysm* develops following rupture of a recent infarcted segment of the myocardial wall forming a localized hemopericardium confined by adjacent parietal pericardium. It has a mounth that usually is considerably smaller than the maximal diameter of the aneurysm and it was the rupture site at the time of the acute myocardial infarction; its wall is composed of parietal pericardium and never contains residual myocardial fibers.

From a practical point of view, the distinction of these three types of aneurysms is very important. A functional aneurysm is a dyskinetic segment of the ventricular wall, and is potentially reversible. The akinetic or dyskinetic movement of a true anatomic aneurysm is never reversible and the risk of thrombus formation in its cavity is high. The false aneurysm represents an uncommon survival after rupture of the ventricular free wall, always containing thrombotic material in its cavity, and had a marked tendency for rupture.

Because of the ability to image tomographically through the apex of the heart from various transducer positions, two dimensional echocardiography is well suited for the recognition of the different types of left ventricular aneurysms, the identification of its contents and the assessment of its movements as well as the contraction of the remaining ventricular wall.

Although left ventricular aneurysm is considered as one of the most common complications of myocardial infarction, aneurysms of the right ventricular wall have seldom been described [14, 72]. Functional right ventricular aneurysms, however, may be found in a high percentage (over 20% in our experience) of patients with acute right ventricular infarction; there is a good correlation between the functional aneurysm and the severe forms of right ventricular dysfunction and, in most cases, the dyskinetic movement disappears after few days or weeks [27].

The anatomic right ventricular aneurysms are far less common than in the left ventricle. In a series of 50 consecutive patients surviving an episode of right ventricular infarction we could only find five with a true right ventricular aneurysm [73] (Figure 12). The segments involved included always the right

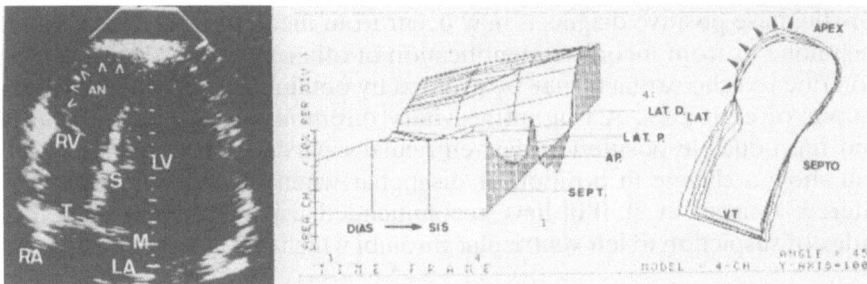

Figure 12. Right ventricular aneurysm (AN) in a patient with acute right ventricular infarction. Protrusion of the right ventricular apex (RV) and distal portion of the right ventricular wall are present through the cardiac cycle (arrows). LA: left atrium; LV: left ventricle; RA: right atrium; S: interventricular septum; T: tricuspid valve.

ventricular apex and in two cases a thrombus was identified inside its cavity. It is interestig to observe that all cases presented a persistent ST segment elevation in lead V_{4R} during several days or weeks of follow up after the infarct, which is an unusual electrocardiographic abnormality after a right ventricular infarction; however, the specificity of this electrocardiographic alteration during the first days of the infarct is low [73].

The formation of a false aneurysm after rupture of the right ventricular free wall is a very unusual complication but some cases have been described after trauma [74] and after acute right ventricular infarction [75, 76]. Although the possibilities of such complication should be the same as after rupture of the left ventricular free wall, rupture of the right ventricular wall after infarction is less common [77, 78]. Nevertheless, the diagnosis is of practical interest as surgery is the treatment of choice.

Right ventricular thrombi

Intraventricular thrombi formation is a common postmortem finding both after left and right ventricular infarction [67]. However, before the availability of two dimensional echocardiography, the presence of thrombi became clinically apparent only if an embolic event occurred or if detection was made by contrast ventriculography. Two dimensional echocardiography is a sensitive method for identifying intraventricular thrombi which are imaged as an occupying mass inside the ventricular cavity with a density usually greater than that of the adjacent myocardium [79–81]. Intraventricular thrombi are almost always located at the apex and the segment of the ventricular wall adjacent to the thrombus always presents contraction abnormalities, mainly akinesia or dyskinesia. The surface of the thrombus may be smooth or irregular, protruding inside the ventricular cavity. Sometimes a pediculum may be identified with free motion of the thrombus in the ventricular cavity during the cardiac cycle. Variations may be noted in serial echocardiographic examinations. Although the echocardiographic features of a thrombus may be characteristic, false positive diagnosis may occur from incomplete or faulty imaging technique or from incorrect identification of other structures. Misinterpretation due to echo artifacts may be avoided by obtaining multiple sector orientations of each area. A true intracavitary thrombus should have a constant and reproducible position in the ventricular cavity whereas spurious echoes will show a change in position or disappear when the sector orientation is altered. Asinger et al. [80] have recommended using a grading scale as an index of suspiction to left ventricular thrombi which can also be applied to the

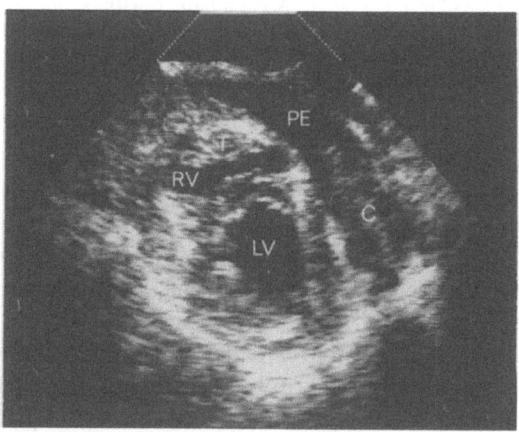

Figure 13. Subcostal short axis view from a patient with right ventricular infarction, right ventricular thrombus (T) and free right ventricular wall rupture. Observe the presence of a large pericardial effusion (PE) with the pericardial cavity partially occupied by a high density echogenic mass. C: clot.

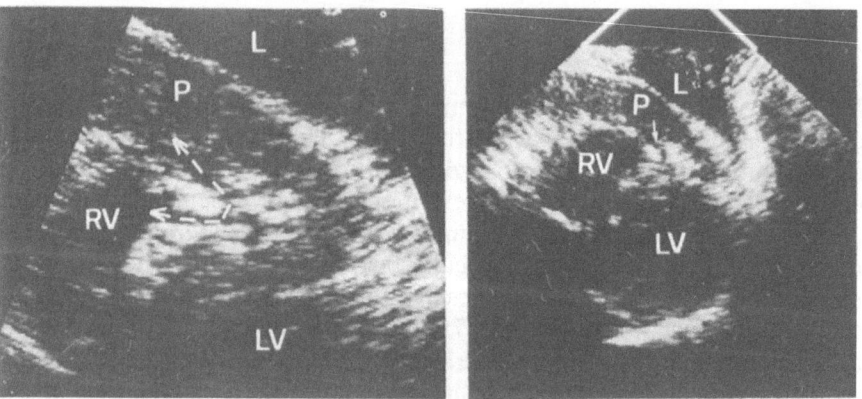

Figure 14. Subcostal short axis view from a patient with rupture of the posterior right ventricular wall adjacent to the interventricular septum (findings at surgery). A defect of echoes, persistent through the echocardiographic study, was identified at the level where the ventricular rupture was identified at surgery (arrows). Observe also the large pericardial effusion (P) with the pericardial cavity partially filled with high density echoes. L: liver; LV: left ventricle; RV: right ventricle.

right ventricle. Cardiac structures that may be mistaken as thrombi include papillary muscles, chordal structures and, specially important in the right ventricle, muscle trabeculae.

Right ventricular thrombosis is considered as a frequent complication of right ventricular infarction but few echocardiographic descriptions have been made [17, 20, 82–84]. Its identification may have therapeutical amplications as many of these patients subsequently develop pulmonary embolism. Jugdutt et al. [20], found right ventricular thrombi in 7 of 12 patients with acute right ventricular infarction studied by two dimensional echocardiography and 5 of them developed pulmonary embolism. False positive diagnosis are more easily made than in the left ventricle due to the characteristic trabeculation of the right ventricular wall, and only class III and IV of Asinger classification should be considered as true positives (Figure 13). Accordingly, we could only found 6 cases in a series of 50 patients with acute right ventricular infarction studied by two dimensional echocardiography.

Right ventricular free wall rupture

Free wall ventricular rupture is one of the most frequent lethal complication of acute myocardial infarction. It is usually followed by sudden death but a significant number of patients survive for hours or even days allowing the relieve of cardiac tamponade and the surgical correction of the myocardial tear [78, 85–89]. Rupture of the right ventricular free wall is observed far less frequently than in the left ventricle but cases surviving surgical correction have been described [75, 77, 78, 87, 90, 91].

The direct diagnosis of free wall ventricular rupture by identification of the myocardial tear (Figure 14) is extremely difficult because, in those cases surviving the acute episode of rupture, the orifice through the myocardium is anfractuous and is occupied by coagulated blood and thrombi. In all patients with subacute ventricular rupture the pericardial cavity is filled with blood in different stages of coagulation. Experimental studies have demonstrated the echogenicity of fluid as well as coagulated blood in the pericardial cavity [92], and patients with hemopericardium secondary to subacute ventricular rupture present high density echoes partially or completely filling the distended pericardial cavity [77, 78, 88, 93] (Figure 13–14). These findings, as well as the presence of hemodynamic signs of cardiac tamponade undoubtedly are useful for the diagnosis of subacute cardiac rupture, and their accuracy in patients with acute myocardial infarction has been determined [76].

Interventricular septal rupture

Interventricular septal rupture is a relatively common complication of biventricular infarction [94, 95]. Although its diagnosis may be made in presence of simple hemodynamic data [96], two dimensional echocardiography allows the direct identification of the myocardial tear [97–99] (Figure 15) and may also

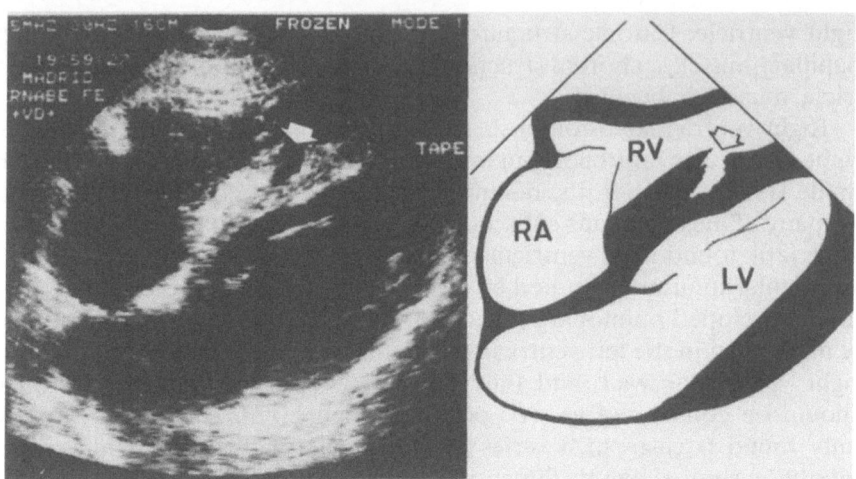

Figure 15. Subcostal four chamber view from a patient with a large biventricular infarction. Rupture of the interventricular septum, (angiographic and postmortem findings), imaged as a line free of echoes (arrows). LV: left ventricle; RA: right atrium; RV: right ventricle.

provide information about other structures and ventricular function which may conditionate a surgical indication as well as prognosis.

The identification of the myocardial tear is possible due to the existence of a left to right shunt and, obviously, the ventricular septal defect is occupied by flowing, nonechogenic blood. The ventricular septal defect may be imaged as an irregular line of echoes or as an ample space free of echoes along the interventricular septum. Nevertheless, the defect cannot be directly identified in all cases. Smyllie [100] imaged the site and location of ventricular septal defect with two dimensional echocardiography in only 14/38 patients with postinfarction ventricular septal defect. However, in other studies the sensitivity of 2D echocardiography to identify the myocardial tear within the interventricular septum was higher [101]. Injection of contrast in a peripheral vein may demonstrate the existence of a small right to left shunt but in most cases, and specially when the ventricular septal defect is not directly visualized, the diagnosis is supported by the wash out of the contrast in the right ventricle produced by the left to right shunt [97].

Many investigators reported the usefulness of pulsed Doppler echocardiography in the diagnosis of ventricular septal rupture [101–104]. The shunt is detected by the presence of the turbulence generated within the ventricular septum and in the right ventricular cavity. This technique has shown a greater sensitivity than two dimensional echocardiography alone to diagnose ventricular septal rupture [102]. Color coded flow mapping shows significant advantages over the standard Doppler for the location of the defect as well as the width and direction of the jet [100] (Figure 16).

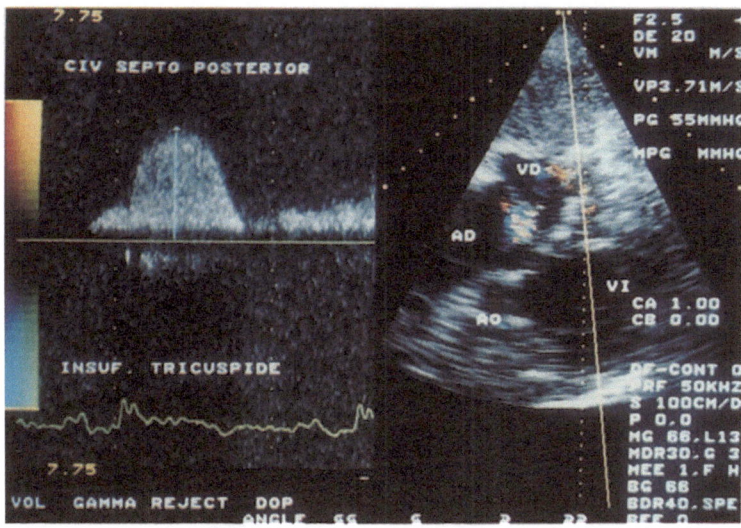

Figure 16. Subcostal four chamber view. Color coded flow mapping in a case with rupture of the interventricular septum. We can detected a jet across the interventricular posterior area. The simultaneous study with continuous wave Doppler allow identified the gradient between both cavities (55 mmhg). There was also a tricuspid regurgitation (arrows).

Ischemic tricuspid valve dysfunction

Tricuspid regurgitation is a common complication after right ventricular infarction [14, 18, 20, 105–107]. In such cases, tricuspid insufficiency may be produced by several mechanisms including tricuspid valve annular dilatation secondary to right ventricular dysfunction, ischemic dysfunction of the tricuspid papillary muscles, asyneresys of the right ventricular wall and finally, rupture of one or several papillary muscles. Although all the aforementioned causes may play an important role in the genesis of tricuspid regurgitation after acute right ventricular infarction, probably the most common cause of tricuspid incompetence is the dilatation of the tricuspid valve anulus secondary to right ventricular dysfunction, as tricuspid regurgitation is always accompanied by right ventricular dilatation and also because the tricuspid valve is anatomically more prone to functional incompetence than the mitral valve [108–109]. Rupture of a papillare muscle has been described in several cases of right ventricular infarction [20, 95, 110–114], and although it may be considered as a rarity, in spite that many cases remain undiagnosed, its identification may be of practical importance.

The combination of echocardiographic image, standard Doppler and color coded flow mapping (Figure 17) is the most reliable method for detecting the presence of tricuspid regurgitation and define its severity [115–124], also it is well known that the continuous wave Doppler can be used to determine right ventricular systolic pressure in patients with tricuspid regurgitation [125–129].

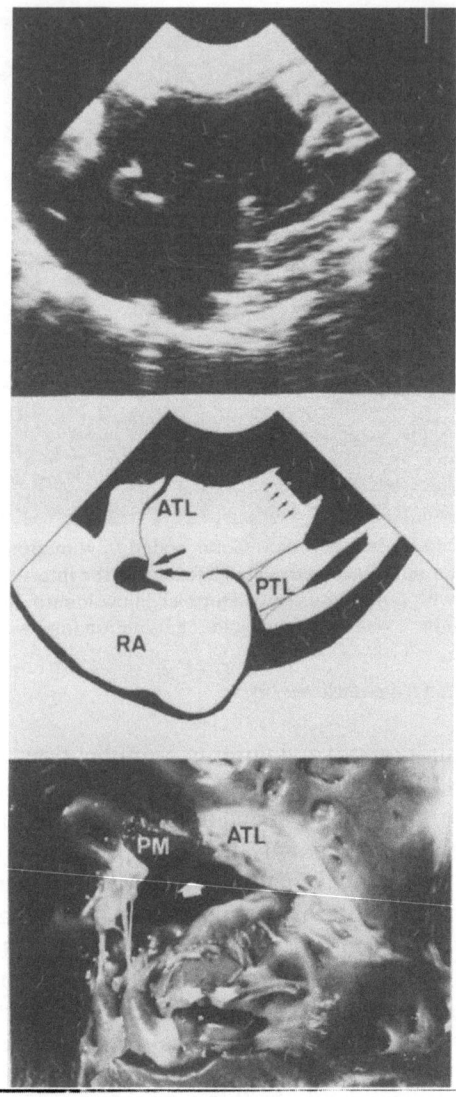

Figure 17. Long axis view of the right ventricle in a dog with surgical section of the anterior tricuspid papillary muscle (PM). Observe the sharp cut in the papillary muscle (small arrow) and the echo free image of the tip of the papillary muscle attached to the anterior tricuspid leaflet (ATL). PTL: posterior tricuspid leaflet. RA: right atrium.

We have found that 66% of patients with acute right ventricular disfunction had tricuspid regurgitation; 55% corresponding to mild and 45% moderate to severe. In cases of rupture of a papillary muscle there are some especific findings that could support this diagnostic according to studies in dogs [130]: absent tip of a papillary muscle, tricuspid valve flail and detection of a movile mass between both right cavities (Figure 17).

References

1. Henry WL, De Maria An, Gramiak R, King DL, Kisslo JA, Popp RL (1980) Report of the American Society of Echocardiography Committee on nomenclature and standards in two dimensional echocardiography. *Circulation* 62: 212–217.
2. Yuste P, García-Fernandez MA (1982) PLanos de estudio, en: *Atlas de ecocardiografia bidimensional y Doppler*, pp 27–61. Ediciones Norma, Madrid.
3. García-Fernandez MA (1983) Estudio de la patología cardiaca mediante ecocardiografia bidimensional, en: *Avances en cardiología*, pp 393–421. Sociedad Española de Cardiología, Ed. Científico Médica, Barcelona.
4. Isner JN (1988) Right ventricular myocardial infarction, in: *The Right Ventricle*, pp 89–129. Boston: Kluwer Academic Publishers.
5. López-Sendón J, García-Fernandez MA, Coma-Canella I, Moreno Yangüela M, Bañuelos F (1983) Segmental right ventricular function after acute myocardial infarction. Two dimensional echocardiographic study in 63 patients. *Am J Cardiol* 51: 390–396.
6. Hutchins GM, Bilkley BH, Ridolfi RL, Griffith LSC, Lohr FT, Piasio MA (1977) Correlation of coronary arteriograms and left ventriculograms with postmortem studies. *Circulation* 56: 32–37.
7. Reduto LA, Berger HJ, Cohen LS, Gottschalk A, Zaret BL (1978) Sequential radionuclide assessment of left and right ventricular performance after acute transmural myocardial infarction. *Ann Inter Med* 89: 441–447.
8. Weiss JL, Bulkley BH, Hutchins GM, Mason SJ (1981) Two dimensional echocardiographic recognition of myocardial injury in man. Comparison with postmortem studies. *Circulation* 63: 401–408.
9. Lieberman AN, Weiss JL, Judgut BI, et al. (1981) Two dimensional echocardiography and infarct size. Relationship of regional wall motion and thickening to the extent of myocardial infarction in the dog. *Circulation* 63: 739–746.
10. Marmor A, Geltman EM, Biello DR, Sobel BE, Siegel BA, Roberts R (1981) Functional response of the right ventricle to myocardial infarction. Dependence on the site of left ventricular infarction. *Circulation* 64: 1005–1011.
11. Starling MR, Dell'Italia LJ, Chaudhuri TK, Boros BL, O'Rourke RA (1984) First transit and equilibrium radionuclide angiography in patients with transmural myocardial infarction: Criteria for the diagnosis on associated hemodynamically significant right ventricular infarction. *J Am Coll Cardiol* 4: 923–930.
12. Lorell B, Leinbach RC, Pohost GM, et al. (1979) Right ventricular infarction. Clinical diagnosis and differentiation from pericardial tamponade and pericardial constriction. *Am J Cardiol* 43: 465–471.
13. Yung-Dae P, Shintaro B, Seiki N, et al. (1980) Assessment of asynergy in right ventricular infarction with real time two dimensional echocardiography. *Circulation* 62: III: 329.
14. D'Arcy BJ, Nanda NC (1982) Two-dimensional echocardiographic features of right ventricular infarction. *Circulation* 65: 167–173.
15. Vannuci A, Cecchi F, Zuppiroli A, Marchionni N, Pini R, Di Bari M, Calamandrei M, Conti A, Ferrucci L, Greppi B, De Alfieri W (1983) Right ventricular infarction: Clinical, hemodynamic; mono and 2D echocardiographic features. *Eur Heart J* 4: 854–864.
16. Baigrie RS, Haq A, Morgan C, Rakowski H, Drobac M, McLaughlin P (1983) The spectrum of right ventricular involvement in inferior wall myocardial infarction: A clinical, hemodynamic and noninvasive study. *J Am Coll Cardiol* 1: 1396–1340.
17. Panidis IP, Ren JF, Kotler MN, Mintz G, Iskandrian A, Ross J, Kane S (1983) Two-dimensional echocardiographic estimation of right ventricular ejection fraction in patients with coronary artery disease. *J Am Coll Cardiol* 2: 911–918.
18. Daubert JC (1983) Etude prospective des critères diagnostiques et prognostiques de l'atteinte ventriculaire droite à la phase aiguë des infarctus inféro-postérieurs. *Arch Mal Coeur* 76: 991–1003.

19. Panidis IP, Kotler MN, Mintz GS, Ross J, Ren JF, Herling I, Kutalek S (1984) Right ventricular function in coronary artery disease assessed by two dimensional echocardiography. *Am Heart J* 107: 1187–1194.
20. Jugdutt BI, Sussex BA, Sivaram CA, Rosall RE (1984) Right ventricular infarction. Two dimensional echocardiographic evaluation. *Am Heart J* 107: 505–518.
21. Dell'Italia, Starling MR, Crawford MH, Boros BL, Chaudhuri TH, O'Rourke RA (1984) Right ventricular infarction: Identification by hemodynamic measurements before and after volume loading and correlation with noninvasive techniques. *J Am Coll Cardiol* 4: 931–939.
22. Strasberg B, Pinchas A, Arditti A, Lewin RF, Sclarousky S, Hellman C, Zafrir N, Agmon J (1984) Left and right ventricular function in inferior acute myocardial infarction and significance of advanced atrioventricular block. *Am J Cardiol* 54: 985–987.
23. Doyle T, Troup PJ, Wann LS (1985) Mid-diastolic opening of the pulmonary valve after right ventricular infarction. *J Am Coll Cardiol* 5: 366–368.
24. Pais F, de Sá EP, Diogo AN, et al. (1984) Sensibilidade e especificidade da ecocardiografia no diagnóstico do enfart do ventrículo direito. *Rev Port Cardiol* 3: 241–245.
25. Arditti A, Lewin RF, Hellman C, Sclarowski S, Strasberg B, Agmon (1985) Right ventricular dysfunction in acute inferior myocardial infarction. An echocardiographic and isotopic study. *Chest* 87: 307–314.
26. Wolf JE, Fagret D, Page E, Machecourt J, Bourlard P, Reboud JP, Denis B (1985) A prospective study of the value of echo and myocardial scintigraphy with 99MTC pyrophosphate in the acute stage of right ventricular infarction. *Arch Mal Coeur* 78: 1464–1471.
27. Bellamy GR, Rasmussen HH, Nasser FN, Wiseman JC, Cooper RA (1986) Value of two dimensional echocardiography and clinical signs in detecting right ventricular infarction. *Am Heart J* 112: 304–309.
28. Godenir JP (1985) Infarction of the right ventricle. Value of 2D echocardiography. *Ann Cardiol Angeiol* 7: 461–466.
29. López-Sendón J, Coma-Canella I, Gamallo C (1981) Sensitivity and specificity of hemodynamic criteria in the diagnosis of acute right ventricular infarction. *Circulation* 64: 515–525.
30. Haines DE, Beller GA, Watson DD, Nygaard TW, Craddock GB, Cooper AA, Gibson RS (1985) A prospective clinical, scintigraphic, angiographic and functional evaluation of patients after inferior myocardial infarction with and without right ventricular dysfunction. *J Am Coll Cardiol* 6: 995–1003.
31. Wyat HL, Forrester JL, DaLuz PL, Diamong GA, Chagrasolis R, Swan HJC (1976) Functional abnormalities in nonoccluded regions of myocardium after experimental coronary occlusion. *Am J Cardiol* 37: 366–370.
32. Parodi O, Marzullo P, Neglia D, et al. (1984) Transient predominant right ventricular ischemia caused by coronary vasospasm. *Circulation* 70: 170–177.
33. Maurer G, Nanda NC (1981) Two dimensional echocardiographic evaluation of exercise induced left and right ventricular asynergy. Correlation with tallium scaning. *Am J Cardiol* 48: 720–727.
34. Kaul S, Hopkins JM, Shah PM (1983) Chronic effects of myocardial infarction on right ventricular function: A non invasive assessment. *J Am Coll Cardiol* 2: 607–615.
35. Ramanathan K, Bodenheimer MM, Banka VS, Helfat RH (1981) Natural history of contractile abnormalities after acute myocardial infarction in man. Severity and response to nitroglycerin as a function of time. *Circulation* 63: 731–738.
36. Holman BL, Wynne J, Idoine T, Neill RT (1980) Disruption in the temporal sequence of regional ventricular contraction. *Circulation* 61: 1075–1083.
37. Weyman AE, Franklin JD Jr, Hogan RD, et al. (1984) Importance of temporal heterogeneity in assessing the contraction abnormalities associated with acute myocardial ischemia. *Circulation* 70: 102–109.

38. Gillan LD, Hogan RD, Foale RA, Franklin T Jr, Newell JB, Guyer DE, Weyman A (1984) A comparison of quantitative echocardiographic methods for delineating infarct induced abnormal wall motion. *Circulation* 70: 113–122.
39. Erhardt LR, Sjogren A, Whalberg I (1976) Single right-sided precordial lead in the diagnosis of right ventricular involvement inferior myocardial infarction. *Am Heart J* 91: 571–576.
40. López-Sendón J, Coma-Canella I, Alcasena S, Seoane C, Gamallo C (1985) Electrocardiographic findings in acute right ventricular infarction. Sensitivity and specificity of electrocardiographic alterationsin right precordial leads V4R, V3R, Vi, V2, V3. *J Am Coll Cardiol* 6: 1273–1279.
41. Banka V, Agarwall JB, Bodenheimer MM, Helfant RH (1981) Intraventricular septal motion. Biventricular angiographic assessment of its contribution to left and right ventricular contraction. *Circulation* 64: 992–996.
42. Kaul S (1986) The interventricular septum in health and disease. *Am Heart J* 112: 568–581.
43. Lima JA, Guzman PA, Yin FCP, Brawley RK, Humphrey L, Traill TA, Lima SD, Marino P, Weisfeldt ML, Weiss JL (1986) Septal geometry in the unloaded living human heart. *Circulation* 74: 463–468.
44. Candell Riera J, Gutierrez Palau L, Valle Tudela V, Rius Garriga J (1980) Estudio ecocardiográfico del infarto agudo de miocardio inferior propagado a ventrículo derecho. *Rev Esp Cardiol* 33: 403–408.
45. Coma-Canella I, López-Sendón J, Oliver J (1981) Premature pulmonicvalve opening and inverted septal convexity in acute ischemic rightventricular dysfunction. *Am Heart J* 101: 684–685.
46. López-Sendón J, Coma-Canella I, Lombera F, Benito F (1982) Diagnosis of ischemic right ventricular dysfunction by M-Mode echocardiography. *Eur Heart J* 3: 230–237.
47. Sharkey SW (1985) M-mode and 2D echo analysis of the septum in experimental right ventricular infarction: Correlation with hemodynamic alterations. *Am Heart J* 110: 1210–1218.
48. Kingma I, Tyberg JV, Smith ER (1983) Effects of diastolic transeptal pressure gradients on ventricular septal position and motion. *Circulation* 68: 1304–1214.
49. Goto Y, Yamamoto J, Saito M, Haze K, Sumiyoshi T, Fukami K, Hiramori K (1985) *Circulation* 72: 1104–1114.
50. Beppu S, Izumi S, Nagata S (1984) Ventricular interdependence reflected in interventricular septal motion. With special reference to right ventricular pressure overload. *J Cardiogr* 14: IV: 53–62.
51. Agata Y (1985) Two-dimensional echocardiographic determinants of interventricular septal configuration in right or left ventricular overload. *Am Heart J* 110: 819–825.
52. Feneley M, Gavaghan T (1986) Paradoxical and pseudoparadoxical interventricular septal motion in patients with right ventricular volume overload. *Circulation* 74: 230–238.
53. Kaul S, Tei C, Hopkins JM, Shah PM (1984) Assessment of right ventricular function using two dimensional echocardiography. *Am Heart J* 107: 526–531.
54. Rushmer RF, Crystal DK, Wagenr C (1953) The functional anatomy of ventricular contraction. *Circ Res* 162–175.
55. García-Fernandez MA, Eizaguirre J, Moreo Yangüela M, Bañuelos F (1983) Normal patterns of wall motion of the right ventricle. Two dimensional echocardiographic study, in: Martin G (ed), *The Application of Computers in Cardiology*, pp 213–216. Elsevier Science Publ.
56. Sharpe DN, Botvinik EH, Shames DH, et al. (1978) The noninvasive diagnosis of right ventricular infarction. *Circulation* 57: 483–491.
56. Gomez G, Fresh D, Grismer J, Tristani F, Keelan M (1973) Hemodynamic and echocardiographic correlation of right ventricular disfunction in acute myocardial infarction, (abstracts). *Clin Res* 21: 240.

57. Bommer W, Weinert L, Newman A, Neef J, Mason DT, De Maria A (1979) Determination of right atrial and right ventricular size by two dimensional echocardiography. *Circulation* 60: 91–100.

58. Saito A, Ueda K, Nakano H (1981) Right ventricular volume determination by two dimensional echocardiography. *J Cardiogr* 11: 1159–1167.

59. Ninomiya K, Duncan WJ, Cook DH, Rowe RD (1981) Right ventricular ejection fraction and volumes after Mustard repair. Correlation of two dimensional echocardiograms and cineangiograms. *Am J Cardiol* 48: 317–324.

60. Watanabe R, Katsume H, Marsukubo H, Furukawa K, Ihichi H (1982) Estimation of right ventricular volume with two dimensional echocardiography. *Am J Cardiol* 49: 1946–1953.

61. Starling MR, Crawford MH, Sorensen SG, O'Rourke RA (1982) A new two dimensional echocardiographic technique for evaluating right ventricular size and performance in patients with obstructive lung disease. *Circulation* 66: 612–620.

62. Hiraishi S, DiSessa TG, Jarmakani JM, Nakanishi T, Isabel-Jones JB, Friedman WF (1982) Two dimensional echocardiographic assessment of right ventricular volume in children with congenital heart disease. *Am J Cardiol* 50: 1368–1375.

63. Levine RA, Gibson TC, Aretz T, et al. (1984) Echocardiographic measurement of right ventricular volume. *Circulation* 69: 497–505.

64. Linker DT, Pearlman AS, Moritz WE, Huntsman LH (1982) A new method for right ventricular volume calculation from a three dimensional echocardiographic reconstruction. *Circulation* 66: II–338.

65. Linker DT, Moritz WE, Pearlman AS (1986) A new three dimensional echocardiographic method of right ventricular volume measurement. In vitro validation. *J Am Coll Cardiol* 8: 101–106.

66. Wann LS, Stickels KR, Bamrah VS, Gross CM (1984) Digital processing of contrast echocardiograms: A new technique for measuring right ventricular ejection fraction. *Am J Cardiol* 53: 1164–1168.

67. Cabin HS, Roberts WC (1980) Left ventricular aneurysm, intraaneurismal thrombus and systemic embolus in coronary heart disease. *Chest* 75: 586–590.

68. Starling MR, Crawford MH, Walsh O, Rourke RA (1980) Value of tricuspid valve echogram for estimating right ventricular end diastolic pressure during vasodilatador therapy. *Am J Cardiol* 45: 966–972.

69. Legrand V, Rigo P (1981) Premature opening of the pulmonary valve in right ventricular myocardial infarction. *Acta Cardiol* 36: 289–293.

70. Coma canella I, López Sendón J, Oliver J (1981) Premature valve opening and inverted septal convexity in acute ischemic right ventricular disfunction. *Am Heart J* 101: 684–685.

71. Benito F, López Sendón J, García-Fernandez MA, Coma I, Lombera F (1984) Premature pulmonic valve opening. An echocardiographic finding indicative of reduced right ventricular compliance. *Am H J* 107: 1029–1032.

71. bis. Cohn JN, Guiha NH, Broder MI, Limas CJ (1974) Right ventricular infarctium. *Am J Cardiol* 33: 209–214.

72. García-Fernandez MA, López-Sendón J, Moreno Yangüela M, Jadraque L, Bañuelos F (1983) Aneurisma de ventrículo derecho. Presentación de un caso diagnosticado mediante ecocardiografía bidimensional. *Rev Esp Cardiol* 36: 255–257.

73. Lombera F, López-Sendón J, García-Fernandez MA, et al. (1982) Alteraciones de la contractilidad del ventrículo derecho en el infarto agudo de miocardio. Correlación con V4R. *Rev Esp Cardiol* 35: I–34.

74. Manga P, King J (1985) Trauma induced pseudopaneurysm of the right ventricle: Diagnosis by two-dimensional echocardiography. *Am J Cardiol* 55: 1658–1659.

75. Chiariello L, Macrina F, Caretta Q, Cattolica FL, Papalia U, Marino B (1985) Extracar-

diac left to right shunt in a patient with biventricular postinfarction rupture and pseudo-aneurysm. *J Am Coll Cardiol* 6: 246–249.

76. Hamilton K, Ellenbogen K, Lowe JE, Kisslo J (1985) Ultrasound diagnosis of pseudo-aneurysm and contiguous ventricular septal defect complicating inferior myocardial infarction. *J Am Coll Cardiol* 6: 1160–1163.
77. Gonzalez Maqueda I, López-Sendón J, Iglesias A, Pabon, Osuna C, Martin Luengo E, Martin Jadraque L (1984) Rotura de parel libre del ventrículo derecho postinfarto agudo de miocardio. Presentación de un caso. *Rev Esp Cardiol* 37: 72–74.
78. López-Sendón J (1985) Rotura cardiaca subaguda post infarto de miocardio. Estudio de la precisión diagnóstica de parámetros clínicos, ecocardiográficos y hemodinámicos. Thesis, Universidad Complutense de Madrid, Madrid.
79. García-Fernandez MA, Moreno Yangüela M, Sobrepera JL, Forteza JF, Rossi PN, Bañuelos F (1983) Estudio de los trombos ventriculares izquierdos con ecocardiografía bidimensional. *Rev Esp Cardiol* 36: 35–42.
80. Asinger R, Mikell F, Sharma B, Hodges M (1981) Observations on detecting left ventricular thrombus with two dimensional echocardiography. Emphasis on avoidance of false positive diagnosis. *Am J Cardiol* 47: 145–156.
81. Mikell FL, Asinger RW, Elsperger KJ, Anderson WR, Hodges M (1982) Do the tissue acoustic properties of fresh left ventricular thrombi limit their visualization by two dimensional echocardiography? Experimental observations. *Am J Cardiol* 49: 1157–1165.
82. Stowers SA, Leiboff RH, Wasserman AG, Katz RJ, Bren GB, Hsu I (1983) Right ventricular thrombus formation in association with acute myocardial infarction: Diagnosis by two dimensional echocardiography. *Am J Cardiol* 52: 912–913.
83. Almeria C, García-Fernandez MA (1982) Diagnóstico con ecocardiografía bidimensional de los trombos del ventrículo derecho. Ultrasonidos 1: 345.
84. Nesser HJ, Markt B, Baumgartner G, Davogg S (1984) Transienter rechtsventriculaer Thrombus nach Hinterwand myocardinfarkt. Diagnostic mittels zweidimensionaler Echocardiographie. Zeitschrift für Kardiol. 73: 472–474.
85. O'Rourke MF (1973) Subacute heart rupture following myocardial infarction. Clinical features of a correctable condition. *Lancet* 2: 124–127.
86. Coma-Canella I, López-Sendón J, Nuñez Gonzalez L, Ferrufino O (1983) Subacute left ventricular free wall rupture following acute myocardial infarction. Bedside hemodynamics, differential diagnosis and treatment. *Am Heart J* 106: 278–294.
87. Cobbs BW, Hatcher ChR, Robinson PH (1973) Cardiac rupture. Three operations with two long term survivals. *JAMA* 223: 532–536.
88. López-Sendón J, Calvo Orbe L, Cabrera A, Oliver J, Larrea JL, Martín Jadraque L (1984) Utilidad de la ecocardiografía bidimensional en el diagnóstico de la rotura cardiaca. Presentación de un caso. *Rev Esp Cardiol* 37: 70–71.
89. Mestres CA, Murtra M, Igual A, Martinez Gutierrez F, Batalla J, Petit M (1984) Siete años de seguimiento de una rotura postinfarto de ventrículo izquierdo tratada quirurgicamente con éxito. *Rev Esp Cardiol* 37: 67–69.
90. King TC, Saffitz JE (1985) Acute right ventricular infarction resulting from intracardiac infusion of hyperosmotic hyperalimentation solutions. *Am J Cardiol* 55: 1659–1660.
91. Hubbard JF, Girod DA, Caldwell RL, Hurwitz RA, Mahony LA, Waller BF (1983) Right ventricular infarction with cardiaca rupture in an infant with pulmonary valve atresia with intact ventricular septum. *J Am Coll Cardiol* 2: 263–268.
92. López-Sendón J, García-Fernandez MA, Coma-Canella I, Silvestre J, De Miguel E, Martín Jadraque L (1984) Identification of blood in the pericardial cavity by two dimensional echocardiography. *Am J Cardiol* 53: 1194–1197.
93. García-Fernandez MA, Moreno Yangüela M, Rossi PN, López-Sendón J, Bañuelos F (1984) Echocardiographic features of hemopericardium. 107: 1035.
94. Erhardt LR (1974) Clinical and pathological observations in different types of acute myocardial infarction. A study of 84 patients deceased after treatment in a coronary care unit. *Acta Med Scand* 560: 1–78.

95. Fananapazir L, Bray CL, Dark JF, Moussalli H, Deiranilla AK, Lawson RAM (1983) Right ventricular dysfunction and surgical outcome in postinfarction ventricular septal defect. *Eur Heart J* 4: 155–167.
96. López-Sendón J, Coma-Canella I (1981) Valoración de la función ventricular en la unidad coronaria. Monitorización hemodinámica, in: Martín Jadraque L, Coma-Canella I, Maqueda I, López-Sendón J (eds), *Ediciones Norma*, pp 401–429.
97. Farcot JC, Boisante L, Rigaud M, Bardet J, Bourdarias JP (1980) Two dimensional echocardiographic visualization of ventricular septal rupture after acute myocardial infarction. *Am J Cardiol* 45: 370–377.
98. Bishop HL, Gibson RS, Stamm BR, Beller GA, Martin RP (1981) Role of two dimensional echocardiography in the evaluation of patients with ventricular septal rupture after acute myocardial infarction. *Am Heart J* 102: 965–971.
99. Mintz GS, Victor MF, Kotler MN, Parry WR, Segal BL (1981) Two dimensional echocardiographic identification of surgically correctable complications of acute myocardial infarction. *Circulation* 64: 91–96.
100. Smyllie J, Sutherland GR, Roelandt J (1988) Postinfarct ventricular septal defects the value of colour flow mapping. *Eur Heart J* 9 (suppl I): 106.
101. Recusani F, Raisaro J, Sgalambro A, Tronconi L, Venco A, Salerno J, Ardissino D (1984) Ventricular septal rupture after myocardial infarction. Diagnosis by two dimensional and pulsed Doppler echocardiography. *Am J Cardiol* 54: 277–281.
102. Richards KL, Hoekenga DE, Leach JK, Blaustein JC (1979) Doppler-cardiographic diagnosis of interventricular septal rupture. *Chest* 76: 101–103.
103. Keren G, Sherez J, Roth A, Miller H, Laniado S (1984) Diagnosis of ventricular septal rupture from acute myocardial infarction by combined two-dimensional and pulsed Doppler echocardiography. *Am J Cardiol* 53: 1202–1203.
104. García-Fernandez FA, Moreno Yangüela M, Graña N (1985) Eco bidimensiona-Doppler en la rotura septal post infarto de miocardio. *Ultrasonidos* 4: 37–38.
105. López-Sendón J, García-Fernandez MA, Coma-Canella I, Moreno Yangüela M, Martín Jadraque L, Bañuelos F (1982) Segmental right ventricular function after acute myocardial infarction. IX World Congress of Cardiology. Moscow.
106. Ohagon J, et al. (1984) Infarction of the right ventricle and major tricuspid regurgitation, Case report. *Coeur* 771–774.
107. Onoyama H, Iwasaka T, Sugiura T, et al. (1986) Tricuspid valve regurgitation associated with right ventricular infarction, p 460. X World Congress of Cardiology.
108. Hollman A (1957) The anatomical appearance in rheumatic tricuspid valve disease. *Br Heart J* 19: 211–220.
109. Ubago JL, Figueroa A, Ochoteco A, Colman T, Duran RM, Duran C (1983) Analysis of the amount of tricuspid valve annular dilatation required to produce functional tricuspid regurgitation. *Am J Cardiol* 52: 155–158.
110. Eissenberg S, Suyemoto J (1964) Rupture of a papillary muscle of the tricuspid valve following acute myocardial infarction. *Circulation* 30: 588–591.
111. Perrault MA, Leclerq JF, Masquet Ch, Nitenberg G, Slama R, Bouvrain Y (1977) Infarctus massif biventriculaire avec rupture d'un pilier mitral et d'un pilier trcuspidien. Etude anatomique. *Arch Mal Coeur* 70: 1091–1095.
112. Daubert JC, Langella B, de Place C, et al. (1980) Frequence et prognostic de l'atteinte ventriculaire droite à la phase aigüe de l'infarctus du myocarde. *Arch Mal Coeur* 73: 785–794.
113. Grosse R, Spindola-Franco H (1981) Right ventricular infarction in acute ventricular septal defect. *Am Heart J* 101: 67–74.
114. Lader E, Colvin S, Tunick P (1983) Myocardial infarction complicated by rupture of both ventricular septum and right ventricular papillary muscle. *Am J Cardiol* 52: 423–424.
115. García-Fernandez MA, Moreno Yangüela M (1986) Ecocardiografía Doppler en la insuficiencia tricúspide. *Rev Esp Cardiol* 39: 18–25.

116. García-Fernandez MA (1988) Valoracion con tecnica de contraste y doppler de la insuficienciua tricuspide. Tesis Doctoral, Universidad Complutense de Madrid.
117. Waggoner AD, Quinones MA, Young JB, Brandon TA, Shah AA, Verani M, Miller RR (1981) Pulsed Doppler echocardiographic right sided valve regurgitation. Experimental results and clinical significance. *Am J Cardiol* 47: 279–286.
118. García Dorado D, Falzgraf S, Almazan A, Delcan JL, López Bescós L, Menarguez L (1982) Diagnosis of functional tricuspid insufficiency by pulsed-waved Doppler ultrasound. *Circulation* 66: 1315–1321.
119. Miyatake K, Okamoto M, Kiroshita N, Ohta T, Kozuka T, Sakakibara H, Nimura Y (1982) Evaluation of tricuspid regurgitation by pulsed Doppler and two dimensional echocardiography. *Circulation* 66: 777–783.
120. DePace NL, Ross J, Iskandrian AS, et al. (1984) Tricuspid regurgitation. Noninvasive techniques for determining causes and severty. *J Am Coll Cardiol* 3: 1540–1550.
121. García-Fernandez MA, López-Sendón JL, Coma-Canella I (1988) Significance of laminar flow detected by Doppler echocardiography in tricuspid regurgitation: Experimental and clinical study. *J of Cardiovas Ultason* 7: 3–8.
122. García-Fernandez MA (1989) Etxebeste Doppler Color en Cardiologia. Madrid: Mc Graw Hill Inter.
123. Roelandt J (1985) Color coded flow imaging: What are the prospects? *Eur Heart J* 7: 184–189.
124. Miyatake K, Okamoto M, Kinoshita N, Izumi S, Owa M, Takao S, Sakakibara H, Nimura Y (1984) Clinical application of a new type of real-time two dimensional Doppler flow imaging system. *Am J Cardiol* 54: 857–868.
125. Hatle L, Brubakk A, Tromsdal A, Angelsen B (1978) Noninvasive assessment of pressure drop in mitral stenosis by Doppler ultrasound. *Brit Heart J* 40: 3–40.
126. García-Fernandez MA, Chapman CV, López-Sendón J, Sotillo J, Fantidis P, Gonzalez A (1986) Cálculo de la presión sistólica ventricular derecha con Doppler continuo. Estudio experimental en perros. *Rev Port Cardiol* 5 (suppl I): 83.
127. Skjaerpe T, Hatle L (1981) Diagnosis and assessment of tricuspid regurgitation by Doppler ultrasound, in: Rijsterborg H (ed), *Echocardiology*, pp 299–304. Boston: Martinus Nijhoff.
128. Yock PG, Popp RL (1984) Noninvasive estimation of right ventricular systolic pressure by Doppler ultrasound in patients with tricuspid incompetence. *Circulation* 70: 657–662.
129. Currie PJ, Seward JB, Chan KL, et al. (1985) Continuous wave Doppler determination of right ventricular pressure. A simultaneous Doppler catheterization study in 127 patients. *J Am Coll Cardiol* 750–756.
130. García-Fernandez MA, López-Sendón J, Coma-Canella I, Silvestre (1987) Echocardiographic findings after rupture of the tricuspid subvalvular apparatus: Experimental study in dogs. *J of Cardiovas Ultrason* 6: 9.
131. Mintz GS, Kotler MN, Parry WR, Iskandrian AS, Kane SA (1981) Real time inferior vena cava ultrasonography. Normal and abnormal findings and its use assessing right heart function. *Circulation* 64: 1018–1024.
132. Coma-Canella I, López-Sendón J, Nunez L (1983) Subacute left ventricular free wall rupture following acute myocardial infarctium. Bedside hemodynamic, differential diagnosis and treatment. *Am Heart J* 106: 278–284.
133. Lopéz de SA E, López-Sendón J, Pare J, et al. (1988) Shape of the interauricular septum in right ventricular infarction. Hemodynamic correlations. *Eur Heart J* 9 (suppl I): 153.

16. The role of cardiac ultrasound in the diagnosis of the 'surgical' complications of acute myocardial infarction

JOHN H. SMYLLIE, PATRICIA E. ASSMANN, GEORGE R. SUTHERLAND, ALAN G. FRASER and JOS R.T.C. ROELANDT

Introduction

Two-dimensional echocardiography is a useful technique for the diagnosis of patients presenting with myocardial infarction. It can rapidly differentiate acute myocardial infarction from other causes of acute severe chest pain such as thoracic aortic dissection, pericarditis and aortic valve disease. The technique has also become a major diagnostic tool for the detection of the mechanical complications of myocardial infarction which in many cases can be corrected by surgical intervention. In addition Doppler echocardiography and more particularly color Doppler flow mapping help to assess the hemodynamic and blood flow abnormalities resulting from these complications so that their presence and severity can be readily evaluated at the bedside in the coronary care unit. The diagnostic potential of both methods may be extended by the transesophageal approach offering an alternative window to the heart when the precordial windows provide poor quality images. This is especially true in immobile, supine patients on ventilators or with an intra aortic counterpulsation in situ. However, at the present time, the reported experience with transesophageal echocardiography in the assessment of the acute complications of myocardial infarction is limited.

Rupture of the free wall

Acute presentation – tamponade

The incidence of left ventricular free wall rupture is between 5–24% of fatal acute myocardial infarctions [1–4]. It is more common than rupture of a papillary muscle or the interventricular septum [1, 5]. Rupture of the free wall usually leads to acute tamponade and death, but prompt diagnosis has occasionally allowed successful surgical treatment [5–8].

Cardiac tamponade should be suspected in the presence of hemodynamic collapse and/or electromechanical dissociation which is often preceded by

S. Iliceto et al. (eds.), Ultrasound in Coronary Artery Disease, 183–196.
© 1991 *Kluwer Academic Publishers.*

recurrent chest pain. Two-dimensional echocardiography may be useful for making a prompt bedside diagnosis [8–12]. The hemopericardium in cardiac tamponade resembles pericardial effusion. A more specific echocardiographic sign of tamponade is abnormal diastolic right ventricular free wall motion, as well as the more sensitive right atrial inversion [13–17].

In acute tamponade, where urgent intervention is required, two-dimensional echocardiography can sometimes be helpful in guiding the pericardiocentesis aspiration needle and for visualising the degree of any penetration of the needle into the myocardium and ventricular cavity. Two-dimensional echocardiography can also rapidly assess the immediate results of pericardiocentesis.

Subacute presentation – pseudoaneurysm

Cardiac rupture following myocardial infarction may sometimes lead to the development of a left ventricular false or pseudoaneurysm. In this situation the wall of the pseudoaneurysm is formed by adherent pericardium which has prevented fatal tamponade. Due to the propensity for pseudoaneurysms to rupture [18], early diagnosis is essential so that subsequent surgical repair can be performed.

In 1975 we reported the two-dimensional echocardiographic signs of a left ventricular pseudoaneurysm [19]. Since then, several investigators have con-

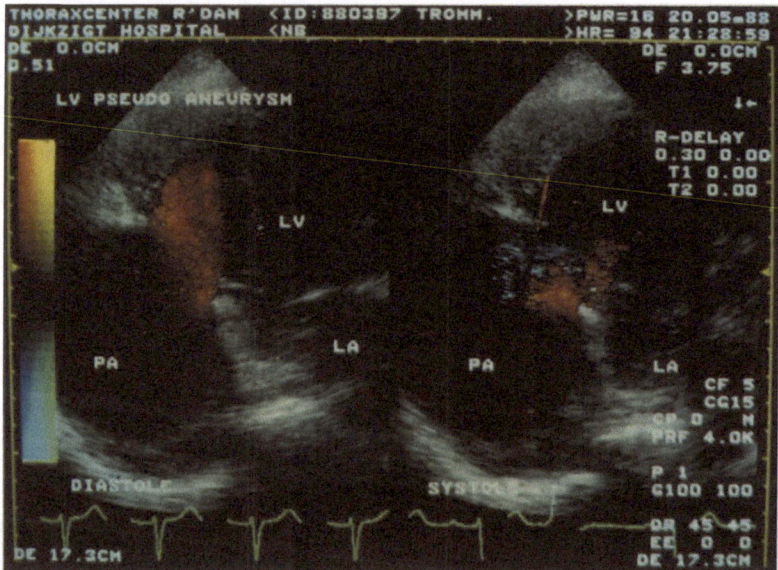

Figure 1. A posterior left ventricular pseudoaneurysm recorded from a modified apical long axis view. The color flow map, in diastole and systole, demonstrates blood flow traversing a myocardial defect between the left ventricle and the pseudoaneurysm cavity. LV = left ventricle, LA = left atrium, PA = pseudoaneurysm.

firmed those findings [20–26]. They are an extra myocardial cavity which is delineated by pericardium and/or extracardiac tissue and an orifice size which is small compared to maximal cavity dimension [19, 23–26]. Like a true left ventricular aneurysm, pseudoaneurysms exhibit akinetic or dyskinetic motion and frequently contain thrombus [21, 23, 26].

Color Doppler flow mapping highly facilitates the diagnosis of a pseudoaneurysm by demonstrating transmyocardial blood flow passing to and fro across the free wall defect (Figure 1), [26–28]. This is particularly important when the myocardial rupture is small and cannot be visualized by two-dimensional imaging along [28]. In this instance the differential diagnosis of an extramyocardial cavity would be between a pseudoaneurysm, a loculated pericardial effusion, a simple haematoma or a pericardial cyst. Color Doppler flow mapping by demonstrating turbulent blood flow passing between the left ventricle and the extramyocardial cavity, thus confirming the diagnosis of a communication and hence a pseudoaneurysm [28].

The role of transesophageal echocardiography in the diagnosis of left ventricular pseudoaneurysm is as yet untested. Our initial experience has indicated that some myocardial rupture sites can be difficult to directly visualise from the esophageal approach [28].

Ventricular septal rupture, papillary muscle rupture and dysfunction

Two-dimensional echocardiography is of particular value in the management of patients who develop a new systolic murmur and congestive heart failure following acute myocardial infarction. Early detection of structural complications such as interventricular septal rupture, papillary muscle rupture or papillary muscle dysfunction is important as these conditions often require urgent surgical intervention.

Ventricular septal rupture

Rupture of the ventricular septum occurs in about 2% of patients following myocardial infarction and usually develops within the first week [29]. The mortality of this condition is high and early surgery remains the treatment of choice. Echocardiographic evidence of inferior wall infarction and combined right ventricular and septal dysfunction appear to be predictive for a higher surgical mortality. The echocardiographic diagnosis of ventricular septal rupture can be difficult. The septum may show an echo free area, dyskinesis or aneurysm formation, however, these signs are not always diagnostic for ventricular septal rupture [30–36]. Furthermore small defects may be impossible to visualize and in some series only 50% of defects were readily visualized by two-dimensional echocardiography alone. An injection of peripheral contrast can visualize right-to-left flow by the appearance of microbubbles within the left ventricle, while negative echocontrast in the right ventricle demonstrates left-to-right shunting which predominates in these patients [30, 33, 37, 38].

Simultaneous pulsed Doppler and two-dimensional echocardiographic examination may provide the diagnosis when a ventricular septal rupture is suspected, by detecting the high velocity right ventricular systolic flow disturbance which occurs in these patients [39–32]. However repeated interrogation of the interventricular septum is often required to detect any left to right shunt and this can be time consuming. Also the pulsed Doppler technique is inaccurate at predicting the precise septal rupture site in some cases [43].

Color Doppler flow mapping has been found to be highly sensitive for the diagnosis of postinfarction ventricular septal rupture (Figure 2) and by demonstrating the area of transseptal flow can give an accurate prediction of the defect site or multiple sites [43]. The combination of two-dimensional echocardiography and color Doppler flow mapping can provide detailed information regarding left ventricular function, the presence and site of the septal rupture and the presence and grading of any co-existing mitral and tricuspid regurgitation. Thus left ventricular cineangiography prior to surgical repair can be avoided as this may be a potentially hazardous procedure in these patients [44].

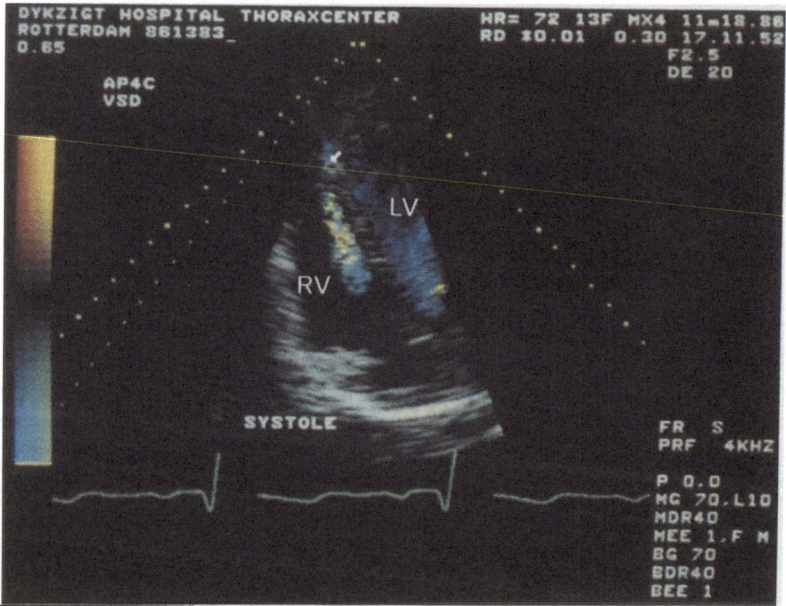

Figure 2. An apical postinfarction ventricular septal defect recorded from the apical four chamber view. The color flow map depicts a high velocity 'mosaic' jet crossing the apical septum (arrow). This defect was not visualised by imaging alone. LV = left ventricle, RV = right ventricle.

Transesophageal echocardiography with color Doppler flow mapping has been reported in the diagnosis of postinfarction ventricular septal rupture [45] and may provide an alternative technique in patients in whom precordial echocardiography has been unsatisfactory.

Postinfarction mitral regurgitation

Papillary muscle rupture or dysfunction may cause acute mitral and tricuspid regurgitation after myocardial infarction. In our experience the incidence of papillary muscle rupture is much less frequent than ventricular septal rupture although papillary rupture has been reported as being the cause of up to 5% of fatalities after acute myocardial infarction. Papillary muscle rupture usually develops between 2 to 7 days after onset of myocardial infarction [46–47] and a median survival of 3 days. Immediate diagnosis is therefore mandatory so that mitral valve replacement can be performed.

The echocardiographic diagnosis of papillary muscle rupture is not simple. Apart from relative left ventricular hyperkinesis this condition may be recognized by rupture of the trunk of one of the papillary muscles, a mobile mass appearing during systole in the left atrium and in diastole in the left ventricle, by noncoaptation of the mitral leaflets or by accentuated holosystolic prolapse [47–51].

Myocardial dyskinesis may cause mitral regurgitation by papillary muscle dysfunction. Two-dimensional echocardiography reveals a unique pattern of incomplete mitral leaflet closure in the majority of patients with de novo mitral regurgitation after prior infarction [52]. Also dyskinesis involved the left ventricular myocardium beneath one of the papillary muscles, thus producing increased tension on the mitral leaflets and preventing normal closure.

Patients with papillary muscle dysfunction may present with late post-infarction congestive heart failure. Two-dimensional echocardiography is the technique of choice of detecting the cause of mitral regurgitation. However, Doppler echocardiography and color Doppler flow mapping are highly sensitive techniques for detecting the presence of mitral regurgitation and both can be used to give a semi-quantitative assessment of severity. This usually involves delineating the extension of the regurgitant velocities into the left atrium [53–55] or by mapping the regurgitant area and expressing it as a ratio of the left atrial size [56]. It should be noted, that these methods have been performed on patients with chronic mitral regurgitation. Our observations suggest this method is not always reliable in the grading of acute mitral regurgitation encountered after myocardial infarction. We would advise that no single Doppler technique should be used to assess the severity of mitral regurgitation but a combination of the left ventricular function, the appearance of the mitral valve, the velocity of forward flow, the dynamics of retrograde flow and the regurgitant area should all be used to assess severity.

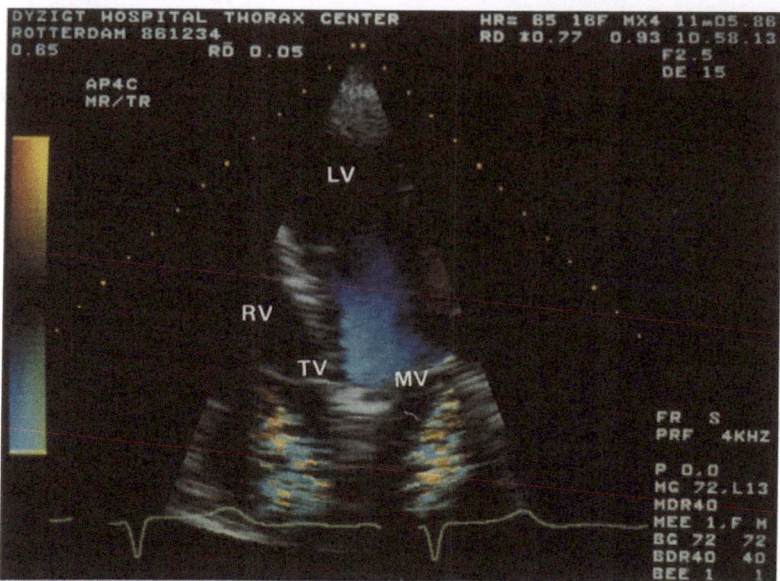

Figure 3. Combined mitral and tricuspid regurgitation following inferior wall infarction record-ed from the apical four chamber view in systole. Two central regurgitant 'mosaic' jets are present in both atria. LV = left ventricle, RV = right ventricle, MV = mitral valve, Tricuspid Valve, RA = right atrium, LA = left atrium.

The simultaneous occurrence of ventricular septal defect and mitral regur-gitation secondary to myocardial infarction has been reported [57–61]. The association of mitral regurgitation with ventricular septal rupture is usually due to the site of rupture. In one surgical series 10% of ventricular septal ruptures were associated with mitral regurgitation due to papillary muscle infarction [62]. Pulsed Doppler echocardiography has been used to differen-tiate ventricular septal defect from mitral regurgitation [63] or to diagnose their combination [64]. Color coded Doppler flow mapping can now be con-sidered to be the best technique in detecting and excluding these complica-tions since it has the capability to visualize the different jets simultaneously within the two-dimensional image (Figure 3).

Right-to-left shunting at atrial level

Right ventricular infarction produces elevation of right ventricular diastolic pressure, transmitted to the right atrium and creating a gradient favorable for right-to-left shunting through a patent foramen ovale, which may exist in up to 27% of adults [65]. This is a possible cause of hypoxemia [66, 67] or para-doxical embolism in the presence of right ventricular infarction [68]. Contrast echocardiography rapidly establishes the diagnosis [67, 69, 70]. The potential of color Doppler flow imaging has not yet been tested in this situation.

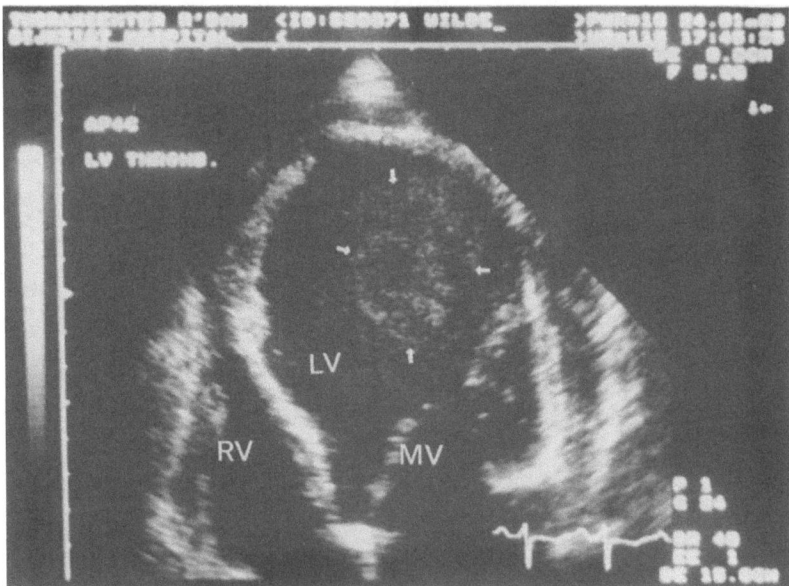

Figure 4. A true aneurysm at the apex of the left ventricle with swirling spontaneous echo contrast within it's cavity (arrows). LV = left ventricle, RV = right ventricle, MV = mitral valve.

True left ventricular aneurysm

Two-dimensional echocardiography accurately detects true left ventricular aneurysm, whereas clinical sign may be of limited value for its diagnosis. It is defined as a well demarcated bulge in the contour of the left ventricular wall demonstrating dyskinesis or akinesis [71–72] (Figure 4). Two-dimensional echocardiographic study indicates that left ventricular aneurysm formation depends on a critical imbalance of myocardial forces where strong left ventricular segments cause bulging of weakened ones [74]. The incidence of aneurysm formation in patients with a first acute myocardial infarction is about 22%, with those following anterior infarction developing in the first 5 days [75]. In patients with an aneurysm treated either medically or surgically mortality is largely determined by size and function of nonaneurysmal myocardium as estimated with two-dimensional echocardiography [76, 77).

Thrombus

Left ventricular thrombus

The incidence of postinfarct mural thrombi recognized by two-dimensional echocardiography ranges from 17 to 34%. Its diagnosis is often dramatic and

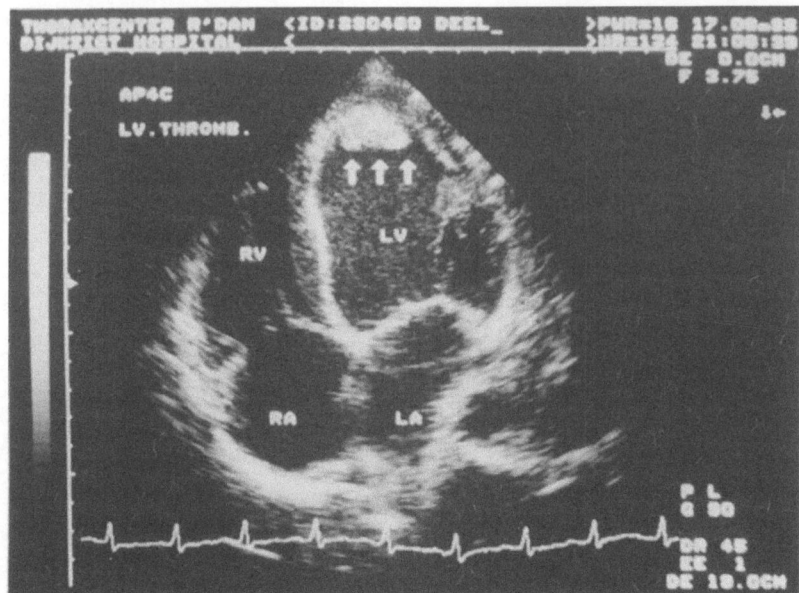

Figure 5. Apical thrombus (arrows) following apical myocardial infarction. LV = left ventricle, RV = right ventricle, RA = right atrium, LA = left atrium.

raises therapeutic questions. Previous studies using surgical or autopsy findings for comparison, have shown that two-dimensional echocardiography is both a sensitive (90%) and specific (90%) means of noninvasively detecting left ventricular thrombi (Figure 5), [78–82].

False positive echocardiographic diagnosis may be avoided if left ventricular thrombus is defined as an echo-dense mass within the left ventricular cavity which is seen adjacent to and can be distinguished from the asynergic myocardium in more than one echocardiographic view [77, 78]. Several investigators have shown that two-dimensional echocardiography is superior to contrast ventriculography and radionuclide methods in assessing thrombi [78, 79, 82, 83]. However, sensitivity and specificity of indium-111 platelet imaging is comparable to that of echocardiography [84]. This expensive non-bedside, time-consuming method, which identifies thrombus activity rather than thrombus mass can be helpful in patients with technically inadequate echocardiograms. Left ventricular thrombi that develop within 2 days of acute myocardial infarction occur in patients with the most extensive myocardial infarction and is predictive of high mortality [85]. Patients with large anterior myocardial infarction and apical akinesis are at high risk for developing left ventricular thrombosus, even when receiving oral anticoagulant therapy [86], while those with inferior myocardial infarction will seldom have thrombus [82, 87–89]. However, the large majority of left ventricular thrombi do not cause a clinically detectable embolic event [85, 87]. Some investigators have found that left ventricular thrombi which project into the lumen and which have inceased mobility are at high risk for embolization [90, 91]. However, others suggest that tissue characteristics of the thrombus and not clot mobility are predictive of systemic embolization [92].

Right atrial and right ventricular thrombus

Thrombus in the right atrium or ventricle after acute myocardial infarction, though rare, must be considered as the cause of paradoxical embolization [68] and can be detected echocardiographically [92, 93–95].

Conclusion

Two-dimensional echocardiography in combination with Doppler and color Doppler flow mapping is now considered the technique of choice for the early diagnosis and assessment of the 'surgical' complications of acute myocardial infarction. It has the advantage of being a rapid, safe technique with ease of portability and repeatability, at relatively low cost. Transesophageal echo-cardiography may provide an alternative 'window' for imaging cardiac structure and function, but as yet its value in the diagnosis of the complications of myocardial function is not proven.

Two dimensional echocardiography is the most sensitive method to diagnose right ventricular infarction and provides information predictive of early and late postinfarct complications. In the acute phase, two-dimensional echocardiography can diagnose the cause of hemodynamic deterioration by distinguishing primary pump failure from the mechanical complications discussed in this chapter. In the subacute phase, complications including left ventricular true and false aneurysms and mural thrombus may be detected by two-dimensional echocardiography and this information allows optimal management decisions to be made. Thus, echocardiography has become an indispensable technique on the coronary care unit. It provides a complete picture of cardiac structure and function making it superior to other methods in the clinical situation of an acute myocardial infarction which has such a volatile and unpredictable course.

Acknowledgement

J. H. Smyllie was supported in part by The Royal College of Physicians of Edinburgh's 'Glaxo Travelling Fellowship'. P. E. Assmann was supported by grant 84093 from the Dutch Heart Foundation.

References

1. Zeman FD, Rodstein M (1960) Cardiac rupture complicating myocardial infarction in the aged. *Arch Int Med* 105: 121–132.
2. Lewis AJ, Burchell HB, Titus JL (1969) Clinical and pathologic features of postinfarction cardiac rupture. *Am J Cardiol* 23: 43–53.
3. Naeim F, De la Moza LM, Robbins SL (1972) Cardiac rupture during myocardial infarction: A review of 44 cases. *Circulation* 45: 1231–1239.
4. Bates RJ, Beutler S, Reskenov L, Anagnastopoulos CE (1977) Cardiac rupture-challenge in diagnosis and management. *Am J Cardiol* 40: 429–437.
5. Windsor HM, Chang VP, Shanahan MX (1982) Postinfarction cardiac rupture. *J Thorac Cardiovasc Surg* 84: 755–761.
6. Desoutter P, Halphen C, Haiat R (1984) Two-dimensional echocardiographic visualization of free ventricular wall rupture in acute myocardial infarction. *Am Heart J* 108: 1360–1361.
7. Hochreiter C, Goldstein J, Borer JS, Tyberg T, Goldberg HL, Subramanian V, Rosenfeld I (1982) Myocardial free-wall rupture after acute infarction: Survival aided by percutaneous intra-aortic balloon counterpulsation. *Circulation* 65: 1279–1282.
8. Balakumaran K, Verbaan CJ, Essed CE, Nauta J, Bos E, Haalebos MMP, Penn O, Simoons ML, Hugenholtz PG (1984) Ventricular free wall rupture: Sudden, subacute, slow, sealed and stabilized varieties. *Eur Heart J* 5: 282–288.
9. Hagemeijer F, Verbaan CJ, Sonke PCF, de Rooy CH (1980) Echocardiography and rupture of the heart. *Br Heart J* 43: 45–46.
10. Qureshi SA, Rissen T, Gray KE (1982) Survival after subacute cardiac rupture. *Br Heart J* 47: 180–182.
11. Matangi MF, Norris RM, Hill DG (1983) Subacute cardiac rupture: A surgical emergency. *NZ Med J* 96: 1003–1005.
12. Hermoni Y, Engel PJ (1986) Two-dimensional echocardiography in cardiac rupture. *Am J Cardiol* 57: 180–181.
13. Schiller NB, Botvinick (1977) Right ventricular compression as a sign of cardiac tamponade. *Circulation* 56: 774–779.
14. Armstrong WF, Schilt BF, Helper DJ, Dillon JC, Feigenbaum H (1982) Diastolic collapse of the right ventricle with cardiac tamponade: An echocardiographic study. *Circulation* 65: 1491–1496.
15. Gillam LD, Guyer DE, Gibson TC, King ME, Marshall JE, Weyman AE (1983) Hydrodynamic compression of the right atrium: A new echocardiographic sign of cardiac tamponade. *Circulation* 68: 294–301.
16. Kronzon I, Cohen ML, Winer HE (1983) Diastolic atrial compression: A sensitive echocardiographic sign of cardiac tamponade *J Am Coll Cardiol* 2: 770–775.
17. Fast J, Wielenga RP, Janssen E, Schuurmans Stekhoven JH (1986) Abnormal wall movements of the right ventricle and both atria in patients with pericardial effusion as indicators of cardiac tamponade. *Eur Heart J* 7: 431–436.
18. Vlodaver Z, Coe JI, Edwards JE (1975) True and false aneurysms: Propensity of the latter to rupture. *Circulation* 51: 567–72.
19. Roelandt J, Brand M vd, Vletter WB, Nauta J, Hugenholtz PG (1975) Echocardiographic diagnosis of pseudoaneurysm of the left ventricle. *Circulation* 52: 466–472.
20. Morcerf FP, Duarte EP, Salcedo EE, Siegel W (1976) Echocardiographic findings in false aneurysm of the left ventricle. *Cleve Clin Q* 43: 71–76.
21. Sears TD, Ong YS, Starke H, Forker AD (1979) Left ventricular pseudoaneurysm identified by cross-sectional echocardiography. *Ann Int Med* 90: 935–936.
22. Katz RJ, Simpson A, DiBianco R, Fletcher RD, Bates HR, Sauerbrunn BJL (1979) Noninvasive diagnosis of left ventricular pseudoaneurysm. *Am J Cardiol* 44: 372–377.
23. Catherwood E, Mintz GS, Kother MN, Parry WR, Segal BL (1980) Two-dimensional echocardiographic recognition of left ventricular pseudoaneurysm. *Circulation* 60: 294–303.

24. Gatewood RP, Nanda NC (1980) Differentiation of left ventricular pseudoaneurysm from true aneurysm with two dimensional echocardiography. *Am J Cardiol* 46: 869–878.

25. Zijlstra F, Roelandt J (1985) The left ventricular false aneurysm. *Ned Tijdschr Geneesk* 129: 1473–1478.

26. Brabandt H v, Piessens J, Stalpeart J, de Geest H (1985) Pseudoaneurysm of the left ventricle following cardiac surgery. Report of 3 cases and review of the literature. *Thor Cardiovasc Surg* 33: 118–124.

27. Roelandt JRTC, Sutherland GR, Yoshida K, Yoshikawa J (1988) Improved diagnosis and characterisation of left ventricular pseudoaneurysm by Doppler colour flow imaging. *J Am Coll Cardiol* 85: 807–811.

28. Sutherland GR, Smyllie JH, Roelandt JTC (1989) Advantages of colour flow imaging in the diagnosis of left ventricular pseudoaneurysm. *Br Heart J* 61: 59–64.

29. Moore CA, Nygaard TW, Kaiser DL, Cooper AA, Gibson RS (1986) Postinfarction ventricular septal rupture: The importance of location of infarction and right ventricular function in determining survival. *Circulation* 74: 45–55.

30. Scanlan JG, Seward JB, Tajik AJ (1979) Visualization of ventricular septal rupture utilizing wide-angle two-dimensional echocardiography. *Mayo Clin Proc* 54: 381–384.

31. Bishop HL, Gibson RS, Stamm RB, Bellen GA, Martin RP (1981) Role of two-dimensional echocardiography in the evaluation of patients with ventricular septal rupture postmyocardial infarction. *Am Heart J* 102: 965–971.

32. Mintz GS, Victor MF, Kotler MN, Parry WR, Segal BL (1981) Two-dimensional echocardiographic identification of surgically correctable complications of acute myocardial infarction. *Circulation* 64: 91–96.

33. Drobac M, Gilbert B, Howard R, Baigrie R, Rakowski H (1983) Ventricular septal defect after myocardial infarction: Diagnosis by two-dimensional contrast echocardiography. *Circulation* 67: 335–341.

34. Rogers EW, Glassman RD, Feigenbaum H, Weyman AE, Godley RW (1980) Aneurysms of the posterior interventricular septum with postinfarction ventricular septal defect. *Chest* 78: 741–746.

35. Stephens JD, Giles MR, Banim SO (1981) Ruptured postinfarction ventricular septal aneurysm causing chronic congestive cardiac failure. *Br Heart J* 46: 216–219.

36. Hodsden J, Nanda NC (1981) Dissecting aneurysm of the ventricular septum following acute myocardial infarction: Diagnosis by real time two-dimensional echocardiography. *Am Heart J* 101: 671–672.

37. Meltzer RS, Schwartz J, French J, Popp RL (1979) Ventricular septal defect noted by two-dimensional echocardiography. *Chest* 76: 455–457.

38. Farcot JC, Boisante L, Rigaud M, Bardet J, Bourdarius JP (1980) Two-dimensional echocardiographic visualization of ventricular septal rupture after acute anterior myocardial infarction. *Am J Cardiol* 45: 370–377.

39. Recusani F, Raisaro A, Sgalambro A, Tronconi L, Venco A, Salerno J, Ardissino D (1984) Ventricular septal rupture after myocardial infarction: Diagnosis by two-dimensional and pulsed Doppler echocardiography. *Am J Cardiol* 54: 277–281.

40. Keren G, Sherez J, Roth A, Miller H, Laniado S (1984) Diagnosis of ventricular septal rupture from acute myocardial infarction by combined 2-dimensional and pulsed Doppler echocardiography. *Am J Cardiol* 53: 1202–1203.

41. Miyatake K, Okamoto M, Kinoshita N, Park YD, Nagata S, Izumi S, Fusejima K, Sakakibara H, Nimura Y (1985) Doppler echocardiographic features of ventricular septal rupture in myocardial infarction. *J Am Coll Cardiol* 5: 182–187.

42. Smith G, Endresen K, Swersstsen E, Semb G (1985) Ventricular septal rupture diagnosed by simultaneous cross-sectional echocardiography and Doppler ultrasound. *Eur Heart J* 6: 631–636.

43. Smyllie JH, Dawkins K, Conway N, Sutherland GR (1989) The diagnosis of ventricular septal defect following myocardial infarction: the value of colour flow mapping. *Br Heart J* 62: 260–7.

44. Kaplan MA, Harris CN, Kay JH, Parker DP, Magidson O (1976) Postinfarction ventricular septal rupture. Clinical approach and surgical results. *Chest* 69: 734–738.
45. Koenig K, Kasper W, Hofman T, Meinertz T, Just H (1987) Transesophageal echocardiography for the diagnosis of rupture of the ventricular septum or left ventricular papillary muscle rupture during myocardial infarction. *Am J Cardiol* 59: 362.
46. Wei JY, Hutchins GM, Bulkley BH (1979) Papillary muscle rupture in fatal acute myocardial infarction: A potentially treatable form of cardiogenic shock. *Ann Intern Med* 90: 149–152.
47. Nishimura RA, Schaff HV, Shub C, Gersh BJ, Edwards WD, Tajik AJ (1983) Papillary muscle rupture complicating acute myocardial infarction: Analysis of 17 patients. *Am J Cardiol* 51: 373–377.
48. Erbel R, Schweizer P, Bardos P, Meyer J (1981) Two-dimensional echocardiographic diagnosis of papillary muscle rupture. *Chest* 79: 595–598.
49. Scully RE, Mark EJ, McNeely BU (1982) Case records of the Massachusetts General Hospital. *N Engl J Med* 307: 873–880.
50. Come PC, Riley MF, Weintraub R, Morgan JP, Nakao S (1985) Echocardiographic detection of complete and partial papillary muscle rupture during acute myocardial infarction. *Am J Cardiol* 56: 787–789.
51. Ballester M, Foale R, Presbitero P, Yacoub M, Rickards A, McDonald L (1983) Cross-sectional echocardiographic features of ruptured chordae tendineae. *Eur Heart J* 4: 795–802.
52. Godley RW, Wann LS, Rogers EW, Feigenbaum H, Weyman AE (1981) Incomplete mitral leaflet closure in patients with papillary muscle dysfunction. *Circulation* 3: 565–571.
53. Abbasi AS, Allen MW, DeCristofaro D, Ungar I (1980) Detection and estimation of the degree of mitral regurgitation by rangegated pulsed Doppler echocardiography. *Circulation* 61: 143–147.
54. Ascah KJ, Stewart WJ, Jiang L, Guerrero JL, Newell JB, Gillam LD, Weyman AE (1985) A Doppler two-dimensional echocardiographic method for quantitation of mitral regurgitation. *Circulation* 2: 377–383.
55. Veyrat C, Ameur A, Bas S, Lessana A, Abitbol G, Kalmanson D (1984) Pulsed Doppler echocardiographic indices for assessing mitral regurgitation. *Br Heart J* 51: 130–138.
56. Helmcke F, Nanda NC, Hsiung MC et al. (1987) Color Doppler assessment of mitral regurgitation with orthogonal planes. *Circulation* 75: 175–183.
57. Skoulas A, Beier RL (1967) Dissecting perforation of infarcted interventricular septum with associated posterior papillary muscle involvement. *Am J Med* 43: 461–464.
58. Rawlins MD, Medel D, Braimbridge MV (1972) Ventricular septal defect and mitral regurgitation secondary to myocardial infarction. *Br Heart J* 34: 322–324.
59. Fleming HA (1973) Ventricular septal defect and mitral regurgitation secondary to myocardial infarction. *Br Heart J* 35: 344–346.
60. Gowda KS, Loh CW, Roberts R (1976) The simultaneous occurrence of a ventricular septal defect and mitral insufficiency after myocardial infarction. *Am Heart J* 92: 234–236.
61. Zaidi SA (1977) The simultaneous occurrence of a ventricular septal defect and mitral insufficiency after myocardial infarction. *Am Heart J* 94: 538–539.
62. Radford MJ, Johnson RA, Daggett WM, Fallon JT, Buckley MJ, Gold HK, Leinbach R (1981) Ventricular septal rupture: A review of clinical and physiologic features and an analysis of survival. *Circulation* 3: 545–553.
63. Stevenson JG, Kawabori I, Guntheroth WG (1977) Differentiation of ventricular septal defects from mitral regurgitation by pulsed Doppler echocardiography. *Circulation* 56: 14–18.
64. Eisenberg PR, Barzilai B, Perez JE (1984) Noninvasive detection by Doppler echocardiography of combined septal rupture and mitral regurgitation in acute myocardial infarction. *J Am Coll Cardiol* 4: 617–620.
65. Hagen PT, Scholz DG, Edwards WP (1984) Incidence and size of patent foramen ovale during the first 10 decades of life: An autopsy study of 965 normal hearts. *Mayo Clin Proc* 59: 17–20.

66. Morris AL, Donen M (1978) Hypoxia and intracardiac right-to left shunt: Complicating inferior myocardial infarction with right ventricular extension. *Arch Intern Med* 138: 1405–1406.
67. Rietveld AP, Merrman L, Essed CE, Trimbos JB, Hagemeyer F (1983) Right to left shunt, with severe hypoxemia, at the atrial level in a patient with hemodynamically important right ventricular infarction. *J Am Coll Cardiol* 2: 776–779.
68. Meister SG, Grossmann W, Dexter L, Dalen JE (1972) Paradoxical embolism: Diagnosis during life. *Am J Med* 53: 292–298.
69. Manno BV, Bemis CE, Carver J, Mintz GS (1983) Right ventricular infarction complicated by right to left shunt. *J Am Coll Cardiol*: 554–557.
70. Bansal RC, Marsa RJ, Holland D, Bechler C, Gold PM (1985) Severe hypoxemia due to shunting through a patent foramen ovale: A correctable complication of right ventricular infarction. *J Am Coll Cardiol* 5: 188–192.
71. Weyman ES, Peskoe SM, Williams ES, Dillon JC, Feigenbaum H (1976) Detection of left ventricular aneurisms by cross-sectional echocardiography. *Circulation* 54: 936–944.
72. Visser CA, Kan G, David GK, Lie KI, Durrer D (1982) Echocardiographic-cineangiographic correlation in detecting left ventricular aneurysm: A prospective study of 422 patients. *Am J Cardiol* 50: 337–340.
73. Baur HR, Daniel JA, Nelson RR (1982) Detection of left ventricular aneurysm on two-dimensional echocardiography. *Am J Cardiol* 50: 191–196.
74. Arvan S, Badillo P (1985) Contractile properties of the left ventricle with aneurysm. *Am J Cardiol* 55: 338–341.
75. Visser CA, Kan G, Meltzer RS, Koolen JJ, Dunning AJ (1986) Incidence, timing and prognostic value of left ventricular aneurysm formation after myocardial infarction: A prospective, serial echocardiographic study of 158 patients. *Am J Cardiol* 57: 729–732.
76. Barrett MJ, Charuzi Y, Corday E (1980) Ventricular aneurysm: Cross-sectional echocardiographic approach. *Am J Cardiol* 46: 1133–1137.
77. Visser CA, Kan G, Meltzer RS, Moulyn AC, David GK, Dunning AJ (1985) Assessment of left ventricular aneurysm resectability by two-dimensional echocardiography. *Am J Cardiol* 56: 857–860.
78. Asinger RW, Mikell FL, Sharma B, Hodges M (1981) Observations on detecting left ventricular thrombus with two-dimensional echocardiography: Emphasis on avoidance of false positive diagnosis. *Am J Cardiol* 47: 145–156.
79. Visser CA, Kan G, David GK, Lie KI, Durrer D (1983) Two-dimensional echocardiography in the diagnosis of left ventricular thrombus. *Chest* 2: 228–232.
80. Visser CA, Kan G, Lie KI, Durrer D (1983) Left ventricular thrombus following acute myocardial infarction: A prospective serial echocardiographic study of 96 patients. *Eur Heart J* 4: 333–337.
81. Weinreich DJ, Burke JF, Pauletto FJ (1984) Left ventricular mural thrombi complicating acute myocardial infarction. *Ann Int Med* 100: 789–794.
82. Stratton JR, Lighty GW, Pearlman AS, Ritchie JL (1982) Detection of left ventricular thrombus by two-dimensional echocardiography: Sensitivity, specificity and causes of uncertainly. *Circulation* 6: 156–166.
83. Van Meurs-van Woezik H, Meltzer RS, Brand M vd, Essed CE, Michels RHM, Roelandt J (1980) Superiority of echocardiography over angiocardiography in diagnosing a left ventricular thrombus. *Chest* 3: 321–323.
84. Ezekowitz MD, Wilson DA, Smith EO, Burow RD, Harrison LH, Parker DE, Elkins RC, Peyton M, Taylor FB (1982) Comparison of indium-111 platelet scintigraphy and two-dimensional echocardiography in the diagnosis of left ventricular thrombi. *N Engl J Med* 306: 1509–1513.
85. Spirito P, Bellotti P, Chiarella F, Domenicucci S, Sementa A, Vecchio C (1985) Prognostic significance and natural history of left ventricular thrombi in patients with acute anterior myocardial infarction: A two-dimensional echocardiographic study. *Circulation* 72: 774–780.

86. Visser CA, Kan G, Meltzer RS, Lie KI, Durrer D (1984) Long-term follow-up of left ventricular thrombus after acute myocardial infarction. *Chest* 86: 532–536.
87. Johannessen KA, Nordrehaug JE, Lippe G vd (1984) Left ventricular thrombosis and cerebrovascular accident in acute myocardial infarction. *Br Heart J* 51: 553–556.
88. Asinger RW, Mikell FL, Elsperger J, Hodges M (1981) Incidence of left ventricular thrombosis after acute transmural myocardial infarction. *N Engl J Med* 305: 297–302.
89. Bhatnagar SK, Hudak A, Al-Yusuf AR (1985) Left ventricular thrombosis, wall motion abnormalities, and blood viscosity changes after first transmural anterior myocardial infarction. *Chest* 88: 40–44.
90. Visser CA, Kan G, Meltzer RS, Dunning AJ, Roelandt J (1985) Embolic potential of left ventricular thrombus after myocardial infarction: Two-dimensional echocardiographic study of 119 patients. *J Am Coll Cardiol* 5: 1276–1280.
91. Metzer RS, Visser CA, Kan G, Roelandt J (1984) Two-dimensional echocardiographic appearance of left ventricular thrombi with systemic emboli after myocardial infarction. *Am J Cardiol* 53: 1511–1513.
92. Lloret RL, Cortada X, Bradford J, Metz MN, Kinney EL (1985) Classification of left ventricular thrombi by their history of systemic embolization using pattern recognition of two-dimensional echocardiograms. *Am Heart J* 110: 761–765.
93. Come PC (1983) Transient right atrial thrombus during acute myocardial infarction: Diagnosis by echocardiography. *Am J Cardiol* 51: 1228–1229.
94. Stowers SA, Leiboff RH, Wasserman AG, Katz RJ, Bren GB, Hsu I (1983) Right ventricular thrombus formation in association with acute myocardial infarction: Diagnosis by 2-dimensional echocardiography. *Am J Cardiol* 52: 912–913.
95. Tenet W, Missri J, Clark B, Jaskolka D (1985) Right ventricular thrombus complicating right ventricular infarction. *J Cardiovasc Ultrasound* 4: 197–199.

17. Prognostic information obtained by 2D-echo-Doppler evaluation in acute myocardial infarction

CEES A. VISSER, BEN J. DELEMARRE
and AREND J. DUNNING

Introduction

The immediate and long-term prognosis of patients with acute myocardial infarction depends mainly on the extent of the infarcted myocardium. Although some prognostic information can be obtained from the M-mode echocardiogram by measurements of left ventricular internal dimensions and an abnormality in mitral valve closure [1], or by mapping the extent of left ventricular asynergy using multiple transducer positions [2], M-mode echocardiography remains a poor method for quantitating the involved myocardium due to the restricted field of vision.

Two-dimensional echocardiography is capable of displaying the contractile behavior of the entire left ventricle, however, and application in animals, in the late 1970s, to estimate infarct size, demonstrated a good correlation between the extent of abnormally moving myocardium and the histologically measured infarct size [3, 5]. It has also been possible to demonstrate pharmacologic alteration of infarct size in serial examinations [6]. In humans, infarcted areas can also be recognized and localized by two-dimensional echocardiography [7, 8], even in nontransmural infarction [9]. The correlative two-dimensional echocardiographic-pathologic study by Weiss et al. has shown that quantification of infarcted tissue is possible [10]. Other studies have correlated two-dimensional echocardiographic infarct size with scintigraphy [11] (both thallium 201 and technetium 99 m-pyrophosphate) and peak CK-MB values [12, 13], Table 1).

Animal studies, however, suggest that the extent of two-dimensional echocardiographic wall motion abnormalities exceeds pathologic infarct size because abnormally contracting myocardium may affect the function of adjacent normal myocardium. This non-ischemic dysfunction may partly be the result of a tethering effect [14]. Correlation with postmortem findings in humans has also shown that the degree of wall motion abnormality roughly correlates to the transmural extent of infarction [10]. Normal regional wall motion excludes transmural infarction but occasionally it may be associated

S. Iliceto et al. (eds.), Ultrasound in Coronary Artery Disease, 197–211.
© 1991 *Kluwer Academic Publishers.*

Table 1. Results of studies correlating two-dimensional echocardiographic infarct size with other methods of infarct quantification.

Author	No. of subjects	Echo method	Standard	r
Weiss et al. [10]	20	% a/dyskinesis	Pathology	0.90
Nixon et al. [11]	19	Segment core	Thallium 201	0.87
	21	Segment score	^{99m}Tc-PYP[a]	0.74
Visser et al. [12]	66	Asynergic area	Peak CK-MB	0.87
Visser et al. [13]	48	Asynergic area	Peak CK-MB	0.81

[a] Technetium 99m-pyrophosphate.

with subendocardial infarction. Regional akinesis or dyskinesis, on the other hand, usually signifies transmural extent of infarction.

It has recently been shown in animal studies, on the other hand, that regional thickening achieves better separation of normal from infarcted myocardium than wall motion analysis. Though zones adjacent to infarcted areas frequently show abnormal endocardial motion, they less often show systolic thinning [15, 16]. However, there is a poor correlation between the transmural extent of infarction and the percentage systolic thickening. Instead, a threshold phenomenon seems to exist: when less than 20% of the thickness in a given segment is infarcted, it shows reduced thickening. Systolic thinning is seen if infarction involves more than 20% of wall thickness. Above this value there is no correlation between the degree of systolic wall thinning and the transmural extent of infarction. Thus, regional wall thickening cannot be used to estimate histologic infarct size.

In humans, wall motion abnormalities also tend to exceed, by approximately 14%, the amount of myocardial circumference involved by injury. Notwithstanding this, the severity of left ventricular dysfunction can be assessed using quantitative or semiquantitative methods, and has been shown to correlate with clinical signs of pump failure and risk of death.

Two-dimensional echocardiography and pump failure

Using a wall motion scoring system Hegar et al. [17] were the first who measured left ventricular dysfunction by two-dimensional echocardiography. Of 44 patients with acute transmural infarction, 39 could be studied adequately. The left ventricle was divided into 9 segments. Normokinesis was graded 0, hypokinesis 1, akinesis 2, and dyskinesis 3, whereas hyperkinesis was assigned −1. All segmental values were summed and the result was divided by the number of segments to give the wall motion score index. The results were correlated with Forrester class [18]: patients with signs of pulmonary congestion (class II) had higher wall motion score indexes than did patients without (class I); patients with signs of peripheral hypoperfusion (class III) or a combination of hypoperfusion and congestion (class IV) had even higher values.

Gibson et al. [19] studied 75 patients with acute myocardial infarction. In 59 patients, all 11 left ventricular segments could be evaluated, using the scoring system of Hegar et al. [17] described above. Of all 825 segments (75×11), 795 (96%) could be assessed. The wall motion score index showed, in relation to admission Killip class, an increase from 1.08 ± 0.38, class I, to 1.79 ± 0.10, class IV. However, one patient from class I and 8 patients from class II subsequently developed cardiogenic shock, and these patients had higher wall motion score indexes than the patients who showed no hemodynamic deterioration. Because the echocardiograms were obtained a mean of 7.9 ± 3.1 h (SD) after admission, bad risk patients could be identified early. These authors developed a discriminant function analysis, incorporating admission Killip class (I or II) and wall motion score index, that was able to predict correctly whether development of cardiogenic shock would occur in 91% of cases. Age, previous infarction, infarct site, peak CK-MB level, and roentgenographic findings did not provide a significant additional contribution to the prediction of cardiogenic shock.

Nishimura and co-workers [20] also showed a correlation between a wall motion score index and admission Killip class in a study of 61 patients with acute infarction undergoing echocardiographic examination with 12 h from admission and within 24 h from the onset of symptoms. Their scoring system used a number of 14 segments and a scale ranging from 0 for hyperkinesis through +4 for dyskinesis, with an extension to +5 for aneurysmal deformation. Again a wall motion score index was obtained by dividing the summed segmental scores by the number of segments visualized. These authors found significantly higher wall motion score indexes in patients developing congestive heart failure than in those without (2.4 ± 0.5 versus 1.6 ± 0.5), and in patients with ventricular arrhythmias and those without (2.4 ± 0.5 versus 1.8 ± 0.6).

Only little change is known to occur in the extent of asynergy over the first days of infarction [12, 20]. Even between wall motion score indexes obtained on the first day(s) and predischarge there is little change [20, 21]. Thus, a strong case can be made for early echocardiography in acute infarction. We confirmed this in a study of 90 patients with acute infarction, studied within 24 h from admission [22]. Patients were grouped according to worst Killip class during hospital stay (Figure 1). There was a progressive decline in ejection fraction, the higher the Killip class was. All 6 patients developing cardiogenic shock were only in class I or II on admission, again underlining the potential of early echocardiography in recognizing these patients, who subsequently died. Using an ejection fraction of 30% or less as a cutoff value, sensitivity was 4/6 (67%) and specificity 82 (92%).

More recently, Jaarsma et al. [23] compared admission values of a wall motion score and hemodynamic monitoring in 77 patients without clinical signs of heart failure. Progression into Killip class III or IV was found in 16 of

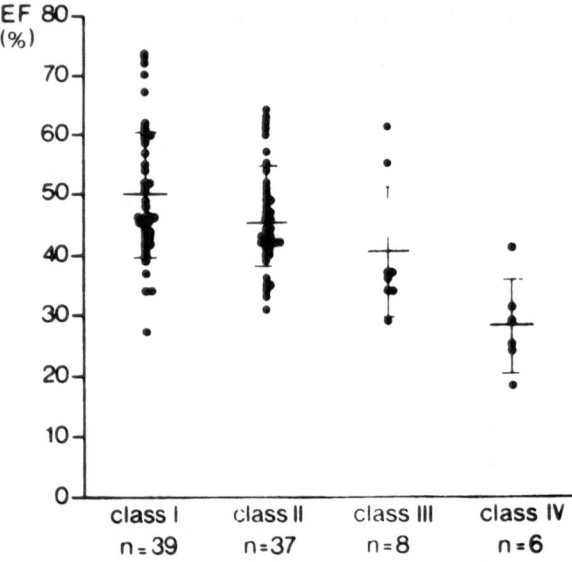

Figure 1. Diagram showing two-dimensional echocardiographically derived left ventricular ejection fraction (EF) according to Killip class.

77 patients (21%) within 32 ± 6 h after admission. Mean wall motion score, left ventricular stroke work index, and pulmonary capillary pressure in those 16 patients were significantly different from those who did not develop severe pump failure. A wall motion score of >7 and stroke work index of <35 gm/m^2 had a sensitivity of 88% and 94%, respectively, in predicting the development of Killip class III or IV, and a specificity of 57% and 87%, respectively. This underlines the value of early two-dimensional echocardiography, once again, for identification of low-risk patients.

In-hospital mortality

Studies employing wall motion scores obtained from echocardiograms recorded during the first day(s) of infarction show that it is possible to separate a group with a high (all cause) mortality. The results of these studies are summarized in Table 2.

Van Reet et al. [21] performed echocardiography in 93 patients within 48 h of admission. Their scoring system used 13 segments (4 walls divided into thirds + the apex) and a scale ranging from +4 for hyperkinesis to −1 for dyskinesis. The scoring system used by Nishimura et al. [20] has been described above. Our group used a 13-segment score (6 walls divided into halves + the apex) with a grading system ranging from − for hyperkinesis to +3 for dyskinesis and +4 for aneurysm [24]. Echoes were obtained within 12 h from admission.

Table 2. Studies using wall motion score indices (WMSI) to predict in-hospital death.

Author	Time (h)	n	WMSI value	Cutoff value	Sensi-tivity	Specif-icity	Predictive value		
							Positive	Negative	Overall
Nishimura et al. [20]	<12	61	1	≤2.0	10/12 (83%)	32/49 (65%)	10/27 (37%)	32/34 (94%)	42/61 (69%)
Van Reet et al. [21]	<48	93	1[a]	≥0.5[a]	10/12 (83%)	67/81 (83%)	10/25 (40%)	67/68 (98%)	77/93 (83%)
Kan et al. [22]	<12	90	0	≤0.77	27/31 (87%)	241/314 (76%)	27/100 (27%)	241/245 (98%)	268/345 (78%)

[a] Scale reversed.

It appears that even semiquantitative assessment of left ventricular function is quite sensitive for *in-hospital* mortality, but positive predictive value (or the chance that a patient with a bad left ventricle will die) is disappointing at first sight. However, when the patients who are classified as false positives as to *in-hospital* mortality remain bad risks in that they show a high 1-year mortality (see below). Even so, an analysis of wall motion score values according to the cause of death shows that by far the highest values were obtained in those patients who died from cardiogenic shock; patients dying from ruptures had significantly lower wall motion scores (see Table 3). Especially in ventricular septal rupture or papillary muscle rupture, the infarct may be only modest or small, and these patients die 'by accident' rather than from the extent of left ventricular damage. Only in a few of these patients, where rupture was present on admission, decreased afterload may have resulted in reactive segmental hyperkinesis, yielding spuriously low wall motion score values.

Segmental hyperkinesis may provide prognostic information as well, as does remote asynergy of the non-infarcted myocardium. Jaarsma et al. [25] studied 113 patients during the early hours after onset of isolated, acute infarction, and found that regional hyperkinesis was more frequently seen in patients with one- and 2-vessel coronary artery disease than in patients with

Table 3. Wall motion score (WMS) of patients dying in hospital in the study by Kan et al. [24] according to cause of death.

Cause of death	n	WMS	
Primary cardiogenic shock	15	19.2 ± 4.2	p < 0.05
All ruptures	16	13.5 ± 6.1	
Free wall rupture	9	15.7 ± 6.9	p < 0.05
VSR or PSR[a]	7	8.5 ± 5.3	

[a] PSR, papillary muscle rupture; and VSR, ventricular septal rupture.

Table 4. Regional hyperkinesis and remote asynergy in relation to peak creatine kinase-MB, wall motion scorek, myocardial infarct site and mortality [25].

	Regional hyperkinesis				Remote asynergy			
	Present (n = 66)			Absent (n = 32)	Present (n = 32)			Absent (n = 81)
CK-MB (U/l)	142 ± 83		NS	118 ± 96	166 ± 87		NS	128 ± 87
WMS	7.5 ± 6		*	11.6 ± 8	15 ± 5		*	7.5 ± 7
Site AMI								
Anterior	44			21	11			54
Inferior	22			11	6			27
Mortality	5 (7.5%)		**	15 (47%)	9 (53%)			11 (14%)

* p < 0.01; ** p < 0.001.
AMI = acute myocardial infarction; NS = not significant; WMS = wall motion score.

3-vessel coronary disease (87 and 72% versus 25%, p < 0.001) (Table 4). In addition, absence of this type of wall motion pattern was significantly associated with a higher wall motion score.

Absence of regional hyperkinesis, in particular in anterior infarcts, was associated with a higher mortality rate, 13 of 19 patients (68%). Asynergy not adjacent to the infarct area and supposed to be related to another vascular region, i.e. remote asynergy, was only present in patients with multivessel disease and was highly related to a higher wall motion score. Also, the presence of remote asynergy was associated with a higher mortality rate, 9 of 17 patients (53%). This in keeping with Gibson et al. [19], who demonstrated that wall motion abnormalities outside the infarct zone was correlated with a higher prevalence of cardiogenic shock, postinfarction angina, reinfarction and death.

Purely quantitative measurements of left ventricular function (i.e. ejection fraction) were used in two studies, one being the study by Van Reet et al. [21] and another performed at our own institution [22]. The former study used a cutoff value of < 35% and the latter study a value of < 30%. This resulted in a higher sensitivity of 83% versus 45%, but in a lower specificity, 77% versus 97%. The greater number of false positives also resulted in a lower figure for positive predictive value, 37% versus 71%, whereas the smaller number of false negatives improved negative predictive value, 97% versus 93%.

Out-of-hospital mortality

Two studies already addressed in the foregoing have dealt with total 1-year (in-hospital + postdischarge) mortality as well, using scores from early two-dimensional echocardiograms. Using a wall motion score index Kan et al. [24] demonstrated a sensitivity, specificity and overall predictive value to predict total one-year mortality of 88%, 86% and 86%, respectively, and Van Reet et al. [21] values of 60%, 85% and 78%, respectively. It appears that patients with severely damaged left ventricles may survive to be discharged from hospital, but still remain at high risk of later death.

Prehospital discharge echocardiography has also been used to detect these high-risk patients. The scoring system employed by Bhatnagar et al. [26], is identical to that of Gibson et al. [19] (11 segments; 0 for normokinesis, +1 for hypokinesis, +2 for akinesis, and +3 for dyskinesis). Follow-up was 5–31 months (mean, 17 months). There were 7 deaths. Using a wall motion score of 8 or more as indicating high risk, all deaths could be predicted (sensitivity, 100%). Specificity was 31/40 (77%). Positive predictive value was 7/16 or 44%, negative predictive value 31/31 (100%), and overall predictive value 38/47 (81%).

In another study by Nishimura et al. [27] of 46 patients undergoing pre-discharge echocardiography, the wall motion score index was significantly higher in patients with complications during a follow-up of 15–28 months (mean, 21 months) than in those without. Complications were death (3 patients), recurrent infarction, congestive heart failure (NYHA class III or IV), and angina (NYHA class III or IV).

Natural history of wall motion abnormalities

We followed the asynergic area over the first 3 days of infarction and found a small increase (worsening) of 0.5 ± 0.2 percentage units between days 1 and 2 [12]. Although statistically significant at the 0.05 level, clinically, with admission values ranging from 0 to 63%, this was of no significance.

Van Reet et al. [21] found a small increase (which in their study means improvement) in wall motion score index between early (with 48 h) and late (approximately 10 days) studies, from 0.74 ± 0.21 to 0.78 ± 0.19 in patients with first infarction. In patients with multiple infarctions, no change occurred. Initially hypokinetic segments showed improvement in 30% of cases and deterioration in 4%. Initially akinetic segments improved in 26% of cases. Normokinetic or hyperkinetic segments remained normal in over 90%.

Kumar et al. [28] using a 17-segment model and a six-point scale (ranging from +1 for dyskinesis through +6 for hyperkinesis), studied 17 infarct patients on days 1, 2, 3 and 5 of their infarction, and at the end of weeks 1, 2, 3, 4, 6 and 8. In 5 of these patients, wall motion abnormalities showed complete normalization after periods of 2–8 weeks. Improvement in wall motion, defined arbitrarily as an increase of two or more points in at least two adjacent segments, occurred in another 5.

We studied changes in ejection fraction between day 1 and day 3 in 30 patients, and between day 1 and 3 months in 35 patients (groups I and II, respectively) [29]. In group I, ejection fraction showed only little change: from $46.7 \pm 9.5\%$ to $49.8 \pm 10.8\%$. When a change of more than 5% (percentage units) is arbitrarily taken as significant, 16 patients were stable. In none of these were complications seen. Likewise, no complications occurred in four patients whose ejection fractions showed decreases between 5 and 10 percentage units. Only two patients showed decreases of more than 10% units (−16% and −12%, respectively). Both had enzymatically confirmed infarct extensions. Increases between 5% and 10% units were seen in 6 patients, and ejection fraction increased by more than 10% units in two (one of the latter two being in pulmonary edema on admission).

In group II ejection fraction was $49.8 \pm 10.8\%$ on day 1 and $46.1 \pm 12.0\%$ (not significant) at 3 months. Only 10 patients showed no 'significant' change. Decrease of between 5% and 10% units occurred in 4 patients, who had an uneventful course. Decreases of more than 10% units were encountered in 11 patients: one had a perioperative infarct, two had enzymatically confirmed reinfarction, 4 had only possible reinfarction (recurrent pain, but no enzymatic confirmation), two developed aneurysms; and two had an uneventful course. However, increases between 5% and 10% units were found in 6 patients: of these, one had an enzymatically confirmed (but small) reinfarction, one developed an angiographically confirmed (but circumscript) aneurysm, and one underwent uneventful bypass surgery for postinfarctional angina. Four patients whose ejection fraction increased more than 10% units had an uneventful course. Thus, even fairly large changes in ejection fraction may occur without complications.

Improvement of contraction abnormalities is likely to be due to improvement of ischemia. Deterioration may be due to reinfarction, silent reinfarction, infarct expansion, or aneurysm formation. Formal assessments of reproducibility by our group [30] and by Gordon et al. [31] in patients with stable coronary artery disease have suggested that ejection fraction changes should amount to 7 or more % units to be considered significant.

Regional left ventricular enlargement

Using serial two-dimensional echocardiography Eaton et al. [32] were the first who demonstrated that regional left ventricular dilation early occurs, and exclusively following anterior infarction. Using a cross-section at the level of the papillary muscles they noted, during the first 2 weeks following infarction, in 6 patients a disproportionate dilation and thinning of the infarct zone which was progressive during this limited follow-up. This regional 'expansion' led to an overall left ventricular enlargement of 25% in these 8 patients compared to 5% in the 20 patients without infarct expansion. In addition, the eight-week mortality was significantly greater in the 8 patients with early regional dilation (4/8), than in those without (0/20). Peak CK-MB levels, however, were not different among these 2 patient groups.

More recently, we found in a prospective study that patients, developing an aneurysm during the acute phase on the coronary care unit (Figure 2), all had anterior infarcts which were biochemically not larger than infarcts leading to aneurysm later, on i.e. after the acute episode [33]. In accord with Eaton et al.

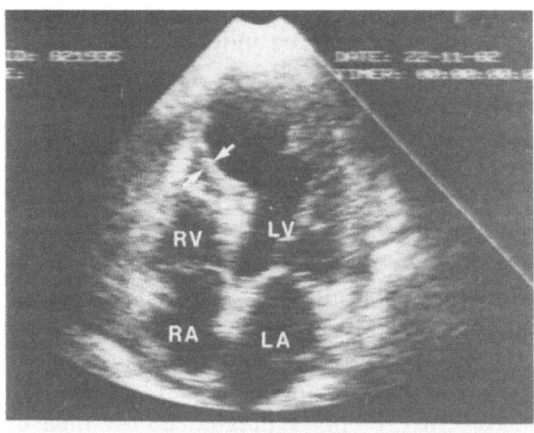

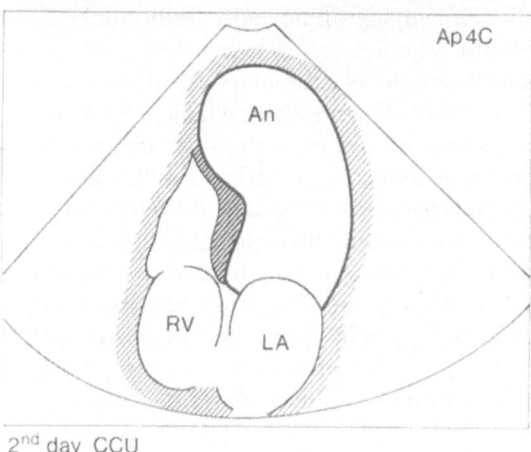

Figure 2. End-diastolic still frame of an apical 4-chamber view obtained on the second day in the coronary care unit in patient with an acute anterior wall infarction and early formation of an aneurysm. There is marked distortion of the apicoseptal area with apparent wall thinning (arrows).

[32] we also found a high early mortality of 67% during the first 3 months in these patients.

Using radionuclide angiography Meitish et al. [34] studied 51 patients with transmural anterior infarction and also found, that the one-year mortality in the patients who developed an early (within 48 h) 'functional aneurysm' was significantly higher than in the patients who did not, 11/18 (61%) versus 3/33 (9%). Furthermore, they found that formation of a functional aneurysm had equal sensitivity and far better specificity and positive predictive accuracy for mortality than left ventricular ejection fraction. With either <30% or "35% used as the cutoff point. Thus, early formation of an aneurysm following infarction occurs after anterior infarction and carries a high risk of death within one year that appears to be independent of left ventricular ejection fraction.

Doppler echocardiography

Diastolic and systolic parameters

Parameters of left ventricular inflow as assessed by radionuclide angiography, such as peak filling rate, have been demonstrated to be subnormal in coronary heart disease, cardiomyopathy and hypertension [35–37]. Doppler echocardiography is another method that can be used to assess left ventricular inflow [38]. Recently, Doppler derived inflow measurements have been correlated with cineangiographic and radionuclide angiographic filling parameters [39, 40]. The left ventricular inflow pattern assessed with pulsed Doppler echocardiography is characterized by two waves: an early (E) wave due to relaxation of the left ventricle and a late (A) wave due to atrial contraction. In absence of mitral valve or aortic valve disease, left ventricular diastolic properties can be estimated by ventricular filling characteristics.

In aging, hypertension, hypertrophic cardiomyopathy, coronary artery disease, and in acute experimental myocardial ischemia, the E-wave velocity may be decreased and the A-wave velocity increased, due to reduced left ventricular compliance [41–46] (Figure 3). As in acute myocardial infarction impairment of left ventricular systolic function is proportionally to infarct size [47], we investigated the potential prognostic value of the E/A ratio as a simple indicator of left ventricular filling abnormalities in acute myocardial infarction.

To this end, we studied 60 selected patients with first acute transmural myocardial infarction and no previous hypertension, by pulsed Doppler echocardiography shortly after admission. The Doppler sample volume was placed at the level of the mitral valve annulus in the apical 4-chamber view.

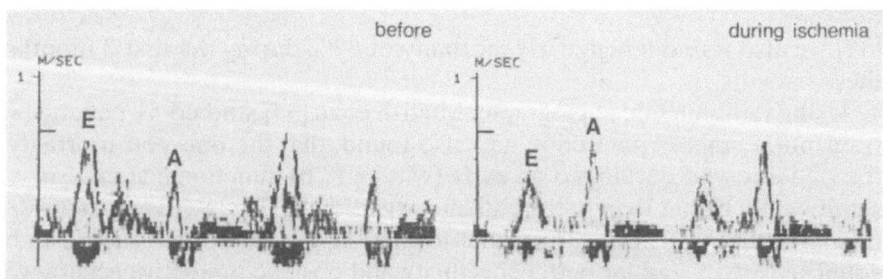

Figure 3. Transmitral flow recordings obtained in an open-chest dog. Occlusion of the left anterior descending artery results in a shift of diastolic filling from early to late diastole (B), and hence decreases the E/A ratio.

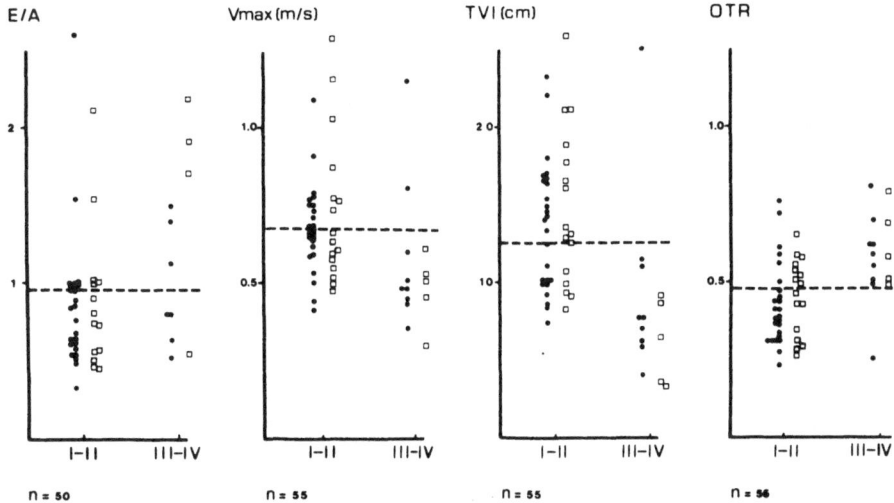

Figure 4. Graphic representation of diastolic and systolic function parameters. Patients with a first infarction (black dots) and previous infarction (open squares) are arranged according to the clinical course. Killip class I and II, mild pump failure and Killip class III and IV, severe pump failure. The mean values of the entire group (dashed lines) were used as cut off values: E/A 0.96, Vmax 66 cm/sec, TVI 12.6 cm and OTR 0.48. n: Numbers of patients in whom a pulsed Doppler signal adequate for analysis was obtained. Other abbreviations as in Table 5.

Table 5. Sensitivity, specificity and positive predictive value of pulsed Doppler derived parameters in identifying acute infarct patients with a mild clinical course [49].

	Sensitivity (%)	Specificity (%)	Pos. pred. value (%)
E/A $\geqslant$ 0.96	36	45	70
Vmax $\geqslant$ 66 cm/s	49	86	91
TVI $\geqslant$ 12.6 cm	59	93	96
OTR $\leqslant$ 0.48	66	93	96

E/A: Peak velocity early (E) inflow wave to peak velocity atrial (A) inflow wave ratio.
Vmax: Maximal velocity of the systolic outflow wave at aortic valve annulus level.
TVI: Time velocity integral of the outflow wave at aortic valve annulus level.
OTR: Outflow tract ratio.

Measurements obtained from 5 cardiac cycles were averaged. Results were correlated with worst Killip class during hospital stay and with mortality.

There was a significant downward trend in the E/A ratio with increasing severity of pump failure, with reversal of the inflow pattern from early to late diastole [48]. The E/A ratio showed a loose but significant correlation with the peak CK-MB value as a biochemical indicator of infarct size (r = 0.65). Again the patients who subsequently developed cardiogenic shock, were only in Killip class I or II on admission. However, we studied more recently an unselected group of patients with first and recurrent myocardial infarction and previous hypertension, and found that the E/A ratio was not of value to identify patients with mild and severe pump failure during subsequent clinical course [49] (Figure 4, Table 5). On the other hand, systolic function parameters such as maximal velocity at the level of the aortic valve annulus and time velocity integral, as well as an outflow tract ratio, i.e. parameter of the functional length of the left ventricular outflow tract, were capable to identify, on admission, patients with subsequent mild clinical course and low mortality (Table 5).

Apical flow pattern

Based on pulsed Doppler recordings made in patients with coronary artery disease, two abnormal apical flow patterns have been recognized that may exist separately or together. Range ambiguity recordings from the apical and mitral valve levels may show, in patients with dilated left ventricles, a delay in onset of blood motion at the apical level; the mitral valve inflow signal consistently precedes the apical signal (Figure 5B), [50]. The delay between onset of the curve from the secondary sample volume (mitral valve) and the motion at the level of the primary sample volume (apex) is consistent with the presence of a 'vortex ring' and reflects the time necessary for this vortex ring to travel from mitral valve level to apical level.

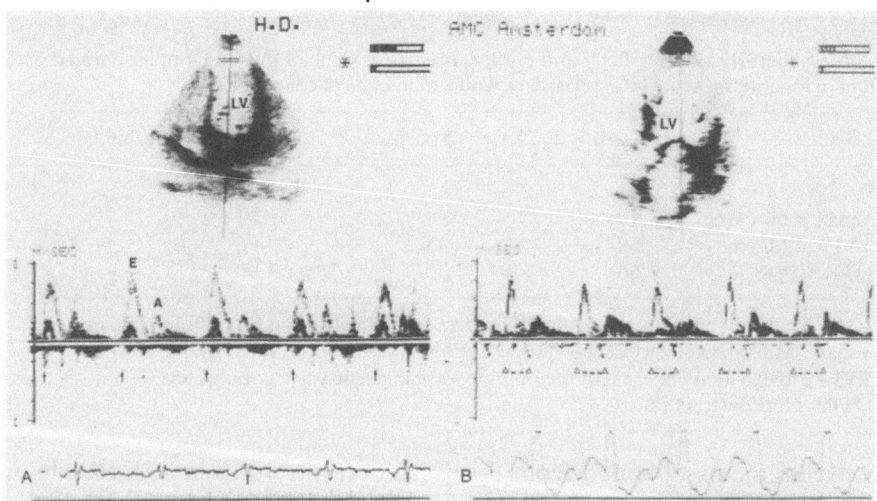

Figure 5(A). Apical 4-chamber view with the sample volume positioned at the level of the apex. Using a high pulse repetition frequency (13.3 KHz) simultaneous flow recording is obtained at the level of the mitral valve leaflets, displaying the early peak flow velocity *(E)* and atrial peak flow velocity *(A)*. There is no delay in onset of both flow recordings (see arrows), in this normal person. LV = left ventricle.
Figure 5(B). This Figure demonstrates an obvious delay (distance between open triangles) between these 2 signals, which were obtained in a patient who sustained multiple infarctions leading to global dilatation of the ventricle.

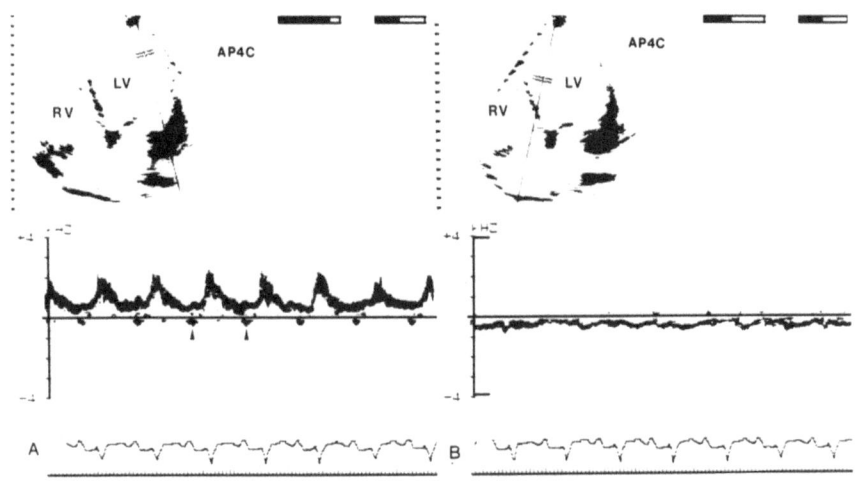

Figure 6(A). Pulsed Doppler recording of abnormal apical flow in the vicinity of the left ventricular free wall. The recording shows a continuous, i.e. during the whole cardiac cycle, positive Doppler shift.
Figure 6(B). Recording of abnormal flow near the interventricular septum. The recording shows a continuous negative signal. Figures 3A and 3B can be explained by a circular flow pattern to be present in the left ventricular apex. LV = left ventricle; RV = right ventricle; Ap 4c = apical 4 chamber view; Arrow heads = 'ghost' signal.

In addition, a circular apical flow pattern can also be found in dilated left ventricles using pulsed Doppler, i.e. a continuous, during entire cardiac cycle, a positive signal near the lateral wall and a continuous negative shift near the interventricular septum (Figure 6) [51]. This flow pattern can be associated with 'spontaneous' intracavitary dynamic echoes [52]. Absence of these abnormal apical flow patterns recently demonstrated a specificity of 84% and positive predictive value of 91% to identify acute infarct patients with subsequent mild clinical course [49]. Furthermore, absence of these flow patterns was never associated with thrombus formation during 3 months following infarction [53].

Conclusion

Two-dimensional echocardiography, and more recently Doppler ultrasound, may, in patients with acute myocardial infarction in its earliest stages, be used as instruments to identify patients at high risk of hemodynamic deterioration and death during the hospital phase and even thereafter. Its non-invasive character and easy applicability at the bedside make them low threshold investigations, the immediacy of its results make it possible to employ measures aimed at preventing subsequent deterioration.

210   C. A. Visser et al.

References

1. Corya BC, Rasmussen S, Knoebel SB, Feigenbaum H (1975) Echocardiography in acute myocardial infarction. *Am J Cardiol* 36: 1–10.
2. Heikkila J, Nieminen M (1975) Echoventriculographic detection, localization, and quantification of left ventricular asynergy in acute myocardial infarction: A correlative echo- and electrocardiographic study. *Br Heart J* 37: 46–59.
3. Weyman AE, Franklin TD, Egenes KM, Green D (1977) Correlation between extent of abnormal wall motion and myocardial infarct size in chronically infarcted dogs (abstracts). *Circulation* 56 (suppl 3): III–72.
4. Heng MK, Lang TW, Wyatt HL, Lee S, Corday E (1977) Quantification of myocardial ischemic damage by 2-dimensional echocardiography (abstracts). *Circulation* 56 (suppl 3): III–125.
5. Meltzer RS, Woythaler JN, Buda AJ, Popp RL (1980) Quantification of experimental canine myocardial infarct size by two-dimensional echocardiography. *Eur J Cardiol* 11: 215–225.
6. Meltzer RS, Buda AJ, Martin RP, Harrison DC, Popp RL (1979) Two-dimensional echocardiographic quantification of infarct size alteration by pharmacologic agents. *Am J Cardiol* 44: 257–262.
7. Hegar JJ, Weyman AE, Wann LS, Dillon JC, Feigenbaum H (1979) Cross-sectional echocardiography of regional left ventricular asynergy. *Circulation* 60: 531–538.
8. Horowitz RS, Morganroth J, Parrotto C, Chen CC, Soffer J, Pauletto FJ (1982) Immediate diagnosis of acute myocardial infarction by two-dimensional echocardiography. *Circulation* 65: 323–329.
9. Loh IK, Charuzi Y, Beeder C, Marshall LA, Ginsburg JH (1982) Early diagnosis of nontransmural myocardial infarction by two-dimensional echocardiography. *Am Heart J* 104: 963–968.
10. Weiss JL, Bulkley BH, Hutchins GM, Mason SJ (1981) Two-dimensional echocardiographic recognition of myocardial injury in man: Comparison with postmortem studies. *Circulation* 63: 401–408.
11. Nixon JV, Narahara KA, Smitherman TC (1980) Estimation of myocardial involvement in patients with acute myocardial infarction by two-dimensional echocardiography. *Circulation* 62: 1248–1255.
12. Visser CA, Lie KI, Kan G, Meltzer R, Durrer D (1981) Detection and quantification of acute, isolated myocardial infarction by two-dimensional echocardiography. *Am J Cardiol* 47: 1020–1025.
13. Visser CA, Lie KI, Kan G, Becker AE, Durrer D (1982) Apex two-dimensional echocardiography: Alternative approach to quantification of acute myocardial infarction. *Br Heart J* 47: 461–465.
14. Kerber RE, Marcus ML (1978) Evaluation of regional myocardial function in ischemic heart disease by echocardiography. *Prog Cardiovasc Dis* 20: 441–451.
15. Lieberman AN, Weiss JL, Jugdutt BI (1981) Two-dimensional echocardiography and infarct size: Relationship of regional wall motion and thickening to the extent of myocardial infarction in the dog. *Circulation* 63: 739–746.
16. Buda AJ, Zotz RJ, Pace DP, Krause LC (1986) Comparison of two-dimensional echocardiographic wall motion and wall thickening abnormalities in relation to the myocardium at risk. *Am Heart J* 111: 587–592.
17. Hegar JJ, Weyman AE, Wann S, Rogers EW, Dillon JC, Feigenbaum H (1980) Cross-sectional echocardiographic analysis of the extent of left ventricular asynergy in acute myocardial infarction. *Circulation* 61: 1113–1118.
18. Forrester JS, Diamond GA, Swan HJC (1977) Correlative classification of clinical and hemodynamic function after acute myocardial infarction. *Am J Cardiol* 39: 135–137.
19. Gibson RS, Bishop HL, Stamm RB, Crampton RS, Beller GA, Martin RP (1982) Value of

early two-dimensional echocardiography in patients with acute myocardial infarction. *Am J Cardiol* 49: 1110–1119.

20. Nishimura RA, Tajk AJ, Shub C, Miller FA Jr, Ilstrup DM, Harrison CE (1984) Role of two-dimensional echocardiography in the prediction of in-hospital complications after acute myocardial infarction. *J Am Coll Cardiol* 4: 1080–1087.
21. Van Reet RE, Quinones MA, Poliner LR, Nelson JG, Waggoner AD, Kanon D, Lubetkin SJ, Pratt CM, Winters WL Jr (1984) Comparison of two-dimensional echocardiography with gated radionuclide ventriculography in the evaluation of global and regional left ventricular function in acute myocardial infarction. *J Am Coll Cardiol* 3: 243–252.
22. Kan G, Visser CA, Lie KI, Durrer D (1984) Early two-dimensional echocardiographic measurement of left ventricular ejection fraction in acute myocardial infarction. *Eur Heart J* 5: 210–217.
23. Jaarsma W, Visser CA, Eenige MJ van, Verheugt FWA, Funke Kupper AJ, Roos JP (1988) Predictive value of two-dimensional echocardiographic and hemodynamic measurements on admission with acute myocardial infarction. *J Am Soc Echo*: 187–193.
24. Kan G, Visser CA, Meltzer RS, Koolen JJ, Dunning AJ (1986) Short- and long-term predictive value of admission wall motion score in acute myocardial infarction: A cross-sectional echocardiographic study of 345 patients. *Br Heart J* 56: 422–427.
25. Jaarsma W, Visser CA, Eenige MJ van, Bes J, Funke Kupper AJ, Verheught FWA, Roos JP (1986) Prognostic implications of regional hyperkinesia and remote asynergy of noninfarcted myocardium. *Am J Cardiol* 58: 394–398.
26. Bhatnagar SK, Moussa MAA, Al-Yusuf AR (1985) The role of prehospital discharge two-dimensional echocardiography in determining the prognosis of survivors of first myocardial infarction. *Am Heart J* 109: 472–477.
27. Nishimura RA, Reeder RS, Miller FA, Ilstrup DM, Shub C, Seward JB, Tajik AJ (1984) Prognostic value of predischarge 2-dimensional echocardiogram after acute myocardial infarction. *Am J Cardiol* 53: 429–435.
28. Kumar A, Minagoe S, Chandrazratna PAN (1986) Two-dimensional echocardiographic demonstration of restoration of normal wall motion after acute myocardiol infarction. *Am J Cardiol* 57: 1232–1236.
29. Kan G, Visser CA, Lie KI, Durrer D (1984) Measurement of left ventricular ejection fraction after acute myocardial infarction: A serial cross-sectional echocardiographic study. *Br Heart J* 51: 631–636.
30. Kan G, Visser CA, Lie KI, Durrer D (1984) Serial left ventricular ejection fraction in acute myocardial infarction by cross-sectional echocardiography: Correlation of changing ejection fraction with clinical course. *Eur Heart J* 5: 470–476.
31. Gordon EP, Schnittger I, Fitzgerald PJ, Williams P, Popp R (1983) Reproducibility of left ventricular volumes by two-dimensional echocardiography. *J Am Coll Cardiol* 2: 506–511.
32. Eaton LW, Weiss JL, Bulkley BH, Garrison JB (1979) Regional cardiac dilatation after acute myocardial infarction: Recognition by two-dimensional echocardiography. *N Engl J Med* 300: 57–64.
33. Visser CA, Kan G, Meltzer RS, Koolen JJ, Dunning AJ (1986) Incidence, timing and prognostic value of left ventricular aneurysm formation after myocardial infarction: A prospective, serial echocardiographic study of 158 patients. *Am J Cardiol* 57: 729–732.
34. Meizlish JL, Berger HJ, Plankey M, Errico D, Levy W, Zaret BL (1984) Functional left ventricular aneurysm formation after acute anterior transmural infarction. *New Engl J Med* 311: 1001–1006.
35. Bonow RO, Bacharach SL, Green MV, Kent KM, Rosing DR, Lipson LC, Leon MB, Epstein SE (1981) Impaired left ventricular diastolic filling in patients with coronary artery disease: Assessment with radionuclide angiography. *Circulation* 64: 315–323.
36. Bonow RO, Rosing DR, Bacharach SL, Green MV, Kent KM, Lipson LC, Maron BJ, Leon MB, Epstein SE (1981) Effects of verapamil on left ventricular systolic function and diastolic filling in patients with hypertrophic cardiomyopathy. *Circulation* 64: 787–796.

37. Inouye I, Massie B, Loge D, Topic N, Silverstein D, Simpson P, Tubdu J (1984) Abnormal left ventricular filling: An early finding in mild to moderate systemic hypertension. *Am J Cardiol* 53: 120–126.

38. Hatle L, Angelsen B (1985) *Doppler Ultrasound in Cardiology*, pp 78–79. Philadelphia: Lea & Febiger.

39. Rokey R, Kuo LC, Zoghbi WA, Limacher MC, Quinones MA (1984) Determination of parameters of left ventricular diastolic filling with pulsed Doppler echocardiography: Comparison with cineangiography. *Circulation* 71: 543–550.

40. Friedman B, Drinkovic N, Miles H, Stipp V, Mazzoleni A, De Maria AE (1985) Assessment of left ventricular diastolic function: Comparison of Doppler and blood pool scintigraphy. *Circulation* 72 (suppl 3): III–429.

41. Miyatake K, Okamoto M, Kinoshita N, Owa M, Nakasone I, Sakakibara H, Nimura Y (1984) Augmentation of atrial contribution to left ventricular inflow with aging as assessed by intracardiac Doppler flowmetry. *Am J Cardiol* 53: 586–589.

42. Bryg RJ, Williams GA, Labovitz AJ (1987) Effect of aging on left ventricular diastolic filling in normal subjects. *Am J Cardiol* 59: 971–974.

43. Kitabatake A, Inoue M, Asao M, Tanouchi J, Masuyama T, Aabe H, Morita H, Senda S, Matsuo H (1982) Transmitral blood flow reflecting diastolic behavior of the left ventricle in health and disease. A study by pulsed Doppler technique. *Jpn Circulation J* 46: 92–102.

44. Fujii J, Yazaki Y, Sawada H, Aizawa T, Watanabe H, Kato K (1985) Noninvasive assessment of left and right ventricular filling in myocardial infarction with a two-dimensional Doppler echocardiographic method. *J Am Coll Cardiol* 5: 1155–1162.

45. Tagagi S, Yokota M, Iwase M, Koide M, Jin HX, Hayashi H, Sotobata I (1986) Evaluation of left ventricular diastolic filling by a pulsed Doppler flowmeter in patients with coronary artery disease, in: Spencer MP (ed), *Cardiac Doppler Diagnosis II*, p 157. Boston: Martinus Nijhoff.

46. Visser CA, Janse MJ, Koolen JJ, Delemarre BJ, Dunning AJ (1986) Comparison of left ventricular systolic and diastolic dysfunction sequence following transient ischemia (abstracts). *Circulation* 74 (suppl 2): II–471.

47. Rackley CE, Russell RO, Mantle JA, Rogers WJ, Papapietro SE (1981) Modern approach to myocardial infarction: Determination of prognosis and therapy. *Am Heart J* 101: 75–85.

48. Visser CA, De Koning H, Delemarre BJ, Koolen JJ, Dunning AJ (1986) Pulsed Doppler-derived mitral inflow velocity in acute myocardial infarction: An early prognostic indicator. *J Am Coll Cardiol* 7: 136A (abstracts).

49. Delemarre BJM, Visser CA, Bot H, Koning HJ De, Dunning AJ (1980) Predictive value of pulsed Doppler echocardiography in acute myocardial infarction. *J Am Soc Echo* (in press).

50. Delemarre BJM, Bot H, Pearlman AS, Visser CA, Dunning AJ (1987) Diastolic flow characteristics of severely impaired left ventricles: A pulsed Doppler ultrasound study. *J Clin Ultrasound* 15: 115–119.

51. Delemarre BJM, Bot H, Visser CA, Dunning AJ (1988) Pulsed Doppler echocardiographic description of a circular flow pattern in spontaneous left ventricular contrast. *J Am Soc Echo*: 114–118.

52. Mikell FL, Asinger RW, Elsperger KJ, Anderson WR, Hodges M (1982) Regional stasis of blood in the dysfunctional left ventricle: Echocardiographic detection and differentiation from early thrombosis. *Circulation* 66: 755–801.

53. Delemarre BJM, Visser CA, Bot H, Koning H De, Dunning AJ (1987) Prediction of apical thrombosis formation in acute myocardial infarction based on abnormal left ventricular spatial flow pattern: A prospective pulsed Doppler echocardiographic study (abstracts). *Circulation* 76 (suppl IV): IV–227.

18. Analysis of left ventricular function in patients with myocardial infarction
Methodological problems and possible solutions

ALAN G. FRASER, JOHN H. SMYLLIE,
PATRICIA E. ASSMANN, GEORGE R. SUTHERLAND
and JOS R.T.C. ROELANDT

Introduction

Reduced left ventricular function is a major determinant of prognosis after myocardial infarction, so many acute interventions including thrombolysis are directed at preventing or reversing acute left ventricular damage. Assessment of the outcome of such therapies is necessary both for clinical decision making and for research, and requires accurate and reproducible methods of identifying or localising regions of abnormal function and of quantifying left ventricular function. Traditionally, the standard for such measurements has been biplane left ventricular cineangiography, but this is neither feasible in all patients in the acute phase after myocardial infarction nor applicable for repeated use during recovery and convalescence.

Alternative techniques for assessing ventricular function after myocardial infarction now include gated isotope ventriculography, gated computed tomography, and gated nuclear magnetic resonance imaging, as well as cross-sectional echocardiography. Of these options, echocardiography is the most practical method for repeated measurements and the least expensive, and of course it is totally non-invasive. It has the potential to be a sensitive detector of ischaemia, since within seconds of coronary occlusion and before the development of electrocardiographic changes, there is a reduction of myocardial wall thickening and of endocardial motion. When combined with pulsed or continuous wave Doppler techniques and colour flow mapping, cross-sectional echocardiography also provides information about intra-cardiac flow patterns and haemodynamic performance, including diastolic function. However, like almost all present methods (and all widely available ones), it has the theoretical disadvantage that it cannot acquire a three-dimensional image instantaneously. From any two-dimensional cross-sectional image or series of images, assumptions must therefore be made, and geometric models applied, in order to extrapolate data about regional and global left or right ventricular function.

This review will discuss the echocardiographic techniques which can be used to assess ventricular function, and their accuracy, variability and

S. Iliceto et al. (eds.), Ultrasound in Coronary Artery Disease, 213–229.
© 1991 *Kluwer Academic Publishers.*

reproducibility. Some possible solutions to the problems which arise will be discussed, and the use of these echocardiographic techniques will be illustrated with some examples of their application in patients with infarction or angina.

Assessment of myocardial function

The function of both ventricles can be analysed using long and short axis cross-sectional views obtained from standard parasternal and apical transducer positions. The apical long axis view is particularly useful for assessing the left ventricle since angulation of the probe towards the outflow tract and aorta defines a plane which is reproducible. Since it does not have equivalent landmarks, the apical two-chamber view is not so reproducible. For optimal short axis views, the transducer is usually angled until a circular cross-section of the left ventricle is obtained, even though such an image may not represent a true cross-section in all patients with infarction. The parasternal long axis view is often used to assess ventricular function from derived M-mode dimensions, but since this plane does not include the left ventricular apex it cannot be used for the calculation of left ventricular volumes by methods based on measurements of area and length. It is now also appreciated that assessment of left ventricular systolic function from M-mode echocardiograms can give significantly different results from two-dimensional analysis [1]. In general, left ventricular function should be assessed in several planes, because a single plane may well not include all regions of abnormal function. Additional short axis views from the sub-xiphoid approach are helpful for the analysis of right ventricular function. In patients with coronary artery disease, the best images are usually produced from the apical rather than the parasternal approach. If good quality images cannot be obtained from the praecordium and there are particular circumstances where it is important to define ventricular function, it is usually possible to get clear short axis images of the left ventricle during transoesophageal echocardiography, as discussed elsewhere in this volume (van Daele et al., pp. 67–81).

Echocardiographic images of the ventricles can be analysed in either a global or a segmental manner, using either qualitative or quantitative criteria. In most clinical circumstances at present, real-time assessment of ventricular function is possible only with qualitative methods, but further developments in automated methods are likely to make on-line or immediate quantitative, objective assessment practical in the future. Video analysis techniques can be improved by using video disc systems rather than standard video recorders, because these allow the echocardiographic image to be updated twice as frequently as normal, and therefore reduce the chance of temporal asynchronicity between different myocardial segments within a single frozen image [2].

Qualitative methods

Qualitative analysis of global myocardial function rapidly establishes a diagnosis of primary pump failure, seen as a grossly dilated and uniformly poorly contracting heart, but without more sophisticated techniques it can be difficult even for an experienced observer to differentiate between ischaemic and non-ischaemic dilated cardiomyopathy. Gross abnormalities of systolic function are not difficult to detect on visual inspection of two-dimensional echocardiograms, as long as any segment of dyskinesis does not exceed 50% of the circumference of the ventricle. Above this level it is impossible without reference to the electrocardiogram to distinguish between true systole and diastole. Another disadvantage of qualitative methods is that subtle changes in function are easily missed, yet it is now appreciated that in ischaemic heart disease systolic function may be abnormal in the first part of systole alone [3], and that diastolic function is sometimes affected by ischaemia while systolic function is still normal. Such abnormalities of cardiac function, and temporal inhomogeneity of contraction and relaxation, cannot be adequately assessed by qualitative methods.

For the qualitative recognition of lesser degrees of wall motion abnormality during systole, the ventricles are divided into segments, which are defined by internal landmarks in order to standardise interpretation. Numerous systems have been developed, and there is little standardisation either of the number of segments which are analysed, or of their nomenclature. All such methods have similar theoretical disadvantages. For example, it may be difficult to find or select a reference area of normal function, against which to compare areas of abnormal function, and significant sampling errors may occur if the two-dimensional cross-sections chosen for analysis do not include all areas of abnormal function. These can be minimised by analysing several cross-sections, the choice being designed to include areas of myocardium supplied by all major coronary arterial branches [4].

The amplitude of motion of each segment is graded by the observer and assigned a score. In the scheme used most often, 0 = hyperkinetic, 1 = normal, 2 = hypokinetic, 3 = akinetic, and 4 = dyskinetic; sometimes hyperkinetic segments are allocated a score of −1. The sum of these numbers is the wall motion score, and it can be divided by the number of segments analysed to give the wall motion score index. With this method, a normally contracting heart has a wall motion score index of one or less.

Abnormal myocardial function can also be detected by assessing regional thickening of the left ventricular wall during systole. Once myocardial blood flow has been reduced by 20% or more, wall thickening is reduced by at least 50%, and this is appreciable on visual inspection. This can be of considerable help in distinguishing between hypokinetic myocardium which thickens during systole, and akinetic myocardium, which does not, since contraction in healthy myocardial segments adjacent to akinetic ones can give the spurious appearance of some contraction in the akinetic segment. Changes in contractile function of the ventricular myocardium are very sensitive indicators of ischaemia, since they occur when coronary blood flow is reduced by as little as 10–20% [5], and because they precede the development of any electro-cardiographic or haemodynamic changes [6].

Interobserver and intraobserver variability in the detection and qualitative grading of regional wall abnormalities can be considerable [7]. The method is subjective, but consistent results can be achieved by highly trained observers [8]. In comparison, reassessment of left ventricular angiograms in the CASS study using qualitative criteria demonstrated significant differences in left ventricular function in 10% of investigations [9].

Quantitative methods

Quantitative analysis of left ventricular function can only be performed if the endocardial contour of the ventricle can be traced. Other more simple methods which do not involve planimetry are feasible but probably give less accurate results [10–12]. However, manual tracing of left ventricular contours is very time consuming, particularly since it is now appreciated that if minor or transient abnormalities of function are to be detected, it is not sufficient to analyse only systolic and end-diastolic frames. When echocardiography is used to analyse the sequence of contraction and relaxation throughout the cardiac cycle, it is 100% sensitive for the detection of ischaemic wall motion abnormalities, and different temporal patterns of dysfunction can be recog-nised [13]. In comparison, analysis of end-diastolic and end-systolic frames alone identified only 80% of abnormalities related to chronic infarction and 56% of those caused by transient ischaemia [13]. The accuracy of quantitative techniques may be improved if digital tracing is performed using an electroni-cally directed cursor and a microcomputer [2, 14]. Automated contour detec-tion systems are not yet widely available for routine clinical application, for example in patients with coronary artery disease, but it is increasingly obvious that they are necessary. Their accuracy has improved from earlier reports [15, 16] but several technical problems remain. Digital analytic techniques were reviewed recently by Grube et al. [17].

Quantitative analysis of global left ventricular function has been performed with several algorithms [18–24]. From single plane apical four chamber views of the left ventricle, the area length method has been used frequently, and cor-relates well with other methods. For geometrical calculations of volume using several cross-sectional images, a truncated cone is the most common model. However, after myocardial infarction the left ventricle can undergo consider-able change in shape, because of asymmetrical expansion of the infarcted seg-ments of myocardium, and so biplane volume algorithms which allow for asymmetric model hearts are required [18–21]. The changes in shape vary according to the site of infarction, with the left ventricle becoming more triangular in shape after occlusion of the left anterior descending coronary artery, and more elongated after circumflex occlusion [25].

Quantitative analysis of segmental left ventricular function is also possible, and several different approaches have been reported [26–32]. The function of each segment can be assessed by measuring the change in length during systole of a radius drawn from a central reference point to that segment, or the change in area of a sector enclosed by two radii and the overlying myocardium on the perimeter of the ventricular contour. The intraobserver variability of both of these methods is less than 10%. If radii are measured at 10° intervals around the circumference of the ventricle, the technique can detect abnormal function of a segment of myocardium as small as 5.6% [2]. Echocardiography can identify damage to as little as 18% of the left ventricular mass, but it may not able to detect smaller infarcts, especially if they are subendocardial [33].

If both the epicardial and the endocardial contours are traced, then regional wall thickening can also be quantified, but since the measurements are small in absolute terms, the percentage changes are high and reproducibility is correspondingly reduced. Nevertheless, in experimental studies the extent of abnormal systolic wall thickening correlated more closely with the region of true infarction, defined by the injection of microspheres, than did the area of abnormal regional fractional shortening [34, 35]. One other technique which has been reported to correlate very well in experimental and clinico-pathological studies with the histological extent of infarction, and which has the advantage of being uninfluenced by assumptions about the shape of the ventricle, is the endocardial mapping technique [36–38]. However, because it is based on the construction of 20 segments derived from 5 cross-sectional images, it may be time consuming and therefore not practical for routine clinical applications.

All of these methods can be used to detect wall motion abnormalities and measure changes in function, particularly in groups of patients. Gordon et al. estimated that mean changes in end-diastolic volume of > 2%, in end-systolic volume of > 5%, and in ejection fraction of > 2% are likely to represent real changes [8]. However, the reproducibility of individual measurements is relatively poor, so that the confidence intervals for detecting true changes in function in individual patients over a period of time are much greater: 15% for end-diastolic volume, 25% for end-systolic volume, and 10% for ejection fraction [8]. Nevertheless, these figures compare quite favourably with those relating to left ventricular angiography in the CASS study: 31% for end-diastolic volume, 43% for end-systolic volume, and 5% for ejection fraction, with > 20% variability between two measurements of the same angiogram [9]. Trobaugh et al. reported the 95% confidence intervals for the echocardiographic estimation of end-diastolic volume to be ± 25 ml/m^2 [39]. An appreciation of these values is important, because in some pharmacological studies the measured changes in echocardiographic parameters have fallen within these limits [40]. The power of any clinical trial to demonstrate real changes in echocardiographic measurements has to be carefully assessed in advance. There is also a very wide range of values in normal subjects. For example, Pandian et al. compared systolic changes in fractional area in different segments in normal subjects, and found that they ranged from 0–100%, while changes in segmental wall thickening ranged from 0–150% [41]. In addition, indices of systolic function when expressed as a percentage of the end-diastolic values, increase in normal subjects from the base towards the apex [42].

All quantitative methods, and particularly those used for segmental wall motion analysis, are limited by the quality of the echocardiographic images to be analysed. It can be difficult to recognise the true endocardial border, for example due to 'drop-out' of echoes from a segment of endocardium or adjacent myocardium, and it may be difficult to distinguish between the endocardium of the true ventricular wall and echoes from trabeculae on its surface [43–45], or from non-structural echoes, when the gain settings are high. In future, it may be possible to use intravenous injections of echo-contrast agents which cross the pulmonary circulation, in order to enhance the myocardial echoes and thus improve endocardial contour detection. It has also been reported that improved border detection can be achieved by using a filtered Fourier reconstruction technique [46].

An important consideration for all quantitative methods is that the whole heart may move during systole or diastole, particularly because of extracardiac motion associated with respiration. This is particularly obvious after cardiac surgery, perhaps because of the loss of normal pericardial constraint. Such motion means that when myocardial function is compared against a fixed reference point, artefactual movement may appear to occur, due to translation or rotation of the whole heart. Using a fixed reference point can lead to the erroneous impression of areas of hypokinesis in a normal heart. In order to overcome this, a floating reference system can be used, in which the reference point in the centre of the heart (the centroid) against which motion in the myocardium is compared, itself moves as the heart moves during respiration. However, this too is not ideal because it will underestimate wall motion abnormalities in patients with infarction [29, 31, 47]. There is in routine practice little translation of a short axis cross-sectional image obtained at the level of the papillary muscles, and so a fixed centroid may be the best option for analysis of short axis images. In an experimental study in which good epicardial and endocardial definition was achieved, the most accurate measurements were obtained using the epicardial contour and a floating reference point, while the worst correlation with true volume was obtained with the endocardial contour and a floating centroid [48]. Thus a floating centroid is an acceptable method when good epicardial images are available for analysis, but in general, fixed reference systems allow more accurate measurements and are preferable if there is little translation of the heart.

Our recent experience suggests that a significant reduction of errors or variability due to movement of the whole heart can be achieved by using cross-sectional echocardiograms recorded at end-expiration. The apical long axis and four-chamber views are most useful for routine quantitative analysis, and can be standardised by the use of internal landmarks for orientation during repeated studies. It is important to record images with the probe at the true apex; otherwise there is a risk of foreshortening the left ventricle in the four-chamber view. In this plane, during normal contraction there is shortening of the long axis of the left ventricle, and alteration of the orientation of the base of the heart which also translates towards the apex, which is relatively stable. A computerised model of compensating for this movement has recently been reported, and allows a correction to be made so that segmental function is analysed more accurately [49]. Fifty segments are analysed between base and apex on each side, and the variability of the measurements is about 10%. An alternative approach to the problems caused by external cardiac motion is to use an index such as the ratio of end-systolic left ventricular cavity radius to wall thickness, which is independent of such motion, and as sensitive and accurate as other methods [50].

At present, the technical problems and time-consuming nature of automated techniques for the analysis of left ventricular function mean that in clinical practice most analyses are qualitative. While such studies can be helpful to recognise major abnormalities of function quickly, they are not accurate or sensitive enough to be used for the evaluation of therapeutic interventions. A practical, accurate and reproducible method of quantifying left ventricular function, preferably using automated techniques, would be invaluable; it is now a realistic prospect because of rapid developments in digital techniques.

Clinical studies using qualitative techniques

Analysis of wall motion using qualitative segmental techniques is possible in most patients with suspected myocardial infarction. Diagnostic images can be obtained in 85–95% of patients, and their accuracy in detecting myocardial infarction is high, since a sensitivity of 94% and a specificity of 84% have been reported [51, 52]. However the method is less sensitive (66%–86%) in patients with non-Q wave infarction [52–54]. When compared with other techniques such as electrocardiography, or when correlated with the extent of infarction at postmortem, two-dimensional echocardiography is a valid method of localising infarction, although it often overestimates the extent of damage [23, 55–59]. Echocardiography may demonstrate abnormal function in myocardial segments adjacent to the zone of infarction, and not just in the area of irreversibly damaged myocardium. Defining infarction by the extent of dyskinesis will tend to underestimate the true extent of myocardial necrosis, while using hypokinesis will tend to overestimate it. Some of this effect is due to 'tethering' of myocardium adjacent to the infarcted muscle, but it is also partly due to the algorithms used during analysis, because a systolic shift in the centre of mass of the left ventricle gives the appearance of systolic expansion of infarcted segments [60]. However, this effect is small and relatively predictable, and the extent of abnormal function demonstrated by echocardiography correlates well with that observed by thallium 201 reperfusion studies, radionuclide angiography, or contrast left ventriculography [55, 61]. The extent of asynergy of the infarct zone has also been reported to correlate well with the peak serum level of the CPK MB isoenzyme [57, 62], although not all investigators have confirmed this [63–65]. Echocardiographic techniques can also be used for repeated studies, and these have been used to detect expansion of infarcted segments of myocardium [66, 67].

Asynergy remote from the primary site of acute infarction has been reported to be an indicator of multiple vessel disease, while compensatory hyperkinesis of unaffected segments occurs in patients with only single vessel disease [59]: 77% of patients with multivessel disease had remote asynergy, compared with none of those with single vessel disease. This may be of value in identifying young patients who should be referred for coronary arteriography after myocardial infarction.

Echocardiographically apparent myocardial damage after acute infarction, assessed by qualitative analysis of wall motion abnormalities, is, as expected, a predictor of subsequent post-infarct angina, cardiac failure, and death [52, 63–65, 68–72]. This observation is in accord with many studies relating the extent of infarction to subsequent prognosis, since echocardiographic parameters also reflect the severity of infarction. For example, Heger et al. [63] reported that patients with uncomplicated infarction had a mean wall motion score of 3.2 ± 2.4, compared with 6.7 ± 1.9 in patients who had acute ventricular septal rupture or acute mitral regurgitation, 9.7 ± 3.1 in those with pulmonary oedema, and 10.6 ± 4.8 in those with both pulmonary oedema and hypotension. The mean wall motion score was also higher in patients who subsequently died, than in those with normal function [63]. The score was less in patients who developed ventricular septal rupture or acute mitral regurgitation than in those with cardiac failure, due to compensatory hyperkinesis of non-infarcted segments and the low left ventricular afterload, but hyperkinesis was in fact predictive of a poor outcome. Similar findings were reported by Nishimura et al., who found that a wall motion index of ≥ 2 identified 88% of patients with acute myocardial infarction who subsequently developed pump failure, severe arrhythmias or death [64]; poor wall motion was also predictive even in patients who had no clinical problems at the time of study.

Qualitative echocardiographic methods have been used to document improvements in wall motion scores in patients who underwent angioplasty after acute myocardial infarction [73].

Right ventricular infarction

Echocardiography has been used to demonstrate that right ventricular infarction occurs in about one third of all patients with infarction, and in all patients with transmural infarction of the inferoposterior wall of the left ventricle or the posterior part of the interventricular septum [74–76]. Although dilatation of the right ventricle is neither sensitive nor specific as an indicator of right ventricular infarction [76–78], wall motion abnormalities on two-dimensional echocardiography are nevertheless more sensitive than haemodynamic criteria [75, 76, 79–81]. Thus in patients with recent infarction who remain hypotensive and fail to respond to conventional therapy, cross-sectional echocardiographic assessment of right ventricular function may help to identify those with significant right ventricular damage and therefore allow appropriate treatment to be initiated.

Clinical studies using quantitative techniques

Measurements of global left ventricular function obtained from echocardiographic methods correlate well with those from contrast ventriculography [24] or radionuclide angiography [19, 71, 82], but echocardiography tends to underestimate left ventricular volumes when compared with ventriculography [20, 23, 24]. This can be explained by differences in the techniques. Even when the papillary muscles are excluded, as usual, and the left ventricular contour is traced outside them, echocardiography tends to define the margin of the ventricular cavity by the inner border of the trabeculae, while the outer border is used in ventriculography because contrast extends between the trabeculae [83].

Left ventricular ejection fraction calculated by echocardiography has been shown to vary considerably during the first twenty four hours after acute infarction [84], although other investigators did not confirm this [85]. As with other techniques, serial echocardiographic assessment of global left ventricular function has shown a gradual improvement in ejection fraction in patients with uncomplicated myocardial infarction, and a deterioration in those with clinical complications.

Quantitative analysis of segmental wall motion abnormalities by cross-sectional echocardiography has been compared with cineventriculography, in patients with suspected coronary artery disease. The sensitivity and specificity of echocardiography for the detection of abnormal anterior wall motion were 68% and 94%, respectively, and for the detection of abnormal posterior wall motion 80% and 96% [86]. Echocardiography is also superior to haemodynamic monitoring or electrocardiography in the detection of ischaemia in patients with variant angina, since a reduction in septal systolic wall thickening occurs first [87].

Numerous pharmacological studies have now been performed using echocardiographic techniques to document changes in ventricular function [88].

Diastolic function

It has been appreciated for many years that diastolic function is abnormal in ischaemic heart disease [89], and recently it has been reported that the onset of left ventricular relaxation is asynchronous during angina pectoris [90]. Previously M-mode recordings of the left ventricle were digitised in order to derive information about peak diastolic filling rates [91], but now more sophisticated analytic techniques need to be applied to the diastolic frames of two-dimensional echocardiographic images in patients with angina pectoris and myocardial infarction, in order to produce information about global patterns of diastolic function and any temporal and regional variations. One new echocardiographic index of diastolic function which has been reported, is the first half filling fraction [92].

Much interest has also been focussed recently on the assessment of left ventricular diastolic function by the analysis of Doppler traces of mitral inflow. Mitral flow velocity patterns are abnormal in patients with poorly compliant ventricles, for example due to ischaemic damage [93], but the appearances in an individual patient may become more normal if the left atrial pressure increases. Thus standard Doppler-derived indices of left ventricular function are influenced by left ventricular preload [94], but a new Doppler echocardiographic filling index, which is independent of preload because the peak filling rate is normalised to the mitral stroke volume, has been described [95]. The clinical potential of such techniques in patients with myocardial infarction has not yet been defined, but may be considerable. In experimental studies of acute myocardial infarction, beneficial effects of angiotensin converting enzyme inhibition on diastolic function have been demonstrated by echocardiography [96].

Stress echocardiography

A detailed discussion of this subject is beyond the scope of this short review, but this expanding field has been reviewed elsewhere [97]. It is now apparent that echocardiographic imaging of ventricular function can be readily performed during either supine exercise on a bicycle ergometer or during isometric exercise with a handgrip dynamometer. The images produced are of good quality and reproducible, and they can be analysed with the methods already outlined. The reproducibility of such images is satisfactory. At the same time, useful information about diastolic function of the left ventricle can be obtained by recording and analysing the pattern of diastolic mitral inflow, using spectral Doppler traces.

Several groups have reported that exercise echocardiography can increase the diagnostic sensitivity of exercise testing in ischaemic heart disease, particularly when it is performed at peak exercise [98–100]. It also improves the predictive power of echocardiography to identify good and poor prognostic groups of patients after acute myocardial infarction [101]. Measurement of left ventricular function during exercise could therefore be considered as a useful adjunct to the routine echocardiographic assessment of post-infarct patients.

Future developments

A consensus is required for the standardisation of methods of qualitative assessment of ventricular function from two-dimensional echocardiograms. This will make it easier to compare the results of different studies, and also to examine changes in function in a particular patient who is examined in different centres.

Other developments are likely to be in the field of automated analysis. All standard echocardiographic machines may incorporate software which gives them the capacity to acquire and smooth multiple images over many beats, by time-gating the acquisition of echocardiographic images, and they should then be able to construct cine loops of the ventricles in the chosen plane. This may not be possible in real-time, but it should be possible to switch from real-time imaging to view a cine loop derived from the newly acquired images. From such images both major and minor abnormalities of function, as well as temporal inhomogeneity of function, should be much more readily identifiable and quantifiable than at present. More sophisticated analytic packages will be available for research, for example better versions of present basic three-dimensional displays [102, 103], and reconstructions of areas of poor function.

Conclusions

Two-dimensional analysis of ventricular function using present echocardiographic techniques is at least as reproducible as other methods such as angiography. Although different methods may give different absolute values for ventricular volumes, this seems relatively unimportant for prospective studies if the method chosen for quantifying left ventricular function is reproducible, especially since it is not known which method represents the true one. Comparisons with subsequent in vitro measurements of volume show that echocardiography is as good as ventriculography; comparisons between the two methods are difficult because they cannot be performed simultaneously [104].

The echocardiographic imaging planes and the methods of analysis to be used will depend on the circumstances. For maximal information, it is necessary to analyse wall motion throughout the cardiac cycle. Qualitative methods are helpful for clinical purposes, and can rapidly provide information of prognostic value. Quantitative methods are now well developed and appropriate for a wide range of research applications. Indeed, with further developments in the processing and analysis of cross-sectional data, echocardiography may come to represent the ideal investigative tool for rapid and serial measurement of left ventricular function.

Acknowledgement

Dr A. G. Fraser was supported by the British Heart Foundation.

References

1. Douglas PS, Reichek N, Plappert T, Muhammad A, St John Sutton MG (1987) Comparison of echocardiographic methods for assessment of left ventricular shortening and wall stress. *J Am Coll Cardiol* 9: 945–951.
2. Mann DL, Gillam LD, Weyman AE (1986) Cross-sectional echocardiographic assessment of regional left ventricular performance and myocardial perfusion. *Prog Cardiovasc Dis* 29: 1–52.
3. Weyman AE, Franklin TD, Hogan RD, Gillam LD, Wiske PS, Newell J, Gibbons EF, Foale RA (1984) Importance of temporal heterogeneity in assessing the contraction abnormalities associated with acute myocardial ischemia. *Circulation* 70: 102–112.
4. Edwards WD, Tajik AJ, Seward JB (1981) Standardized nomenclature and anatomic basis for regional tomographic analysis of the heart. *Mayo Clin Proc* 56: 479–497.
5. Vatner SF (1980) Correlation between acute reductions in myocardial blood flow and function in conscious dogs. *Circ Res* 47: 201–207.
6. Grover-McKay M, Matsuzaki M, Ross J (1987) Dissociation between regional myocardial dysfunction and subendocardial ST segment elevation during and after exercise-induced ischemia in dogs. *J Am Coll Cardiol* 10: 1105–1112.
7. Peart I, Austin A, Hall RJC (1987) Subjective analysis of cross-sectional echocardiograms: Reproducibility and sources of variability. *Eur Heart J* 8: 171–178.
8. Gordon EP, Schnittger I, Fitzgerald PJ, Williams P, Popp RL (1983) Reproducibility of left ventricular volumes by two-dimensional echocardiography. *J Am Coll Cardiol* 2: 506–513.
9. Wexler LF, Lesperance J, Ryan TJ, Bourassa MG, Fisher LD, Maynard C, Kemp HG, Cameron A, Gosselin AJ, Judkins MP (1982) Interobserver variability in interpreting contrast left ventriculograms (CASS). *Cathet Cardiovasc Diagn* 8: 341–355.
10. Erbel R, Schweizer P, Meyer J, Krebs W, Yalkinoglu O, Effert S (1985) Sensitivity of cross-sectional echocardiography in detection of impaired global and regional left ventricular function: Prospective study. *Int J Cardiol* 7: 375–389.
11. Quinones MA, Waggoner AD, Reduto LA, Nelson JG, Young JB, Winters WL, Ribeiro LG, Miller RR (1981) A new, simplified and accurate method for determining ejection fraction with two-dimensional echocardiography. *Circulation* 64: 744–753.
12. Tortoledo FA, Quinones MA, Fernandez GC, Waggoner AD, Winters WL (1983) Quantification of left ventricular volumes by two-dimensional echocardiography: A simplified and accurate approach. *Circulation* 67: 579–584.
13. Zeiher AM, Wollschlaeger H, Bonzel T, Kasper W, Just H (1987) Hierarchy of levels of ischemia-induced impairment in regional left ventricular systolic function in man. *Circulation* 76: 768–776.
14. Borden SG van der, Oomen JAF, Slager CJ, Assmann PE (1988) Computer assisted echocardiographic analysis. A semi-automated approach. *Computers in Cardiology* (IEEE): 425–428.

15. Fuji J, Sawada H, Aizawa T, Kato K, Onoe M, Kuno Y (1984) Computer analysis of cross sectional echocardiogram for quantitative evaluation of left ventricular asynergy in myocardial infarction. *Br Heart J* 51: 139–148.
16. Conetta DA, Geiser EA, Oliver LH, Miller AB, Conti CR (1985) Reproducibility of left ventricular area and volume measurements using a computer endocardial edge-detection algorithm in normal subjects. *Am J Cardiol* 56: 947–952.
17. Grube E, Becher H, Backs B (1987) Automatic contour finding and digital subtraction technique in 2-dimensional echocardiography, in: Roelandt J (ed), *Digital Techniques in Echocardiography*, pp 99–122. Dordrecht: Martinus Nijhoff.
18. Schiller NB, Acquatella H, Ports TA, Drew D, Goerke J, Ringertz H, Silverman NH, Brundage B, Botvinick EH, Boswell R, Carlsson E, Parmley WW (1979) Left ventricular volume from paired biplane two-dimensional echocardiography. *Circulation* 60: 547–555.
19. Folland ED, Parisi AF, Moynihan PF, Jones DR, Feldmann CL, Tow DE (1979) Assessment of left ventricular ejection fraction and volumes by real-time, two-dimensional echocardiography. *Circulation* 60: 760–766.
20. Erbel R, Schweizer P, Meyer J, Grenner H, Krebs W, Effert S (1980) Left ventricular volume and ejection fraction determination by cross-sectional echocardiography in patients with coronary artery disease: A prospective study. *Clin Cardiol* 3: 377–383.
21. Erbel R, Krebs W, Henn G, Schweizer P, Richter HA, Meyer J, Effert S (1982) Comparison of single-plane and biplane volume determination by two-dimensional echocardiography. *Eur Heart J* 3: 469–480.
22. Wahr DW, Wang YS, Schiller NB (1983) Left ventricular volumes determined by two-dimensional echocardiography in a normal adult population. *J Am Coll Card* 1: 863–868.
23. Weiss JL, Eaton LW, Kallman CH, Maughan WL (1983) Accuracy of volume determination by two-dimensional echocardiography: Defining requirements under controlled conditions in the ejecting canine left ventricle. *Circulation* 67: 889–895.
24. Erbel R, Schweizer P, Krebs W, Meyer J, Effert S (1984) Sensitivity and specificity of two-dimensional echocardiography in detection of impaired left ventricular function. *Eur Heart J* 5: 477–489.
25. Marino P, Kass D, Lima J, Maughan WL, Graves W, Weiss JL (1988) Influence of site of regional ischemia on LV cavity shape change in dogs. *Am J Physiol* 254: H547–H557.
26. Moynihan PF, Parisi AF, Feldman CL (1981) Quantitative detection of regional left ventricular contraction abnormalities by two-dimensional echocardiography. I. Analysis of methods. *Circulation* 64: 752–760.
27. Parisi AF, Moynihan PF, Folland ED, Feldman CL (1981) Quantitative detection of regional left ventricular contraction abnormalities by two-dimensional echocardiography. II. Accuracy in coronary artery disease. *Circulation* 63: 761–767.
28. Henschke CI, Risser TA, Sandor T, Hanlon WB, Neumann A, Wynne J (1983) Quantitative computer-assisted analysis of left ventricular wall thickening and motion by 2-dimensional echocardiography in acute myocardial infarction. *Am J Cardiol* 52: 960–964.
29. Grube E, Hanisch H, Zywietz M, Neumann G, Herzog H (1984) Rechnergestutze bestimmung linksventrikularen Kontraktionsanomalien mittels zweidimensionalen Echokardiographie. I. Analyse verschiedener Untersuchungsmethoden und Normalwertbestimmung. *Z Kardiologie* 73: 41–51.
30. Dissmann R, Bruggeman Th, Wegschneider K, Biamino G (1984) Normalbereiche der regionalen linksventrikularen Wandbewegung im zweidimensionalen Echokardiogram. *Z Kardiologie* 73: 686–694.
31. Schnittger I, Fitzgerald PJ, Gordon EP, Alderman EL, Popp RL (1984) Computerized quantitative analysis of left ventricular wall motion by two-dimensional echocardiography. *Circulation* 70: 242–254.
32. Erbel R, Henkel B, Ostlander C, Clas W, Brennecke R, Meyer J (1985) Normalwerte für die zweidimensionale Echokardiografie. *Dtsch Med Wschr* 110: 123–128.

33. Pandian NG, Skorton DJ, Collins SM, Koyanagi S, Kieso R, Marcus ML, Kerber RE (1985) Myocardial infarct size threshold for two-dimensional echocardiographic detection: Sensitivity of systolic wall thickening and endocardial motion abnormalities in small versus large infarcts. *Am J Cardiol* 55: 551–555.

34. Buda AJ, Zotz RJ, Pace DP, Krause LC (1986) Comparison of two-dimensional echocardiographic wall motion and wall thickening abnormalities in relation to the myocardium at risk. *Am Heart J* 111: 587–592.

35. McGillem MJ, Mancini J, DeBoe SF, Buda AJ (1988) Modification of the centerline method for assessment of echocardiographic wall thickening and motion: A comparison with areas of risk. *J Am Coll Cardiol* 11: 861–866.

36. Guyer DE, Gibson TC, Gillam LD, King ME, Wilkins GT, Guerrero JL, Weyman AE (1986) A new echocardiographic model for quantifying three-dimensional endocardial surface area. *J Am Coll Cardiol* 8: 819–829.

37. Guyer DE, Foale RA, Gillam LD, Wilkins GT, Guerrero JL, Weyman AE (1986) An echocardiographic technique for quantifying and displaying the extent of regional left ventricular dyssynergy. *J Am Coll Cardiol* 8: 830–835.

38. Wilkins GT, Southern JF, Choong CY, Thomas JD, Fallon JT, Guyer DE, Weyman AE (1988) Correlation between echocardiographic endocardial surface mapping of abnormal wall motion and pathologic infarct size in autopsied hearts. *Circulation* 77: 978–987.

39. Trobaugh GB, Hallstrom AP, Kennedy JW (1984) Reproducibility of ventricular function measurements by contrast angiography. *Cathet Cardiovasc Diagn* 10: 561–572.

40. Huang H, Scheffers M, Rijsterborgh H, Roelandt J (1988) Does echocardiography allow the monitoring of the cardiac effects of nitrates? *Eur Heart J* 9 (suppl A): 51–55.

41. Pandian NG, Skorton DJ, Collins SM, Falsetti HL, Burke ER, Kerber RE (1983) Heterogeneity of left ventricular segmental wall thickening and excursion in 2-dimensional echocardiograms of normal human subjects. *Am J Cardiol* 51: 1667–1673.

42. Haendchen RV, Wyatt HL, Maurer G, Zwehl W, Bear M, Meerbaum S, Corday E (1983) Quantitation of regional cardiac function by two-dimensional echocardiography. I. Patterns of contraction in the normal left ventricle. *Circulation* 67: 1234–1245.

43. Fenichel NM, Arora J, Khan R, Antoniou C, Ahuja S, Thompson EJ (1976) The effect of respiratory motion on the echocardiogram. *Chest* 69: 655–659.

44. Brenner JI, Waugh RA (1978) Effect of phasic respiration on left ventricular dimension and performance in a normal population: An echocardiographic study. *Circulation* 57: 122–127.

45. Andersen K, Vik-Mo H (1984) Effects of spontaneous respiration on left ventricular function assessed by echocardiography. *Circulation* 69: 874–879.

46. Thomas JD, Hagege AA, Choong CY, Wilkins GT, Newell JB, Weyman AE (1988) Improved accuracy of echocardiographic endocardial borders by spatiotemporal filtered Fourier reconstruction: Description of the method and optimization of filter cutoffs. *Circulation* 77: 415–428.

47. Parisi AF, Moynihan PF, Folland ED, Feldman CL (1981) Quantitative detection of regional left ventricular contraction abnormalities by two-dimensional echocardiography. II. Accuracy in coronary artery disease. *Circulation* 63: 761–767.

48. Zoghbi WA, Charlat ML, Bolli R, Zhu W-X, Hartley CJ, Quinones MA (1988) Quantitative assessment of left ventricular wall motion by two-dimensional echocardiography: Validation during reversible ischemia in the conscious dog. *J Am Coll Cardiol* 11: 851–860.

49. Assmann PE, Slager CJ, Dreysse ST, Borden SG van der, Oomen JA, Roelandt JR (1988) Two-dimensional echocardiographic analysis of the dynamic geometry of the left ventricle: The basis for an improved model of wall motion. *J Am Soc Echo* 1: 393–405.

50. Zoghbi WA, Charlat ML, Bolli R, Kopelen H, Hartley CJ, Roberts R, Quinones MA (1987) End-systolic radius to thickness ratio: An echocardiographic index of regional performance during reversible myocardial ischemia in the conscious dog. *J Am Coll Cardiol* 10: 1113–1121.

51. Weiss JL, Bulkley BH, Hutchins GM, Mason SJ (1981) Two-dimensional echocardiographic recognition of myocardial injury in man: Comparison with postmortem studies. *Circulation* 63: 401–408.
52. Horowitz RS, Morganroth J, Parrotto C, Chen CC, Soffer J, Pauletto FJ (1982) Immediate diagnosis of acute myocardial infarction by two-dimensional echocardiography. *Circulation* 65: 323–329.
53. Loh IK, Charuzi Y, Beeder C, Marshall LA, Ginsburg JH (1982) Early diagnosis of non-transmural myocardial infarction by two-dimensional echocardiography. *Am Heart J* 104: 963–968.
54. Arvan S, Varat MA (1985) Two-dimensional echocardiography versus surface electrocardiography for the diagnosis of acute non-Q wave myocardial infarction. *Am Heart J* 110: 44–49.
55. Nixon JV, Narahara KA, Smitherman TC (1980) Estimation of myocardial involvement in patients with acute myocardial infarction by two-dimensional echocardiography. *Circulation* 62: 1248–1255.
56. Visser CA, Lie KI, Kam G, Meltzer R, Durrer R (1980) Detection and quantification of acute, isolated myocardial infarction by two-dimensional echocardiography. *Am J Cardiol* 47: 1021–1025.
57. Visser CA, Kan G, Lie KI, Becker AE, Durrer D (1982) Apex two-dimensional echocardiography. Alternative approach to quantification of acute myocardial infarction. *Br Heart J* 47: 461–467.
58. Pierard LA, Sprynger M, Gills F, Carlier J (1985) Significance of precordial ST-segment depression in inferior acute myocardial infarction as determined by echocardiography. *Am J Cardiol* 57: 82–85.
59. Stamm RB, Gibson RS, Bishop HL, Carabello BA, Beller GA, Martin RP (1983) Echocardiographic detection of infarct-localized asynergy and remote asynergy during acute myocardial infarction: Correlation with the extent of angiographic coronary disease. *Circulation* 67: 233–244.
60. Force T, Kemper A, Perkins L, Gilfoil M, Cohen C, Parisi AF (1986) Overestimation of infarct size by quantitative two-dimensional echocardiography: The role of tethering and of analytic procedures. *Circulation* 73: 1360–1368.
61. Freeman AP, Giles RW, Walsh WF, Fisher R, Murray IPC, Wilcken DEL (1985) Regional left ventricular wall motion assessment: Comparison of two-dimensional echocardiography and radionuclide angiography with contrast angiography in healed myocardial infarction. *Am J Cardiol* 56: 8–12.
62. Jugdutt BI, Sussex BA, Sivaram CA, Rossal RE (1984) Right ventricular infarction: Two-dimensional echocardiographic evaluation. *Am Heart J* 107: 505–518.
63. Heger JJ, Weyman AE, Wann LS, Rogers EW, Dillon JC, Feigenbaum H (1980) Cross-sectional echocardiographic analysis of the extent of left ventricular asynergy in acute myocardial infarction. *Circulation* 61: 1113–1118.
64. Nishimura RA, Reeder GS, Miller FA, Ulstrup DM, Shub C, Seward JB, Tajik AJ (1984) Prognostic value of predischarge 2-dimensional echocardiogram after acute myocardial infarction. *Am J Cardiol* 53: 429–432.
65. Horowitz RS, Morganroth J (1982) Immediate detection of early high-risk patients with acute myocardial infarction using two-dimensional echocardiographic evaluation of left ventricular regional wall motion abnormalities. *Am Heart J* 103: 814–822.
66. Eaton LW, Weiss JL, Bulkley BH, Garrison JB, Weisfeldt ML (1979) Regional cardiac dilatation after acute myocardial infarction. *N Engl J Med* 300: 57–62.
67. Erlebacher JA, Weiss JL, Weisfeldt ML, Bulkley BH (1984) Early dilation of the infarcted segment in acute transmural myocardial infarction: Role of infarct expansion in acute left ventricular enlargement. *J Am Coll Cardiol* 4: 201–208.
68. Zenker G, Kandlhofer B, Forche G, Harnoncourt K (1983) Risicoeinstufing von akuten Myokardinfarctpatienten mittels zweideimendionaler Echokardiographie. *Wien Klin Wochenschrift* 95: 680–684.

69. Abrams DS, Starling MR, Crawford MH, O'Rourke RA (1983) Value of noninvasive techniques for predicting early complications in patients with clinical class II acute myocardial infarction. *J Am Coll Cardiol* 2: 18–25.
70. Bhatnagar SK, Al-Yusuf AR (1984) Significance of early two-dimensional echocardiography after acute myocardial infarction. *Int J Cardiol* 5: 575–584.
71. Reet RE van, Quinones MA, Poliner LR, Nelson JG, Waggoner AD, Kannon D, Lubethkin SJ, Pratt CM, Winters WL (1984) Comparison of two-dimensional echocardiography with gated radionuclide ventriculography in the evaluation of global and regional left ventricular function in acute myocardial infarction. *J Am Coll Cardiol* 3: 243–252.
72. Kan G, Visser CA, Koolen JJ, Dunning AJ (1986) Short and long term predictive value of admission wall motion score in acute myocardial infarction. A cross sectional echocardiographic study of 345 patients. *Br Heart J* 56: 422–427.
73. Presti CF, Gentile R, Armstrong WF, Ryan T, Dillon JC, Feigenbaum H (1988) Improvement in regional wall motion after percutaneous transluminal coronary angioplasty during acute myocardial infarction: Utility of two-dimensional echocardiography. *Am Heart J* 115: 1149–1155.
74. Ratliff NB, Hackel DB (1980) Combined right and left ventricular infarction: Pathogenesis and clinicopathologic correlations. *Am J Cardiol* 45: 217–221.
75. Lopez-Sendon J, Coma-Canella I, Gamallo C (1981) Sensitivity and specificity of hemodynamic criteria in the diagnosis of acute right ventricular infarction. *Circulation* 64: 515–525.
76. Isner JM, Roberts WC (1978) Right ventricular infarction complicating left ventricular infarction secondary to coronary heart disease. *Am J Cardiol* 42: 885–894.
77. D'Arcy B, Nanda NC (1982) Two-dimensional echocardiographic features of right ventricular infarction. *Circulation* 65: 167–173.
78. Vannucci A, Cerchi F, Zuppiroli A, Marchionni N, Pini R, Di Bari M, Calamandrei M, Conti A, Ferrucci L, Greppi B, De Alfieri W (1983) Right ventricular infarction: Clinical, hemodynamic, mono- and two-dimensional echocardiographic features. *Eur Heart J* 4: 854–864.
79. Kaul S, Hopkins JM, Shah PM (1983) Chronic effects of myocardial infarction on right ventricular function: A noninvasive assessment. *J Am Coll Cardiol* 2: 607–615.
80. Lopez-Sendon J, Garcia-Fernandez MA, Coma-Canella I, Yanguela MM, Banuelas F (1983) Segmental right ventricular function after acute myocardial infarction: Two-dimensional echocardiographic study in 63 patients. *Am J Cardiol* 51: 390–396.
81. Dell'Italia IJ, Starling MR, Crawford MH, Boros BL, Chaudhuri TH, O'Rourke RA, Heyl B, Wray Amon K (1984) Right ventricular infarction: Identification by hemodynamic measurements before and after volume loading and correlation with non-invasive techniques. *J Am Coll Cardiol* 4: 931–939.
82. Starling MR, Crawford MH, Sorensen SG, Levi B, Richards KL, O'Rourke RA (1981) Comparative accuracy of apical biplane cross-sectional echocardiography and gated equilibrium radionuclide angiography for estimating left ventricular size and performance. *Circulation* 63: 1075–1084.
83. Erbel R, Schweizer P, Lambertz H, Henn G, Meyer J, Krebs W, Effert S (1983) Echoventriculography: A simultaneous analysis of two-dimensional echocardiography and cineventriculography. *Circulation* 67: 205–215.
84. Wackers FJ, Berger HJ, Weinberg MA, Zaret BL (1982) Spontaneous changes in left ventricular function over the first 24 h of acute myocardial infarction: Implications for evaluating early therapeutic interventions. *Circulation* 66: 748–754.
85. Kan G, Visser CA, Lie KI, Durrer D (1984) Serial left ventricular ejection fraction in acute myocardial infarction by cross-sectional echocardiography: Correlation of changing ejection fraction with clinical cause. *Eur Heart J* 5: 470–476.
86. Erbel R, Schweizer P, Meyer J, Krebs W, Yalkinoglu O, Effert S (1985) Sensitivity of cross-sectional echocardiography in detection of impaired global and regional left ventricular function: Prospective study. *Int J Cardiol* 7: 375–389.

87. Distante A, Picano E, Moscarelli E, Palombo C, Benassi A, L'Abbate A (1985) Echocardiographic versus hemodynamic monitoring during attacks of variant angina pectoris. *Am J Cardiol* 55: 1319–1322.
88. Erbel R, Zotz R, Henkel B, Schreiner G, Steuernagel C, Zahn R, Kopp H, Clas W, Brennecke R, Schweizer P, Meyer J (1987) Reliability and accuracy of echocardiography for follow-up studies after intervention., in: Roelandt J (ed), *Digital Techniques in Echocardiography*, pp 133–154. Dordrecht: Martinus Nijhoff.
89. Gibson DG, Prewitt TA, Brown DJ (1976) Analysis of left ventricular wall movement during isovolumic relaxation and its relation to coronary artery disease. *Br Heart J* 38: 1010–1019.
90. Dawson JR, Gibson DG (1989) Left ventricular filling and early diastolic function at rest and during angina in patients with coronary artery disease. *Br Heart J* 61: 248–257.
91. Upton MT, Gibson DG, Brown DJ (1976) Echocardiographic assessment of abnormal left ventricular relaxation in man. *Br Heart J* 38: 1001–1009.
92. Zoghbi WA, Rokey R, Limacher MC, Quinones MA (1987) Assessment of left ventricular diastolic filling by two-dimensional echocardiography. *Am Heart J* 113: 1108–1113.
93. Appleton CP, Hatle LK, Popp RL (1988) Relation of transmitral flow velocity patterns to left ventricular diastolic function: New insights from a combined hemodynamic and Doppler echocardiographic study. *J Am Coll Cardiol* 12: 426–440.
94. Choong CY, Herrmann HC, Weyman AE, Fifer MA (1987) Preload dependence of Doppler-derived indexes of left ventricular diastolic function in humans. *J Am Coll Cardiol* 10: 800–808.
95. Bowman LK, Lee FA, Jaffe CC, Mattera J, Wackers FJT, Zaret BL (1988) Peak filling rate normalized to mitral stroke volume: A new Doppler echocardiographic filling index validated by radionuclide angiographic techniques. *J Am Coll Cardiol* 12: 937–943.
96. Mehta PM, Alker KJ, Kloner RA (1988) Functional infarct expansion, left ventricular dilation and isovolumic relaxation time after coronary occlusion: A two-dimensional echocardiographic study. *J Am Coll Cardiol* 11: 630–636.
97. Feigenbaum H (1988) Exercise echocardiography, in: Visser C, Kan G, Meltzer R (eds), *Echocardiography in Coronary Artery Disease*, pp 51–64. Dordrecht: Kluwer.
98. Armstrong WF, O'Donnell J, Dillon JC, McHenry PL, Morris SN, Feigenbaum H (1986) Complementary value of two-dimensional exercise echocardiography to routine treadmill exercise testing. *Ann Intern Med* 105: 829–835.
99. Presti CF, Armstrong WF, Feigenbaum H (1988) Comparison of echocardiography at peak exercise and after bicycle exercise in evaluation of patients with known or suspected coronary artery disease. *J Am Soc Echo* 1: 119–126.
100. Iliceto S, Papa A, D'Ambrosio G, Amico A, Sorino M, Coluccia P, Rizzon P (1987) Prediction of the extent of coronary artery disease with the evaluation of left ventricular wall motion abnormalities during atrial pacing. A cross-sectional echocardiographic study. *Int J Cardiol* 14: 33–45.
101. Applegate RJ, Dell'Italia IJ, Crawford MH (1987) Usefulness of two-dimensional echocardiography during low-level exercise testing early after uncomplicated acute myocardial infarction. *Am J Cardiol* 60: 10–14.
102. Eiho S, Michiyoshi K, Asada N (1987) Left ventricular image processing. *Medical Progress through Technology* 12: 101–115.
103. Fine DG, Sapoznikov D, Mosseri M, Gotsmann MS (1988) Three-dimensional echocardiographic reconstruction: Qualitative and quantitative evaluation of ventricular function. *Computer Methods and Programs in Biomedicine* 26: 33–44.
104. Schnittger I, Fitzgerald PJ, Daughters GT, Ingels NB, Kantrowitz NE, Schwarzkopf A, Mead CW, Popp RL (1982) Limitations of comparing left ventricular volumes by two dimensional echocardiography, myocardial markers and cineangiography. *Am J Cardiol* 50: 512–519.

19. Stress echocardiography for identifying patients at risk after myocardial infarction

SABINO ILICETO, ANTONIO F. AMICO, CARLO CAIATI,
GIOVANNI PICCINNI, FRANCESCO TOTA, VITO
MARANGELLI, CATALDO MEMMOLA and PAOLO RIZZON

Introduction

Several factors contribute to the prognosis of patients surviving acute myocardial infarction [1–3]. Among these, the presence of additional myocardium at jeopardy is felt to be one of the most important. Consequently, many stress tests have been developed and proposed over the last few years for evaluating patients with recent myocardial infarction [1–9]. These tests are based on the combined use of a stress capable of inducing ischemia and a diagnostic technique capable of detecting the direct or indirect signs of acute myocardial ischemia. Among the stress tests used so far for prognostically stratifying patients with recent myocardial infarction, exercise echocardiography (treadmill or bicycle) is certainly the most common.

In recent years there has been an increasing interest in the use of cardiac imaging techniques during stress for the identification of patients at higher risk of future cardiac events after acute myocardial infarction. This is because they provide more sensitive ischemia markers (perfusion defects, regional and/or global left ventricular dysfunction) than the electrical ones obtained by classical exercise stress testing.

Cardiac imaging techniques in the prognostic stratification of patients with recent myocardial infarction

Cardiac imaging techniques have been used for prognostic stratification after myocardial infarction both in the acute phase and at hospital discharge [5–9]. While examinations performed in the acute phase are obviously done in resting conditions in order to evaluate regional and overall left ventricular perfusion defects and/or mechanical dysfunctions related to the occurrence of the acute infarct, exams performed some time after the acute event are usually done during exercise or alternative stresses so as to detect the possible presence of additional myocardium at jeopardy. Recent studies have clearly demonstrated that information derived from stress imaging is prognostically

S. Iliceto et al. (eds.), Ultrasound in Coronary Artery Disease, 231–239.
© 1991 *Kluwer Academic Publishers.*

much better than that obtainable with the traditional exercise stress test or with coronary angiography.

In a large series of patients with recent, uncomplicated myocardial infarction, Gibson [5] has demonstrated that the presence of thallium defects in more than one vascular area is a more accurate predictor of subsequent cardiac events than ST segment depression and/or angina during physical exercise or the extent of coronary artery disease as assessed by coronary angiography. In Gibson's study 94% of patients with subsequent cardiac events after myocardial infarction were correctly identified as high risk by stress thallium, whereas exercise-induced ST segment depression for angina and coronary angiography (presence of multivessel disease) only identified 56% and 71% of patients, respectively.

Until now, radionuclide cardiac imaging techniques have been the most used for this, whereas echocardiography, even if otherwise the most popular and widespread cardiac imaging technique, has been used very little, mainly because of its well-known limitations during physical exercise. The current availability of new stress reviewing systems that make exercise two-dimensional echocardiography (2D Echo) analysis decidedly easier, and alternative stresses that do not alter the 2D Echo quality during stress will certainly increase the role of this imaging technique in the evaluation of patients surviving acute myocardial infarction.

Exercise echocardiography

For over a decade now, some centres have been using exercise echocardiography for the noninvasive diagnosis of coronary artery disease [10–15]. This attractive stress imaging technique can be used not only for diagnostic purposes but also, as has happened for other cardiac imaging techniques, for the prognostic stratification of patients surviving acute myocardial infarction.

Jaarsma and colleagues [16] studied 43 patients after myocardial infarction, performing stress echocardiography within 3 weeks of the acute event. Twelve out of the 16 patients who had major cardiac events during the follow-up had a positive stress echocardiography study (75%) while only 4 of the 27 with a negative exercise 2D Echo presented a complicated follow-up. In this study, the criterion used by the authors to define a positive exercise 2D Echo was the presence of exercise-induced wall motion abnormalities in regions 'remote' from the infarcted area; the authors also correlated the results of exercise 2D Echo with the presence or absence of multivessel disease at coronary angiography: sensitivity was 77% while specificity was 95%. Applegate [17] studied a group of 67 patients with recent myocardial infarction. Echocardiography was performed immediately after treadmill exercise testing: sensitivity and specificity in identifying patients with a subsequent complicated follow-up were 63% and 80%, respectively. More recently, Ryan and colleagues [18] also presented data on a series of patients studied immediately after treadmill exercise testing. Sensitivity and specificity in identifying the ones with future cardiac complications were very good (80% and 95%), better than those obtained by means of the electrocardiographic response to treadmill stress test (55% sensitivity, 65% specificity).

Two-dimensional echocardiography during transesophageal atrial pacing

Atrial pacing was proposed more than 20 years ago by Sowton [19] as a stress for inducing angina in patients with coronary artery disease. More recently, Tzivoni [20, 21] has used atrial pacing to induce ischemic electrocardiographic changes in patients with recent myocardial infarction in order to identify those at risk of future cardiac events. Even if this sort of stress is particularly suitable in these patients (it is considerably safer than exercise and can even be performed shortly after the acute event) it has only been modestly utilized in this clinical setting. This relatively poor utilization can be attributed to the invasive nature of the stress test and the relatively limited sensitivity of the electrocardiographic marker in the detection of myocardial ischemia.

Two-dimensional echocardiography during transesophageal atrial pacing [22, 23] is a stress test, proposed for the diagnosis of coronary artery disease, that overcomes the two above-mentioned major limitations of the classical atrial pacing stress test: it is noninvasive because the atrial stimulation is performed through the oesophagus, and it offers a decidedly more sensitive marker of ischemia (wall motion abnormalities) than the electrocardiographic one. We have used this stress test in patients surviving myocardial infarction within two weeks of the acute event. This test is feasible in practically all patients, even those with specific contraindications to physical exercise, and, because of its safety (if interrupted it allows an immediate return to baseline hemodynamic conditions), it can even be performed shortly after myocardial infarction.

Technique

In Figure 1 the protocol we use in patients with recent myocardial infarction is schematically shown. Once the catheter has been positioned in the distal oesophagus with the help of electrocardiographic monitoring (the best catheter position is achieved when the unipolar atrial electrocardiogram shows the greatest amplitude) atrial stimulation is begun. Pacing is started at 110 beats/min and increased every 2 min by 10 beats/min. Pacing at 140 beats/min is not performed while that at 150 beats/min is maintained for 5 min. Thus, the entire protocol is usually completed in 11 min. 2D Echo is performed before, during the stress test and at peak pacing. Different tomographic planes are used during the test so as to obtain a complete evaluation of left ventricular wall motion. For the purpose of the analysis the left ventricle is divided into 11 segments (Figure 2). Criteria for interruption of the

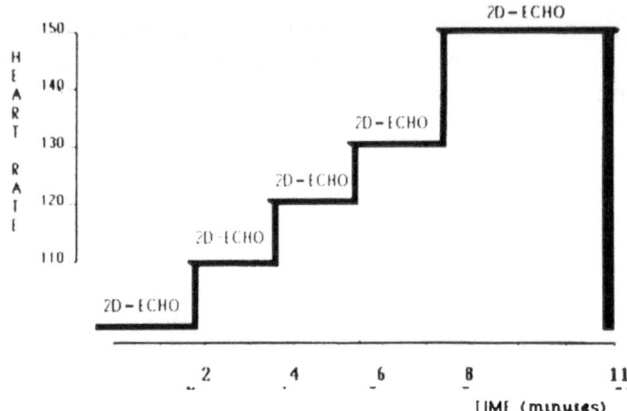

Figure 1. Pacing protocol. Atrial pacing is started at 110 min⁻¹ and increased every 2 min by 10 beats min⁻¹ until a heart rate of 150 beats min⁻¹ is achieved. Two-dimensional echocardiography (2D Echo) is performed at rest, during and after 5 min pacing at highest rate reached.

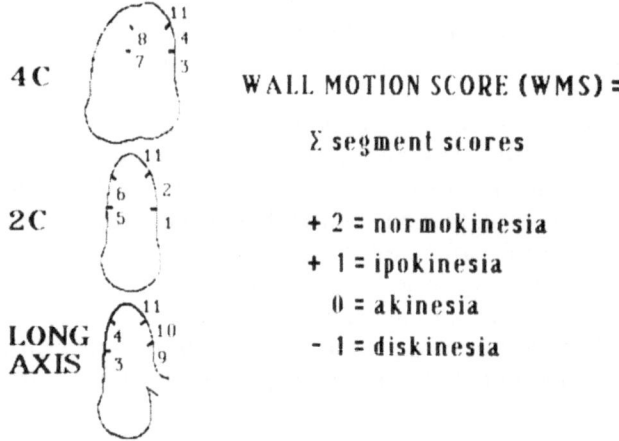

Figure 2. Echocardiographic imaging of the left ventricle is obtained with the apical four-chamber (4C), two-chamber (2C) and long axis views. The left ventricle is divided, for purposes of analysis, into 11 segments. Each segment is assigned a score according to its kinetic. The wall motion score is the sum of the scores of the single segments.

stress test are: occurrence of new, severe wall motion abnormalities, ST depression > 3 mm, or severe chest pain.

Results in patients with recent myocardial infarction

In order to evaluate the prognostic value of this stress test in patients with recent myocardial infarction we performed a prospective study. 83 consecutive patients with recent uncomplicated myocardial infarction entered the study [25]. The inclusion criteria are listed in Table I. All patients underwent

Table 1. Characteristics of a group of 83 consecutive patients studied by transesophageal echo-cardiography: inclusion criteria.

- First acute transmural myocardial infarction
- No cardiac complications
- Capability to undergo physical exercise
- Absence of other concomitant cardiac diseases
- Good quality 2D echo
- Absence of diseases capable to affect the follow-up

---

transesophageal atrial pacing 2D Echo and exercise electrocardiography within 20 days of the acute event. Criteria for test positivity were the following:

- ST-depression ≥ 1 mm for exercise testing and
- development, during pacing, of wall motion abnormalities in regions remote from the infarcted area for transesophageal atrial pacing 2D Echo.

All the patients were followed up after acute myocardial infarction (mean follow-up was 14 ± 5 months). Of the 83 patients, 20 developed cardiac events in the follow-up (new myocardial infarction, angina). In this series of patients transesophageal atrial pacing 2D Echo was much better than stress testing at separating high from low risk patients after uncomplicated myocardial infarction (Figure 3). In fact, the percentage of cardiac events in the group of patients with positive stress 2D Echo was much higher than in the group of patients with positive stress testing (65 vs 32%, $p < 0.005$).

In Figure 4, the survival data are presented in a life table format, according to the results of stress test and atrial pacing 2D Echo. Survival data further underline the greater diagnostic potential of transesophageal atrial pacing 2D Echo as compared to the traditional exercise stress test.

Stress echocardiography for the prognostic stratification of patients surviving myocardial infarction

As with other cardiac imaging techniques, stress 2D Echo can successfully be used to prognostically stratify patients after myocardial infarction. The potential of this diagnostic approach is certainly superior to that of stress testing since the appearance of new, potentially ischemic areas is more reliably identified by cardiac imaging techniques than by traditional stress testing. Furthermore, as previous studies have demonstrated, the prognostic potential of

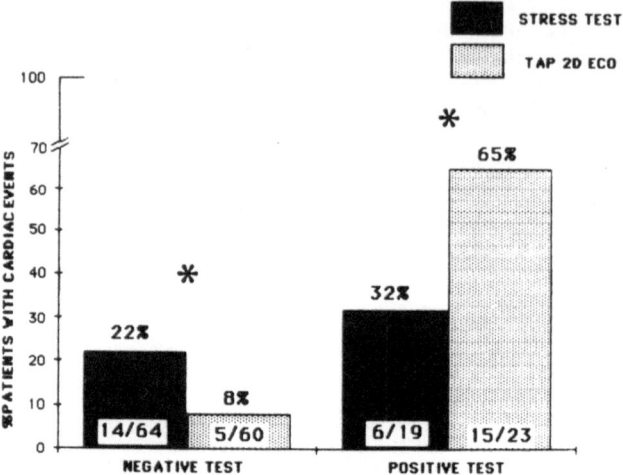

Figure 3. Incidence of cardiac events in a group of 83 patients in the two years following the first myocardial infarct in response to the ECG stress test and the TAP-2D echo. A positive TAP-2D echo meant that the patient entered the group with high incidence of cardiac events; response to the ECG stress test did necessarily predict future risk of cardiac events.

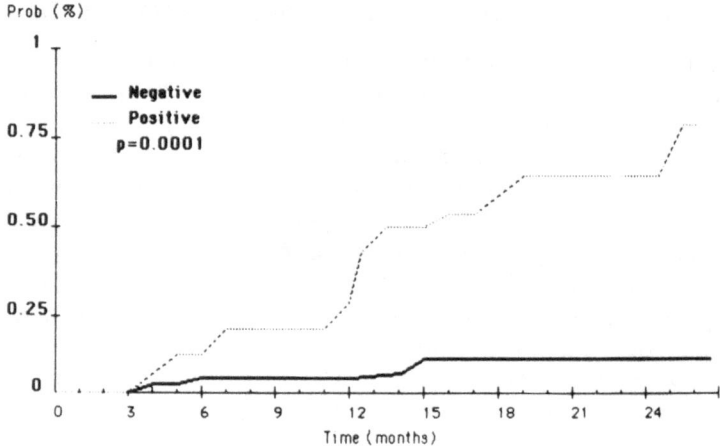

Figure 4. Cumulative probability of cardiac events as a function of transesophageal (TAP) two-dimensional echocardiography (2D Echo). Solid lines indicate patients having negative TAP 2D Echo results, broken line represents patients with positive TAP 2D Echo. The two curves were statistically different at p < 0.0001.

functional parameters is even better than that which can be found from anatomic information supplied by coronary angiography [5]. In other words, the presence of myocardium at jeopardy detected by stress cardiac imaging techniques is a far more reliable indicator of poor prognosis than the presence of multivessel disease. Stress 2D Echo can usefully be used in the stratification of patients with recent myocardial infarction.

The major practical problem when using 2D Echo as an imaging technique is the quality of the images during stress. Lung interposition and chest and muscle mobility strongly affect the quality of echocardiographic images during exercise. This limitation has greatly hampered the adoption of 2D Echo imaging during stress as a diagnostic or prognostic tool. The low acceptance of stress 2D Echo in these clinical settings is mainly due to this major problem. Nowadays, however, the problem of the quality of echocardiographic images during stress can be completely overcome thanks to new advances in digital technology [14, 15] and to the availability of additional kinds of alternative stresses [23–26], not affecting the quality of 2D Echo images, that are as reliable as physical exercise.

A crucial problem that immediately arises when dealing with stress cardiac imaging techniques utilized for the prognostic stratification of patients with myocardial infarction is the definition of a positive test. Since the main purpose, in this context, of stress imaging techniques is the detection of additional myocardium at jeopardy (one of the most important predictors of future cardiac events) a test has been defined positive if wall motion abnormalities, or perfusion defects, are observed in regions 'remote' from the infarcted area. If abnormalities occurring only in 'remote' regions are considered, one can reasonably be sure of only evaluating phenomena related to a possible acutely-induced myocardial ischemia. Vice versa, mechanical alterations in regions 'adjacent' to the infarcted myocardium may simply be due to tethering of myocardial zones that are in close contact with the akinetic infarcted myocardium. In view of this, the importance of accurately defining the site and extent of the 'remote' regions in a patient with myocardial infarction appears obvious. However, consensus on this definition does not yet exist and the definitions used in different studies do not always agree. Despite these limitations, stress echocardiography can be considered a useful tool in the prognostic stratification of patients surviving acute myocardial infarction. Many of the technical limitations affecting feasibility and image quality have been partially or totally overcome (as previously mentioned) by new digital technology and alternative stresses, while conceptual problems related to the difficult accurate definition of 'remote' regions can be more appropriately faced thanks to the multiple tomographic viewing of 2-dimensional echocardiography that allows a complete 3-dimensional reconstruction of left ventricular shape and motion.

References

1. Théroux P, Waters DD, Halphen C, Debaisieux J-C, Mizgala HF (1979) Prognostic value of exercise testing soon after myocardial infarction. *N Engl J Med* 301: 341–345.
2. Williams WL, Nair RC, Higginson LAJ, Baird MG, Allan K, Beanlands DS (1984) Com-

parison of clinical and treadmill variables for the prediction of outcome after myocardial infarction. *J Am Coll Cardiol* 4: 477–486.

3. De Feyter PJ, Eenige MJ van, Dighton DH, Visser FC, Jong J de, Roos JP (1982) Prognostic value of exercise testing, coronary angiography and left ventriculography 6–8 weeks after myocardial infarction. *Circulation* 66: 527–536.

4. Krone RJ, Gillespie JA, Weld FM, Miller JP, Moss AJ and the Multicenter Postinfarction Research Group (1985) Low-level exercise testing after myocardial infarction: Usefulness in enhancing clinical risk stratification. *Circulation* 71: 80–89.

5. Gibson RS, Watson DD, Craddock GB, Crampton RS, Kaiser DL, Denny MJ, Beller GA (1983) Prediction of cardiac events after uncomplicated myocardial infarction: A prospective study comparing predischarge exercise thallium-201 scintigraphy and coronary angiography. *Circulation* 68: 321–336.

6. Morris DD, Rozanski A, Berman DS, Diamond GA, Swan HJC (1984) Noninvasive prediction of the angiographic extent of coronary artery disease after myocardial infarction: Comparison of clinical, bicycle exercise electrocardiographic, and ventriculographic parameters. *Circulation* 70: 192–201.

7. Hung J, Goris ML, Nash E, Kraemer HC, DeBusk RF, et al. (1984) Comparative value of maximal treadmill testing, exercise thallium myocardial perfusion scintigraphy and exercise radionuclide ventriculography for distinguishing high- and low-risk patients soon after acute myocardial infarction. *Am J Cardiol* 53: 1221–1227.

8. Turner JD, Schwartz KM, Logic JR (1980) Detection of residual jeopardized myocardium 3 weeks after myocardial infarction by exercise testing with thallium-201 myocardial scintigraphy. *Circulation* 61: 729–737.

9. Corbett JR, Dehmer GJ, Lewis SE, Woodward W, Henderson E, Parkey RW, Blomquist CG, Willerson JT (1981) The prognostic value of submaximal exercise testing with radionuclide ventriculography before hospital discharge in patients with recent myocardial infarction. *Circulation* 64: 535–544.

10. Wann SL, Faris JV, Childress RH, Dillon JC, Weyman AE, Feigenbaum H (1979) Exercise cross-sectional echocardiography in ischemic heart disease. *Circulation* 60: 1300–1308.

11. Visser CA, Wieken RL van der, Kan G, Lie KI, Busemann-Sokele E, Meltzer RS, Durrer D (1983) Comparison of two-dimensional echocardiography with radionuclide angiography during dynamic exercise for the detection of coronary artery disease. *Am Heart J* 106: 528–534.

12. Maurer G, Nanda NC (1981) Two-dimensional echocardiographic evaluation of exercise-induced left and right ventricular asynergy: Correlation with thallium scanning. *Am J Cardiol* 48: 720–727.

13. Limacher MC, Quinones MA, Poliner LR, Nelson JG, Winters WL, Waggoner AD (1983) Detection of coronary artery disease with exercise two-dimensional echocardiography. *Circulation* 6: 1211–1218.

14. Robertson WS, Feigenbaum H, Armstrong WF, Dillon JC, O'Donnell J, McHenry PW (1983) Exercise echocardiography: A clinically practical addition in the evaluation of coronary artery disease. *J Am Coll Cardiol* 2: 1085–1091.

15. Armstrong WF, O'Donnell J, Ryan T, Feigenbaum H (1987) Effect of prior myocardial infarction and extent and location of coronary disease on accuracy of exercise echocardiography. *J Am Coll Cardiol* 10: 531–538.

16. Jaarsma W, Visser CA, Funke Kupper AJ, Res JCJ, Van Eenige MJ, Roos JP (1986) Usefulness of two-dimensional exercise echocardiography shortly after myocardial infarction. *Am J Cardiol* 57: 86–90.

17. Applegate RJ, Dell'Italia LJ, Crawford MH (1987) Usefulness of two-dimensional echocardiography during low-level exercise testing early after uncomplicated acute myocardial infarction. *Am J Cardiol* 60: 10–14.

18. Ryan T, Armstrong WF, O'Donnell JA, Feigenbaum H (1987) Risk stratification after acute myocardial infarction by means of exercise two-dimensional echocardiography. *Am Heart J* 114: 1305–1316.

19. Sowton GE, Balcon R, Gross G, Frick MH (1967) Measurement of the angina threshold using atrial pacing. *Cardiovasc Res*: 301–307.
20. Tzivoni D, Gottlieb S, Keren A et al. (1984) Early right atrial pacing after myocardial infarction. I. Comparison with early treadmill testing. *Am J Cardiol* 53: 414–417.
21. Tzivoni D, Gottlieb S, Keren A, et al. (1984) Early right atrial pacing after myocardial infarction. II Results in 77 patients with predischarge angina pectoris, congestive heart failure, or age older than 70 years. *Am J Cardiol* 53: 418–420.
22. Chapman PD, Doyle TP, Troup PJ, Gross VM, Wann SL (1984) Stress echocardiography with transesophageal atrial pacing: Preliminary report of a new method for detection of ischemic wall motion abnormalities. *Circulation* 70: 445–450.
23. Iliceto S, D'Ambrosio G, Sorino M, Papa Antonietta, Amico A, Ricci A, Rizzon P (1986) Comparison of postexercise and transesophageal atrial pacing two-dimensional echocardiography for detection of coronary artery disease. *Am J Cardiol* 57: 547–553.
24. Iliceto S, Sorino M, D'Ambrosio G, Papa A, Favale S, Biasco G, Rizzon P (1985) Detection of coronary artery disease by two-dimensional echocardiography and transesophageal atrial pacing. *J Am Coll Cardiol* 5: 1188–1197.
25. Iliceto S, Caiati C, Ricci A, Amico A, D'Ambrosio G, Ferry GM, Izzi M, Lagioia R, Rizzon P (1990) Prediction of cardiac events after uncomplicated myocardial infarction by cross-sectional echocardiography during transesophageal pacing. *Int J Cardiol* 28.
26. Picano E, Lattanzi F, Masini M, Distante A, L'Abbate A (1986) High dose dipyridamole echocardiography test in effort angina pectoris. *J Am Coll Cardiol* 8: 848–854.

20. Two-dimensional echocardiography for the assessment of therapeutic interventions and long-term follow-up of patients with acute myocardial infarction

R. ERBEL, U. NIXDORFF, G. GÖRGE, R. BRENNECKE and J. MEYER

Introduction

Infarct size is the main predictor of prognosis in patients with acute myocardial infarction [1–3]. Dependent on infarct size regional and global left ventricular function is depressed leading to cardiogenic shock, when more than 40% of the myocardium are involved [4]. Thrombolysis therapy has been shown to be effective both preserving ventricular function [5, 6] and survival [7, 8]. For serial measurement of regional and global left ventricular function two-dimensional echocardiography seems to be an ideal bedside noninvasive method. The purpose of study was to establish the long-term effect of thrombolysis therapy on ventricular function dependent on

– time until reperfusion
– completeness of reperfusion and
– additional percutaneous transluminal coronary angioplasty (PTCA), analysed by two-dimensional echocardiography.

Methods

Patients

The study was performed in 206 consecutive patients with acute transmural myocardial infarction with a time interval from onset of symptoms until start of treatment of less than 6 h. Inclusion criteria were

– persistent chest pain of more than 30 min,
– persistent ST-segment elevation of more than 0.3 mV in leads V 1 to V 6 or 0.2 mV in leads I to III. aVL or aVF

Exclusion criteria were:
– resuscitation,
– history of allergic reaction to streptokinase,

S. Iliceto et al. (eds.), Ultrasound in Coronary Artery Disease, 241–254.
© 1991 *Kluwer Academic Publishers.*

- previous cerebral accident,
- surgery in the preceding 10 days,
- history of acute peptic ulcer, and
- history of bleeding problems.

Treatment regimen

All patients received intravenous premedication including 5.000 IU heparine, 250 mg prednisolone, 3 mg/h nitroglycerine and 1 g acetylsalicylate; 250.000 IU streptokinase was infused intravenously within 20 min before cardiac catheterization.

According to the randomization coronary angiography was performed using a 7 F catheter (group I) or 9 F guide catheter (group II). After opacification of the infarct related vessel, 50.000 IU bolus dose of streptokinase dissolved in saline solution followed by a continuous regulated infusion of streptokinase in saline solution at a rate of 4.000 U/min through the coronary artery until a total dose of 200.000 U was reached. After reperfusion infusion rate was increased to 12.000 IU/min. Thus, patients received a total dose of 500.000 IU streptokinase, both intracornary (250.000 IU) and intravenous (250.000 IU). As soon as possible, mechanical recanalization was performed with a 3 F recanalization catheter (group I) or balloon catheter (group II). After application of the full dose of streptokinase, PTCA was performed in group II.

After thrombolytic therapy, left ventricular angiography was performed using a pigtail catheter with injection of 40 ml of urografin 70% (Byk Gulden, Konstanz/Germany) at 14 ml/s. The X-ray equipment was a Siemens biplane Pandoros Optimatic Unit (Berlin, Germany) incorporating a variable mode image intensifier. Before discharge and after 6 months, right and left heart catheterization with coronary angiography and cineventriculography was repeated.

Echocardiography

Two-dimensional echocardiography was performed using a phased-array sector scanner (Diasonics V 3400 R-6400, Toshiba SSH 65A) with 3.25 MHz and 3.5 MHz transducers enabling an echosector of 84–90°. From the apical regional the left ventricle was scanned in the 4-chamber and RAO-equivalent view [9, 10]. Always the heart was scanned in the longest possible axis with a free opening of the mitral valve and aortic valve visible. All echocardiograms were received in depth of the scan field of 15 cm. The echocardiograms were recorded in the catheterization laboratory during the preparation of heart catheterization. The second echocardiogram was recorded after the end of the thrombolytic therapy immediately after the cinventriculogram. At the first and second day on coronary care unit before discharge, after 6, 12, 24, 36, 48 months control studies were performed always in the left lateral position.

Analyses were performed for patients with and without PTCA, with anterior and inferior myocardial infarction, infarct times of less and more than 3 h 30 min and those with open vessels at the first coronary angiogram and persistent occlusion.

Calculation

Left ventricular volumes were determined using a biplane disc method, as previously described [11] with a half automatic computer system (Kontron 200, München, Germany). End-diastole was measured at the peak of the R-wave using a frame signal recorded simultaneously with the electrocardiogram during cineventriculography at a paper speed of 50 mm/s. End-systole was defined as the smallest ventricular silhouette. Stroke volume and ejection fraction were calculated. All volume measurements were corrected for body surface area and expressed as indexes. Normal values were published previously [12].

Echocardiograms in the RAO equivalent view were selected for regional wall motion analysis using a fixed system with the diastolic center of gravity as the center point, creating 32 radii. Percent shortening of the 32 segments calculated and normal values were established in 30 control subjects [13, 14].

Statistics

All values are given as mean values ± standard deviation. Wilcoxon tests were used for paired and unpaired data analysis. A p-value < 0.05 was reported as significant.

Results

A quantitative analysis of left ventricular function was possible in 77% of all ventricular walls. 101 additional studies were not available cause of death of the patients or missing echocardiographic studies related to logistical problems.

Global left ventricular function

Analysis of end-diastolic and endsystolic volume in patients of group with and without PTCA in addition to the thrombolytic therapy demonstrated an continuous increase of volumes during the 3 years follow-up. The increase of changes was more pronounced during the first 3 months and less during the follow-up period afterwards. There seems to be a trend to higher volumes in

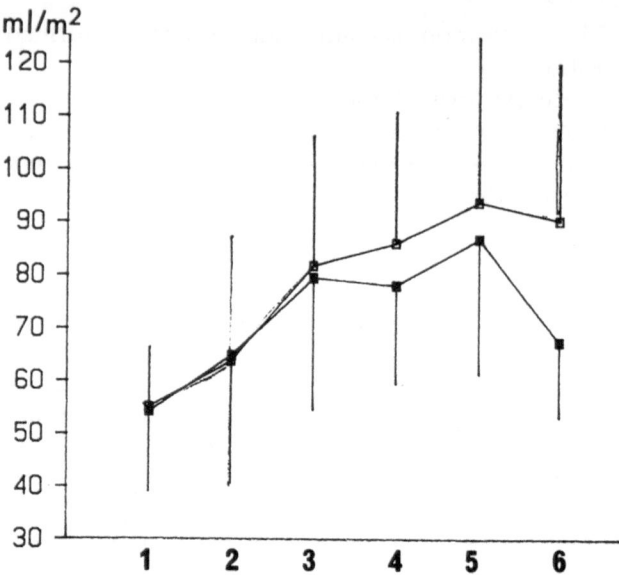

Figure 1. End-diastolic volume index for patients with ▪ and without ▫ PTCA in addition to thrombolytic therapy before therapy (1), before discharge (2), after 3 (3), 12 (4) and 36 (6) months in anterior wall infarction.

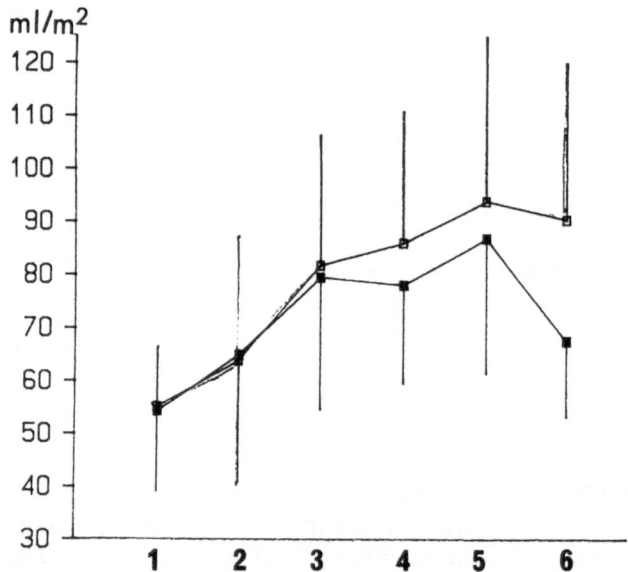

Figure 2. End-systolic volume index for patients with ▪ and without ▫ PTCA in addition to thrombolytic therapy before therapy (1) before discharge (2), after 3 (3), 12 (4) and 36 (6) months in anterior wall infarction.

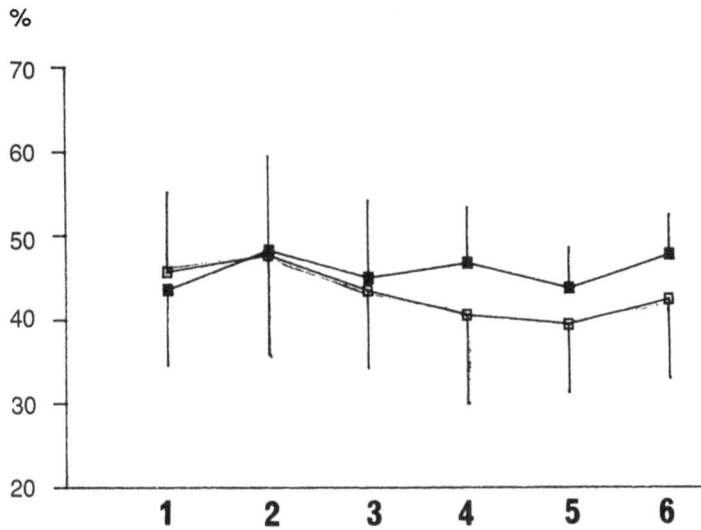

Figure 3. Ejection fraction for patients with ■ and without □ PTCA in addition to thrombolytic therapy before therapy (1), before discharge (2), after 3 (3), 12 (4) and 36 (6) months in anterior wall infarction.

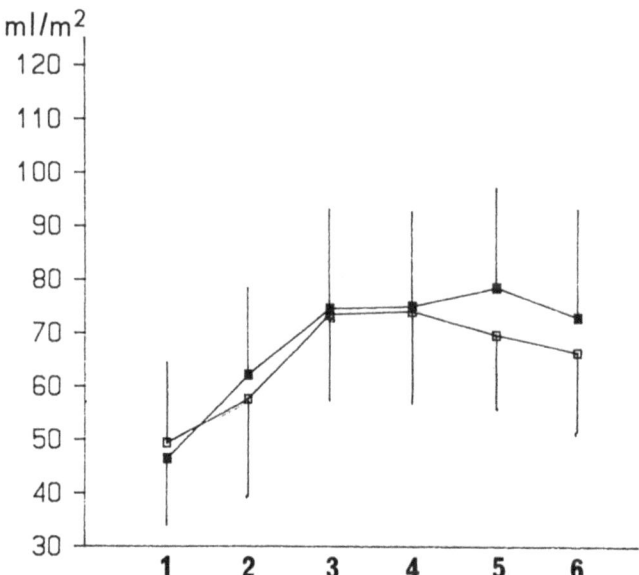

Figure 4. End-diastolic volume index for patients with ■ and without □ PTCA in addition to thrombolytic therapy before therapy (1), before discharge (2), after 3 (3), 12 (4) and 36 (6) months in inferior wall infarction.

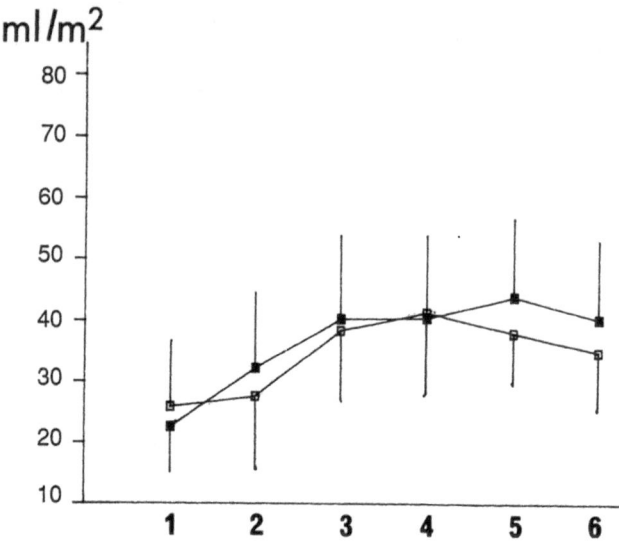

Figure 5. End-systolic volume index for patients with ■ and without ▫ PTCA in addition to thrombolytic therapy before therapy (1), before discharge (2), after (3), 12 (4) and 36 (6) months in inferior wall infarction.

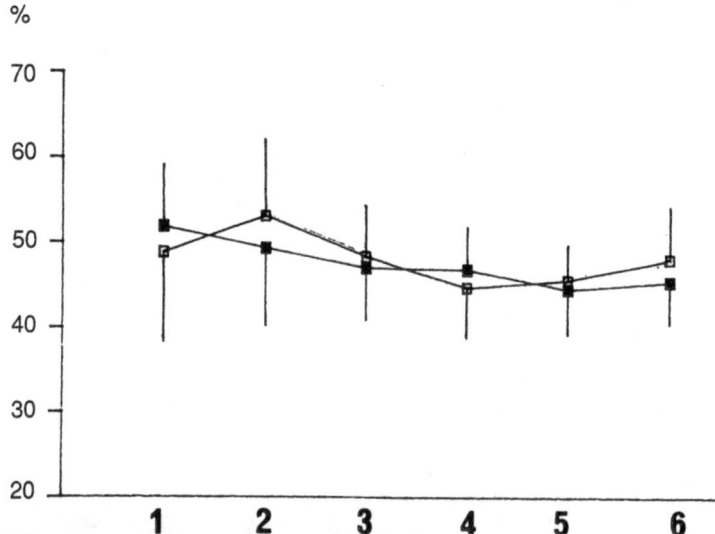

Figure 6. Ejection fraction for patients with ■ and without ▫ PTCA in addition to thrombolytic therapy before therapy (1), before discharge (2), after 3 (3), 12 (4) and 36 (6) months in inferior wall infarction.

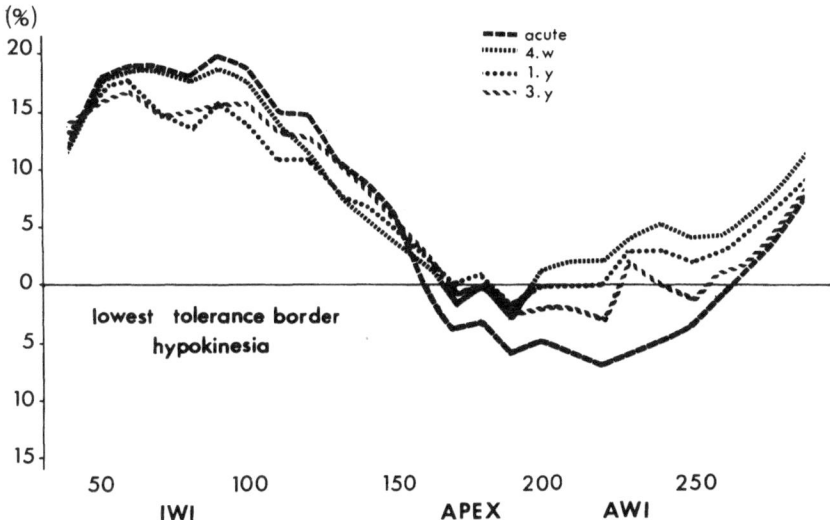

Figure 7. Shortening fraction of 27 radiants in patients with anterior myocardial infarction after thrombolytic therapy with PTCA evaluated by two-dimensional echocardiography (2dE) acute (1), before discharge (4 w), after 1 and 3 years. AW = anterior wall, IW = inferior wall, illustrated as the zero line is the tolerance limit for normal contraction and start of hypokinesia.

patients without PTCA in addition to thrombolytic therapy (Figures 1, 2). Related to left ventricular ejection fraction, there was a continuous slight decrease in patients with thrombolytic therapy but without PTCA in comparison to the group with PTCA (Figure 3).

In patients with inferior myocardial infarction a continuous increase of end-diastolic and end-systolic volume was measured (Figures 4, 5). The volumes in patients with anterior wall infarction were larger than in patients with inferior wall infarction. Between the group with and without PTCA in addition to thrombolytic therapy no significant difference could be detected. During follow-up (Figure 6) for left ventricular ejection fraction there was a continuous but not significant decrease during the follow-up in both patient groups.

Regional wall motion

Regional wall motion demonstrated in patients with anterior wall infarction after thrombolytic therapy a significant decrease only in those with PTCA in addition to the thrombolytic therapy. But also in those without PTCA a decrease of the hypokinetic zone could be demonstrated (Figure 7). In patients with inferior myocardial infarction a slight improvement which was not significant could be demonstrated during the follow-up period more in the group without PTCA and in the group with PTCA. The difference was not significant. In patients with long infarct times regional wall motion demonstrated no improvement during follow-up, whereas in patients with short in-

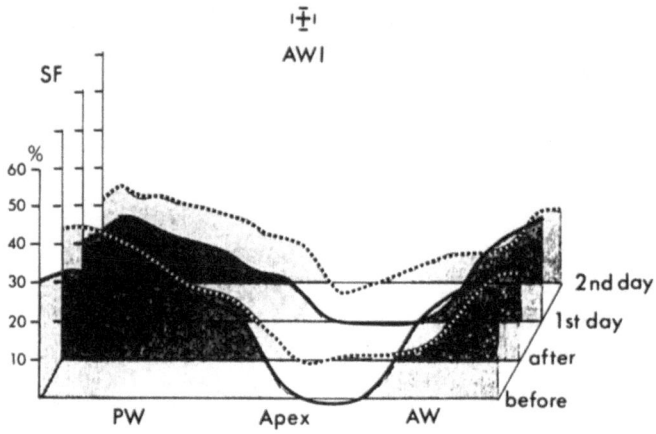

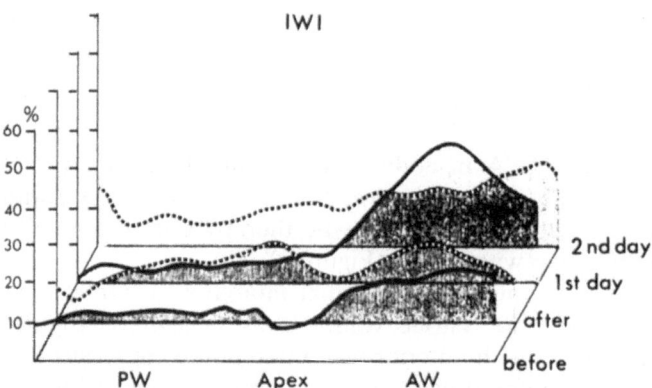

Figure 8. Shortening fraction of 27 radiants in patients with anterior (AW) and inferior myocardial infarction (IWI) after thrombolytic therapy. Results for patients who died during followup. Large wall motion abnormalities are visible.

farct times a decrease could be demonstrated particularly in those with anterior wall infarction. In patients who died during follow-up the early evaluation of regional wall motion demonstrated in anterior as well as in inferior wall infarction extended wall motion abnormalities (Figure 8).

Discussion

Two-dimensional echocardiography has been found to be an accurate method for detection of impaired global and regional left ventricular function with high sensitivity and specificity [16, 17]. Exercise echocardiography seems to increase the sensitivity in patients with coronary artery disease

[18, 19]. The accuracy of echocardiography in determining left ventricular volume was first analysed in heart models yielding high correlations and low standard errors of estimate [11]. Two-dimensional echocardiography was nearly as accurate as radiographic methods. Also in isolated postmortem [20] and formalin fixed hearts [21, 22] the accuracy of two-dimensional echocardiography could be proved. Standard errors of estimate were slightly higher than in model hearts. In patients no golden standard for left ventricular volume determination is available. Therefore comparisons were made to cineventriculography. Numerous studies revealed high correlations between both methods [23].

Obviously two-dimensional echocardiography underestimated left ventricular volumes in comparison to cineventriculography related to the difference between noninvasive and invasive techniques, effects of contrast material, methodological problems – two-dimensional echocardiography is a cross-sectional method and cineventriculography a contour method. The main reason seems to be, however, that the echo transducer position in the apical position of the ventricle didn't image the heart in the full long axis as simultaneous studies demonstrated [23]. Tangential cuts with underestimation of short and long axis and overestimation of wall thickness resulted [23]. These effects were even increased by slice-thickness artefacts [24].

Despite these methodological problems mean rates of ejection fraction were in similar range as for radionuclide studies. The limits of the normal range are for both methods near 50% [12]. Despite differences in absolute values, percentage changes of left ventricular volumes and ejection fraction during atrial pacing [25], after postextrasystolic potentiation [26] and after administration of prenalterol – a positive inotropic agent – were in the same range as for cineventriculography [23].

In the follow-up study, after thrombolytic therapy and before discharge additional cineventriculograms were performed and could be compared to two-dimensional echocardiography [27]. The results demonstrate, that the overall changes of the group were comparable related to the direction and the degree of changes. Cineventriculographic changes of ejection fraction seems to be more pronounced than detected by two-dimensional echocardiography. Similar studies are not available in the literature. Two-dimensional echocardiography can be regarded as a method by which quantitative analyses of left ventricular function can be performed for follow-up studies as for drug intervention studies and after coronary bypass surgery [28].

First cineventriculographic studies suggested significant changes of ejection fraction after thrombolytic therapy [5, 6]. These changes were, however, not confirmed by other studies. Usually significant changes are only observed in subgroups of patients with early reperfusion [29], anterior myocardial infarction [30] and no reperfusion [31].

Our study demonstrated that global left ventricular function was not significant different between the acute and chronic stage. Also between patients with and without PTCA no difference could be observed. Analysing the data

separately for patients with anterior and inferior myocardial infarction significant differences could be demonstrated. In those with thrombolysis and
PTCA a significant increase was found as previously found by cineventriculography [13]. Also Sheehan et al. reported significant changes of ejection
fraction only in patients, who received bypass surgery after thrombolysis
therapy [32]. Continuous increase in end-diastolic and end-systolic volumes
seem to reflect the increase percentage of patients with heart failure which
were found during follow-up studies even after thrombolytic therapy.

Regional wall motion

Regional wall motion improved in patients with anterior myocardial infarction and PTCA. The improvement for patients with PTCA is much more pronounced than for patients without PTCA. These results seems to be based on
experimental data published by Schmidt et al. [33]. After 3 h of ischemia
reperfusion induced salvage of myocardium was limited by underlyning coronary luminal narrowing reducing coronary blood flow to 30% of normal flow.
   Most striking changes were observed between the first and second day in
the control study before discharge. Charuzi et al. [34] followed regional and
global left ventricular function after intracoronary thrombolysis by two-
dimensional echocardiography. Improvement in 18 patients with successful
reperfusion occurred by day 10 but not immediately after reperfusion according to our results. Also previous angiographic studies couldn't demonstrate
significant changes immediately after reperfusion [35, 36]. Control studies
after 10 days showed a significant increase in successful reperfusion as
Reduto et al. [35] and Anderson et al. [37] demonstrated. These results are in
accordance to previous experimental studies [38] demonstrating that left ventricular function requires several weeks to return to normal function after one
hour of coronary artery occlusion. These studies didn't support early reports
of Rentrop et al. [5] and Mathey et al. [6]. Their data were based, however, on
the experience in only a limited number of patients.
   Without reperfusion, experimental studies couldn't find an improvement in
myocardial infarction [39, 40]. Global and regional function were unchanged
in patients with occluded vessels [35–37] as well as control groups [35]. Some
studies even demonstrated a deterioration in these patients [31] with increase
in end-diastolic and end-systolic volume and decrease in ejection fraction.

Influence of infarct time

Improvement of left ventricular function after reperfusion is strongly dependent on infarct time as pointed out previously in experimental studies by
Schaper [41]. Analyses of reperfusion studies in men revealed that beyond in
infarct time of 3–4 h no improvement of left ventricular function will occur
[31] in accordance to our echocardiographic results. In patients with long

infarct time an increase in end-diastolic and end-systolic volume and decrease in ejection fraction was found.

Because prognosis is strongly dependent on ventricular function, mortality was reduced significantly with infarct times of 3 h. Patients with infarct times between 3–6 h showed only slightly reduction of mortality. Patients with infarct times of more than 6 h had no benefit from thrombolysis therapy [42].

Influence of degree of revascularization

After reperfusion, severe residual luminal narrowing is found in 75% of patients [43]. Experimental studies have demonstrated that reduction of coronary blood flow during reperfusion decrease salvage of myocardium achieved by reperfusion [33]. Our randomized controlled study demonstrated in 162 patients an improvement of regional wall motion in anterior myocardial infarction only in those with PTCA but not in those without PTCA [13]. Also analysis of data after coronary bypass surgery after reperfusion by Sheehan et al. [32] demonstrated, that improvement is strongly dependent on completeness of revascularization [32]. The echocardiographic study clearly demonstrated, as independent method, that regional wall motion improvement is dependent on coronary blood flow. But only in anterior wall infarction improvement could be demonstrated as previously reported for cineventriculography [27].

Influence of infarct location

Cause of the infarct size left ventricular volumes are lower and ejection fraction higher in patients with inferior myocardial infarction compared to anterior myocardial infarction according to previous reports [30]. Related to the larger extent reduction of infarct size can be better demonstrated. It cannot be ruled out, that two-dimensional echocardiography and cineventriculography are insensitive to detect changes perhaps occurring in inferior infarctions. These suggestions are supported by the observation that also in inferior myocardial infarction mortality could be reduced by intracoronary application of streptokinase [7]. On the other hand these results could not be explained according to results of left ventricular function [30].

Analyses of right ventricular function revealed significant improvement in patients with right ventricular involvement [14]. Possibly improvement of right ventricular function contributed to the reduction of mortality in patients with inferior infarction.

References

1. Cohn PF, Gorlin R, Cohn H, Collins Jr JJ (1974) Left ventricular ejection fraction as a prognostic guide in the surgical treatment of coronary and valvular heart disease. Am J Cardiol 34: 13.
2. Harris PJ, Harrell FE, Lee KL, Behar VS, Rosati RA (1979) Survival in medically treated coronary artery disease. Circulation 60: 1259.
3. Taylor GJ, O'Neal, Jumphries J, Mellits ED, Pitt B, Schulze RA, Griffith LSC, Aschuff SC (1980) Predictors of clinical course, coronary anatomy and left ventricular function after recovery from acute myocardial infarction. Circulation 62: 960.
4. Page DL, Coulfield JB, Kastor JA, De Sanctis RW, Sanders CA (1971) Myocardial changes associated with cardiogenic shock. N Engl J Med 285: 133.
5. Rentrop P, Blanke H, Karsch KR, Kaiser H, Köstering H, Leitz K (1981) Selective intracoronary thrombolysis in acute myocardial infarction and unstable angina pectoris. Circulation 63: 307.
6. Mathey DG, Kuck KH, Tilsner V, Krebber HJ, Bleifeld W (1981) Nonsurgical coronary artery recanalization in acute transmural myocardial infarction. Circulation 63: 489.
7. Kennedy JW, Ritchie JL, Davis KB, Studius ML, Maynard C, Fritz K (1983) Western Washington randomized trial of intracoronary streptokinase in acute myocardial infarction. N Engl J Med 309: 1477.
8. Simoons ML, Brand M vd, De Zwaan C, Verheugt FWA, Remme W, Serruys PW, Bär F, Res J, Krauss XH, Vermeer F, Lubsen J (1985) Improved survival after early thrombolysis in acute myocardial infarction. Lancet II: 578.
9. Erbel R, Schweizer P, Meyer J, Grenner H, Krebs W, Effert S (1980) Left ventricular volume and ejection fraction determination by cross-sectional echocardiography in patients with coronary artery disease: A prospective study. Clin Cardiol 3: 377.
10. Erbel R, Schweizer P, Krebs W, Pyhel N, Meyer J, Effert S (1981) Monoplane and biplane zweidimensionale echokardiographische Volumenbestimmung des linken Ventrikels. II. Untersuchungen bei koronarer Herzerkrankung. Z Kardiol 70: 436.
11. Erbel R, Krebs W, Henn G, Schweizer P, Richter HA, Meyer J, Effert (1982) Comparison of single-plane and biplane volume determination by two-dimensional echocardiography. I. Asymmetric model hearts. Eur Heart J 3: 469.
12. Erbel R, Henkel B, Ostländer C, Clas W, Brennecke R, Meyer J (1985) Normalwerte für die zweidimensionale Echokardiographie. Dtsch Med Wschr 110: 123.
13. Erbel R, Pop T, Henrichs K v, Olshausen K v, Schuster CJ, Rupprecht HJ, Steuernagel C, Meyer J (1986) Percutaneous transluminal coronary angioplasty after thrombolytic therapy: A prospective controlled randomized trial. J A CC 8: 485.
14. Rupprecht HJ, Erbel R, Schöter KH, Schreiner G, Henrichs HJ, Meyer J Right ventricular infarction: Echocardiographic hemodynamic feature, in: Meyer J, Erbel R, Rupprecht HJ (eds), Improvement of Myocardial Infarction, pp 112. Martinus Nijhoff Publ.
15. Erbel R, Schweizer P, Lambertz, Krebs W, Meyer J, Effert S (1985) Sensitivity and specificity of two-dimensional echocardiography in detection of impaired left ventricular function. Eur Heart J 5: 477.
16. Erbel R, Schweizer P, Meyer J, Krebs W, Yalkinoglu Ö, Effert S (1985) Sensitivity of cross-sectional echocardiography in detection of impaired global and regional left ventricular function: Prospective study. Int J Cardiol 7: 375.
17. Erbel R, Schweizer P, Lambertz W, Meyer J, Effert S (1981) Prognostische Bedeutung der nicht invasiv bestimmten Ejektionsfraktion des linken Ventrikels bei reanimierten Patienten. Intensivmed 18: 102.
18. Heng MK, Simard M, Lake R, Udhoi VH (1984) Exercise two-dimensional echocardiography for diagnosis of coronary artery disease. Am J Cardiol 54: 502.
19. Chapman PD, Timothy P, Doyle P (1984) Stress echocardiography with transesophageal atrial pacing: Preliminary report of a new method for detection of ischemic wall motion abnormalities. Circulation 70: 445.

20. Erbel R, Richter HA, Krebs W, Schweizer P, Massberg I, Zotz R, Meyer J, Effert S (1986) Right ventricular volume determination in isolated human hearts. *J Clin Ultrasound* 14: 89.
21. Wyatt HL, Heng MK, Meerbaum S, Gueret P, Dula E, Corday E (1980) Cross-sectional echocardiography. II. Analysis of mathematical models for quantifying volume of the formalin fixed left ventricle. *Circulation* 61: 1119.
22. Wyatt HL, Meerbaum S, Heng MK, Gueret P, Corday E (1980) Cross-sectional echocardiography. III. Analysis of mathematic models of quantifying volume of symmetric and asymmetric left ventricles. *Am Heart J* 100: 821.
23. Erbel R (1983) Funktionsdiagnostik des linken Ventrikels mittels zweidimensionaler *Echokardiographie*. Darmstadt: Steinkopff.
24. Goldstein A, Madrazo BL (1981) Slice thickness artifacts in gray scale ultrasound. *J Clin Ultrasound* 9: 365.
25. Erbel R, Schweizer P, Krebs W, Langen HJ, Meyer J, Effert S (1984) Effects of heart rate changes on left ventricular volume and ejection fraction: A two-dimensional echocardiographic study. *Am J Cardiol* 53: 590.
26. Erbel R (1985) Funktionsdiagnostik des linken Ventrikels, in: Grube E (Hrsg), *Zweidimensionale Echokardiographie*. Stuttgart: Thieme Verlag, S 345.
27. Erbel R, Steuernagel C, Henrichs KJ, Drexler M, Schreiner G, Henkel B, Mohr-Kahaly S, Meyer J (1988) Evaluation of the effect of thrombolytic therapy on left and right ventricular function by two-dimensional echocardiography and cineventriculography, in: Visser C, Kan G, Meltzer R (eds), *Echokardiography in Coronary Artery Disease*, pp 123–148. Boston: Kluwer.
28. Erbel F, Schweizer P, Bardos B (1981) Long-term control of left ventricular function after aortocornary bypass surgery by two-dimensional echocardiography, in: Rijsterborgh H (ed), *Echocardiology*, p 25. Martinus Nijhoff Publ.
29. Schwarz F, Schuler G, Katus H (1982) Intracoronary thrombolysis in acute myocardial infarction: Duration of ischemia as a major determinant of late results after recanalization. *Am J Cardiol* 50: 433.
30. Ritchie JL, Davis KB, Williams DL, Caldwell J, Kennedy JW (1984) Global and regional left ventricular function and tomographic radionuclide perfusion. The Western Washington Intracoronary Streptokinase in Myocardial Infarction Trial. *Circulation* 70: 867.
31. Erbel R, Pop T, Meinertz T, Kasper W, Schreiner G, Henkel B, Henrichs KJ, Pfeiffer C, Rupprecht HJ, Meyer J (1985) Combined medical and mechanical recanalization in acute myocardial infarction. *Cath Cardiovasc Diagn* 11: 361.
32. Sheehan FH, Mathey DG, Schofer J, Krebber HJ, Dodge HT (1983) Effect of intervention in salvaging left ventricular function in acute myocardial infarction: A study of intracoronary streptokinase. *Am J Cardiol* 52: 431.
33. Schmidt SB, Varghese PJ, Bloom S, Yackee JM, Ross AM (1986) The influence of residual coronary stenosis on size of infarction after reperfusion in a canine preparation. *Circulation* 73: 1354.
34. Charuzi Y, Beeder CI, Lorraine A, Marshall LA, Sasaki H, Pack NB, Geft J, Ganz W (1984) Improvement in regional and global left ventricular function after intracoronary thrombolysis: Assessment with two-dimensional echocardiography. *Am J Cardiol* 53: 662.
35. Reduto L, Smalling R, Freund GC et al. (1981) Intracoronary infusion of streptokinase in patients with acute myocardial infarction: Effects of reperfusion in left ventricular performance. *Am J Cardiol* 48: 403.
36. Kjaha F, Walton J, Brymer F, Lo E, Osterberger L, O'Neill WM, Colter HT, Weiss R, Lee T, Kurian T, Goldberg D, Pitt B, Goldstein S (1983) Intracoronary fibrinolytic therapy in acute myocardial infarction. Report of a prospective randomized trial. *N Engl J Med* 308: 1305.
37. Anderson JL, Marshall HW, Askins JC, Lutz JR, Sroenson SG, Menlove RL, Yanowitz, Hagan AD (1984) A randomized trial of intravenous and intracoronary streptokinase in patients with acute myocardial infarction. *Circulation* 70: 606.

38. Puri PS (1975) Contractile and biochemical effects of coronary reperfusion after extended periods of coronary occlusion. *Am J Cardiol* 36: 244.
39. Constantini C, Corday E, Lang TW, Meerbaum S, Brasch J, Kaplan L, Rubins S, Gold H, Oster J (1985) Revascularization after 3 h of coronary arterial occlusion: Effects on regional metabolic function and infarct size. *Am J Cardiol* 36: 368.
40. Theroux P, Ross J, Franklin D, Kemper WS, Sasayama S (1976) Coronary arterial reperfusion. III. Early and late effects on regional myocardial function and dimensions in conscious dogs. *Am J Cardiol* 38: 599.
41. Schaper W, Frenzel W, Hort W, Winkler B (1979) Experimental coronary occlusion. II. Spatial and temporal evolution of infarcts in dog heart. *Basic Res Cardiol* 74: 233.
42. Group Italiano per la Studio della Streptochinasi nell infarto Miocardico (GISSI) (1986) Effectiveness of intravenous thrombolytic treatment in acute myocardial infarction. *N Engl J Med* 314: 1465.
43. Rutsch W, Schartl M, Mathey D, Kuck K, Merx W, Dörr R, Blanke H, Rentrop P (1981) Percutaneous transluminal coronary recanalization. Procedure, results and acute complications. *Am Heart J* 102: 1178.

21. Possibilities of ultrasonic tissue identification in the heart

N. BOM, H. RIJSTERBORGH, C.T. LANCÉE
and JOS R.T.C. ROELANDT

Introduction

Today the major application of echocardiographic techniques has been a direct diagnostic translation of motional, geometrical and blood velocity parameters to cardiac abnormalities. It can be stated that during the last decade many diagnoses that might be derived from these parameters have been described. In the above quoted 'conventional' echo methods the echo image is based on a fixed setting for the sound velocity and an overall compensation for attenuation as function of depth. With conventional echography small local changes in sound velocity, attenuation and/or backscatter are neglected in the way the data is handled.

Ultrasound signals are created by scattering at small particles compared to the wavelength, such as blood cells and myocardial fibers, as well as by larger reflecting boundaries. Under the assumption that with change of the pathology of the myocardium also the physical parameters in ultrasound change, these changes might become quantifiable with ultrasonic tissue identification. It is the purpose of cardiac tissue identification to

- prove that the changes in ultrasound parameters with changes in cardiac tissue indeed exist, and
- select the optimal parameter or combination of parameters which might be used for in vivo application.

Ultrasonic tissue identification in cardiology aims at direct differentiation of tissue parameters, such as separation between infarcted and normal cardiac tissue; early detection of rejection or early indication of ischaemia. Since the echo information will be distorted by the propagation through intermediate layers of intervening tissue, by angle of incidence variations and above all by motion of the heart itself, it seems obvious that extension to clinical applications is difficult and most present research is carried out in vitro or in animal experimental studies. It will be shown that ultrasonic backscatter is probably the best parameter for future in vivo application.

S. Iliceto et al. (eds.), Ultrasound in Coronary Artery Disease, 255–262.
© 1991 *Kluwer Academic Publishers.*

Examples of early cardiac tissue identification studies

One of the first attempts in cardiac echo amplitude study was carried out by Wild et al. [1] when they demonstrated an infarct as an area of decreased reflection as compared with normal muscle. Gramiak et al. [2] experimented with an amplitude windowing technique. Muscle damage was described by establishing a ratio of signal amplitude in a known infarct to normal myocardium. Their animal experiment revealed that areas of myocardial damage were characterized as regions of high signal amplitude. More recently it has been shown that the results strongly depend on the timing of such measurements after the induced infarct.

Analysis of gated A-mode signal has been tried by a number of research groups. Fitzgerald and Joint [3] based their approach on the concept that echoes from homogeneous cardiac tissue will have a Raleigh distribution and that non-homogeneous tissue returns echoes that are distributed in a Rician manner. They were able to successfully differentiate echoes returning from thrombi, myxomas and specular artifacts in sixteen patients. Leeman et al. [4] calculated the autocorrelation function of the interventricular septum in end-diastole and end-systole. This was compared for a normal and a hypertrophic septum. There seem to be apparent differences.

An angle scanning diffraction has been proposed by Hill [5] and Nicholas [6] this method is based on determination of structural variations at a submillimeter level. Nicholas carried out a post mortem study on four normal human hearts. As a preliminary study of this diffraction technique on the heart he measured in particular fiber orientation versus depth in the heart wall. Since empirical assessment of fiber orientation seemed possible, he suggests that the technique should be capable of detecting local changes in cardiac structure.

It is known that the attenuation of ultrasound increases with frequency. Wells [7] has summarized data from a number of publications. The general trend is the same for, for instance, the cat and the dog heart. Absolute values vary, probably due to different measurement methods. A very important study was carried out by O'Donnell et al. [8]. They measured at 20° Celsius the frequency dependence of the attenuation in normal and in infarcted myocardium. It was found that attenuation slope versus frequency was lower in ischaemic zone up to one day after infarct. Thereafter the situation reversed.

The left ventricular muscle is composed of various layers of fiber. The sound velocity is already different depending on the sound propagation direction. Ultrasound velocity values were reported around 1576 meters/sec perpendicular and around 1592 meters/sec when measured parallel to the fiber direction. Changes in velocity may occur due to increase in muscle stiffness and possible lower blood content during the contractile state. Johnson et al. [9] have broken down the presence of major tissue components of water, protein, and in particular collagen on ultrasonic propagation parameters. It appears that collagen plays an important role in attenuation of sound velocity.

Already in 1975, there was some evidence to suggest that its combination in part determines acoustic contrast during echographic visualization. Cardiac tissue ranges in the medium attenuation categories. Attenuation would decrease with increase of water content. Attenuation of cardiac tissue as well as speed of sound would increase with increased protein content. Since the cardiac tissue after an infarct will pass through a variety of histologically different situations, from edematic with a higher fluid content in a fresh infarct to the fibrotic situation with high collagen content in the old infarct, it becomes clear that any tissue identification result will depend on the time interval between measurement and infarct.

Velocity measurements for tissue identification are carried out with time of flight measurements in vitro studies. Johnson and Greenleaf in the USA [9] and Mol in the Netherlands [10] have tried this approach. Cardiac cross-sections are imaged with a tomographic reconstruction technique. Careful knowledge of velocity as function of temperature for various perfusion fluids must be present. In tomographic reconstruction the shape may influence the reconstruction velocity distribution. Although Mol did not yet study infarcted versus normal tissue, the reconstruction technique allowed induced differences such as a local injection to be clearly visible. Their experimental set-up seemed excellent for further fundamental study of velocity effects in isolated hearts in vitro. The clinical application of tomography for tissue identification on the heart is remote, given the need to have adequate transmission paths in many directions through the heart.

Integrated backscatter

Measurements of the sound velocity requires an acoustic pulse transit time measurement. This is carried out in vitro watertank experiments. The velocity parameter does not seem practical for in vivo studies. Also sound attenuation is usually measured as the resulting loss in a through transmission experiment. Attenuation might be measured in an echo set-up comparing adjacent time gated scattering areas. In the moving heart, however, it does not seem the acoustic parameter of choice.

In myocardial tissue identification two parameters are used to characterize the tissue: the backscattered energy as a function of frequency (frequency transfer function) and the frequency average of the frequency transfer function (integrated backscatter). In practice the actual frequency transfer function of tissue will be blurred by various causes. The frequency response of the ultrasound transducer and the amplifier will distort the actual frequency transfer function. But these can be compensated for. Usually the reflection of a stainless steel reflector, acting as a perfect mirror for ultrasound waves, is recorded in water. This measurement gives the frequency response in transmission and reception as well as the energy reference level.

Another complication affecting the actual frequency transfer function is the frequency dependent ultrasound attenuation of the ultrasound path between the transducer and the sample volume within the tissue under investigation. Theoretically this can be solved by taking the frequency transfer function of adjacent blood as a reference. The red blood cells are excellent scatterers. But to our knowledge this has never been applied in practice.

Measuring integrated backscatter in real time is complicated. First of all one has to calculate frequency transfer function of a wide band high frequency time signal using a Fourier transform. Secondly the obtained frequency transfer function has to be compensated for the various frequency-dependent phenomena such as transducer response and frequency-dependent attenuation. The result has to be averaged to obtain the integrated backscatter. It might be clear that all this cannot be accomplished in real time.

Another possibility is to solve the problem in the time domain and to calculate the energy present in a time signal. A straightforward approach would be to square and to integrate a time signal originating from the tissue. It is difficult, however, to accomplish this with an adequate dynamic range. A practical approach would be to use the acoustic electric effect of cadmium sulfide [11]. Using a digital processor, real-time images can be formed of a continuous signal proportional to the logarithm of integrated backscatter [12]. It should be realized, however, that with these devices no absolute levels of backscatter can be measured, only relative values, or changes of backscatter during the cardiac cycle.

Over the last five years, several review papers have been published on the subject of myocardial tissue characterization [13–15]. Much of this work is credited to the group of the Washington University, St. Louis MO. The various aspects of integrated backscatter measurements of myocardial tissue are summarized here.

– Results which indicated that, averaged over the cardiac cycle, integrated backscatter did increase with time after coronary occlusion [16] and that integrated backscatter, when valued for various levels of ischaemia, showed only a strong increase with severe ischaemia [17] suggesting it to be related to structural damage.
– Studies showed that there exists a relationship between backscatter and collagen content [18].
– Studies of backscatter in open chested dogs and dogs with closed chest under normal and ischaemic conditions showed the increase in mean backscatter under ischaemic conditions. It was also shown possible to compensate for the attenuation effect on the backscatter, but suggested that the attenuation correction be obtained from the scatter data itself [19].
– Studies were undertaken [20] which indicated that integrated backscatter does vary with cardiac cycle. An example obtained in a Rotterdam study is shown in Figure 1.
– The effect of ischaemia on integrated backscatter as function of time in the cardiac cycle and reperfusion effect has been reported [20] and was measured in our laboratory as shown in Figure 1.

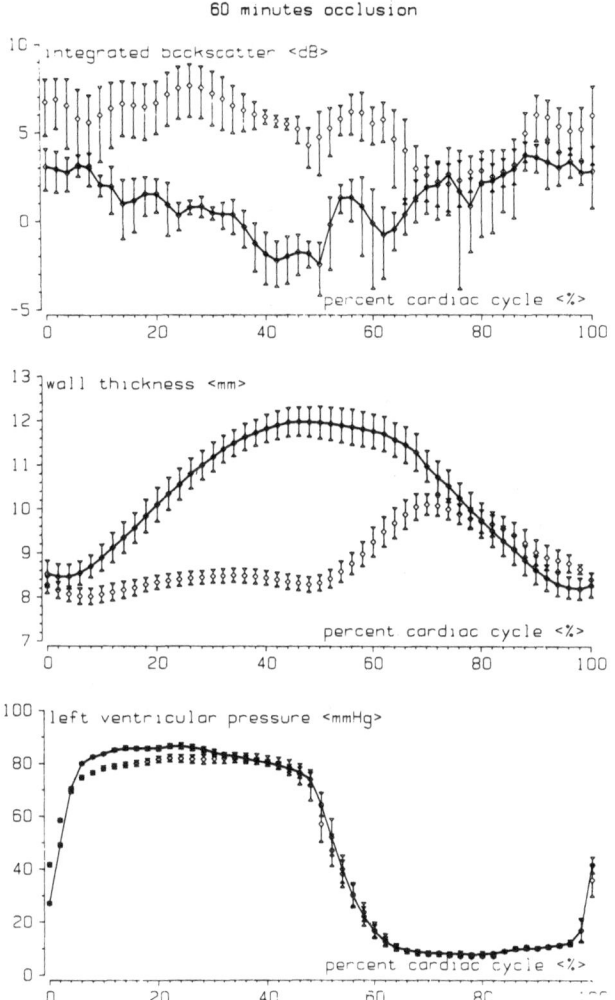

Figure 1. Measurements of integrated backscatter *(top)*, myocardial wall thickness *(middle)* and left ventricular pressure *(bottom)* versus percent cardiac cycle. Shown are the mean values (diamonds) and standard deviations (bars) of ten cardiac cycles in one pig during the reference episode (connected with a solid line) and after 60 min of partial occlusion.

All this indicates the possibilities to quantitate changes in the myocardium through measurements of basic ultrasound parameters such as integrated backscatter.

One of the remaining questions is whether or not simple changes in the cardiac wall thickness (which could be easily measured with M-mode) may not in part be responsible for the measured effect. The following study, will shed light on this particular problem.

In our laboratory we developed a computer-based high-frequency data acquisition system [21]. After processing simultaneous measurements of integrated backscatter, myocardial wall thickness and left ventricular pressure throughout the cardiac cycle are available for further analysis (see Figure 1). With this system in vitro experiments were performed in open-chested pigs during baseline (normal myocardium), during partial occlusion of the left anterior coronary artery (acute ischaemic myocardium) and during subsequent reperfusion. End-systolic and end-diastolic measurements of integrated backscatter and wall thickness taken during the three episodes of the study were compared. End-systolic integrated backscatter measurements were higher during occlusion as compared to the baseline measurements, whereas no statistically significant differences were found in end-diastolic integrated backscatter measurements. End-systolic wall thickness was significantly smaller during occlusion as compared to the baseline measurements. End-diastolic wall thicknesses were comparable during baseline and occlusion.

Since measurements of integrated backscatter and myocardial wall thickness were obtained during the cardiac cycle simultaneously, the relationship between integrated backscatter and wall thickness could be explored. The result is shown in Figure 2, in which the relationship between integrated backscatter and wall thickness during baseline (open circles) as well as during acute ischaemia (closed circles) is depicted. This result suggests a continuous relationship between integrated backscatter and wall thickness. Such a rela-

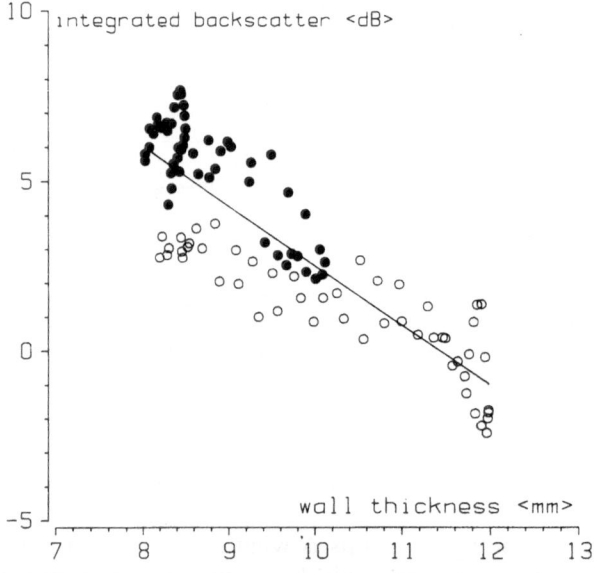

Figure 2. Relationship between myocardial wall thickness and integrated backscatter measurements during the reference episode (open circles) and after 60 min of partial occlusion (closed circles).

tionship would explain the higher level of integrated backscatter in acute ischaemic myocardium as compared to that of normal myocardium. During acute ischaemia two factors that could affect the integrated backscatter level change at the same time: the myocardial wall thickness decreases and the myocardial tissue enters the state of acute ischaemia. These observations have to be explored more systematically.

Discussion

From literature it appears that there is a direct relationship between the echographically measured integrated backscatter and changes in the myocardial tissue such as difference in collagen content and blood volume. This situation changes as function of time after, for instance, an infarct. It has also been proved that the integrated backscatter changes with time within the cardiac style.

When the muscle thickness is measured with an M-mode technique and compared to the measured integrated backscatter from that muscle, it appears that a high correlation exists between the changes in integrated backscatter and the changes in muscle thickness during the cardiac cycle. This is true for normal myocardial tissue as well as during ischaemia. It is not clear yet what creates the fundamental change in integrated backscatter under these circumstances.

In future research will have to be directed towards the study of backscatter as function of frequency if these frequency-dependent parameters follow the same pattern. So far the study has been limited to in-vivo measurements in normal tissue and in ischaemia. It might very well be that these parameters will be of importance in detecting an old infarct or during rejection. This study will have to be carried out to see if such applications might in future avoid the procedure of taking biopsies after cardiac transplantation.

Acknowledgement

These investigations are supported by the Netherlands Technology Foundation (STW).

References

1. Wild JJ, Crawford HD, Reid JM (1957) Visualization of the excised human heart by means of reflected ultrasound or echography. Preliminary report. *Am Heart J* 54: 903–906.
2. Gramiak R, Waag RC, Schenk EA, Lee PPK, Thomson K, Mackintosh P (1979) Ultrasonic imaging of experimental myocardial infarcts, in: Lanceé CT (ed), *Echocardiology*, pp 99–106. The Hague: Martinus Nijhoff Publishers.
3. Fitzgerald PJ, Joynt LF, Green SS, Popp RL (1982) Computerized echocardiographic tis-

sue characterization, in: *Computers in Cardiology 1981*, pp 395–398. IEEE Computer Society Press, Silver Spring MD.

4. Leeman S, Leeks R, Sutton P (1979) Analysis of pulse echo ultrasonic images, in: *Proceedings of the VI International Conference on Information Processing in Medical Imaging*.

5. Hill CR (1974) Interactions of ultrasound with tissues, in: de Vlieger M, White DN, McCready VR (eds), *Ultrasonics in Medicine*, pp 14–20. Amsterdam: Experta Medica.

6. Nicholas D, Nicholas AW, Greenbaum R (1983) An ultrasonic determination of cardiac muscle structures, in: Powers J (ed), *Acoustical Imaging 11*. New York: Plenum Press.

7. Wells PNT (1981) Present status of tissue identification, in: Rijsterborgh H (ed), *Echocardiology*, pp 455–460. The Hague: Martinus Nijhoff Publishers.

8. O'Donnell M, Mimbs JW, Sobel BE, Miller J (1979) Ultrasonic attenuation in normal and ischemic myocardium, in: Linzer M (ed), *Ultrasonic Tissue Characterization II*, pp 63–71. Washington DC: NBS Spec Publ 525, US Government Printing Office.

9. Johnson SA, Greenleaf JF, Samayoa WF, Duck FA, Sjostrand JD (1975) Reconstruction of three-dimensional velocity fields and other parameters by acoustic raytracing. *IEEE Ultrasonics Symp Proc* 75CHP994-4SU: 46.

10. Mol CR (1981) Ultrasound velocity tomography and dynamic cardiac geometry, (thesis, Utrecht).

11. Thomas III LJ, Wickline SA, Perez JE, Sobel BE, Miller JG (1986) A real-time integrated backscatter measurement system for quantitative cardiac tissue characterization. *IEE Trans Ultrasonics* UFFC-33-1: 27–32.

12. Vered Z, Barzilai B, Mohr GA, Thomas III LJ, Genton R, Sobel BE, Shoup TA, Melton HE, Miller JG, Perez JE (1987) Quantitative ultrasonic tissue characterization with real-time integrated backscatter imaging in normal human subjects and in patients with dilated cardiomyopathy. *Circulation* 76: 1067–1073.

13. Miller JG, Perez JE, Sobel BE (1985) Ultrasonic characterization of myocardium. *Prog Cardiovasc Dis* 28: 85–110.

14. Chandraratna PAN, Jones JP, Leeman S, Tak T, Rahimroola SH (1988) *Echocardiography* 5: 183–198.

15. Perez JE, Miller JG, Barzilai B, Wickline S, Mohr GA, Wear K, Vered Z, Sobel BE (1988) Progress in quantitative ultrasonic characterization of myocardium: From the laboratory to the bedside. *J Am Soc Echocardiography*: 294–305.

16. O'Donnell M, Mimbs JW, Miller JG (1981) The relationship between collagen and ultrasonic backscatter in myocardial tissue. *J Acoust Soc Am* 69: 580–588.

17. Mimbs JW, Bauwens D, Cohen RD, O'Donnell M, Miller JG, Sobel BE (1981) Effects of myocardial ischemia on quantitative ultrasonic backscatter and identification of responsible determinants. *Circ Res* 49: 89–96.

18. Mimbs JW, O'Donnell M, Bauwens D, Miller JG, Sobel BE (1980) The dependence of ultrasonic attenuation and backscatter on collagen content in dog and rabbit hearts. *Circ Res* 47: 49–58.

19. Cohen RD, Mottley JG, Miller JG, Kurnik PB, Sobel BE (1982) Detection of ischemic myocardium in vivo through the chest wall by quantitative ultrasonic tissue characterization. *Am J Cardiol* 50: 838–843.

20. Miller JG, Pérez JE, Mottley JG, Madaras EI, Johnston PH, Blodgett ED, Thomas LJ, Sobel BE (1983) Myocardial tissue characterization: An approach based on quantitative backscatter and attenuation. *Proc IEEE Ultrasonics Symp* 83 CH 1947-1: 782–793.

21. Lancée CT, Mastik F, Rijsterborgh H, Bom N (1988) Myocardial backscatter analysis in animal experiments. *Ultrasonics* 26: 155–163.

PART THREE

Evaluation of coronary anatomy and flow

22. Visualization of the coronary arteries by precordial echocardiography

H. FEIGENBAUM

Introduction

Two-dimensional echocardiography is being used to obtain tomographic slices of virtually every segment of the heart and great vessels. It should not be surprising then that one would want to examine all of the vital parts of the cardiovascular system, including the coronary arteries. Trying to obtain a two-dimensional ultrasonic image of the coronary arteries is indeed a challenge. The ostia of the left and right coronary arteries were discovered early in the development of two-dimensional echocardiography. Several early workers demonstrated the left main coronary artery and reported pathology within that vessel [1–4]. Although there was some initial enthusiasm for the possible practical application of this technique, the enthusiasm diminished quickly when the technical difficulties became apparent.

Technical developments

Although the initial goal was to use echocardiography to assess atherosclerotic disease within the coronary arteries [5–7], this application was extremely difficult and did not prove to be very practical [8, 9]. On the other hand the pediatric echocardiographers used this technique to great advantage in detecting aneurysmal dilatation of the coronary arteries in Kawasaki's disease. Thus although the ultrasonic visualization of the coronary arteries for atherosclerosis has been slow in developing, the ultrasonic visualization of the coronary arteries with Kawasaki's disease and to a lesser extent with congenital anomalies has progressed fairly well.

There have been several developments which have renewed interest and optimism in the echocardiographic examination of the coronary arteries utilizing the transthoracic approach. The first of all the ultrasonic instruments have been improving steadily throughout the years. The signal to noise ratio is much better in almost all commercially available equipment. The gray scale in the current instruments is dramatically improved over some of the early two-

S. Iliceto et al. (eds.), Ultrasound in Coronary Artery Disease, 265–268.
© 1991 *Kluwer Academic Publishers.*

dimensional echocardiographs. A major improvement in lateral resolution has occurred with the introduction of annular array technology for cardiology [10, 11]. Lateral resolution is particularly important when looking at small objects, such as coronary arteries. The advantage of annular array focusing is that the beam is narrowed in all dimensions. In order to visualize a 2 mm or 3 mm vessel the beam should be at least as small if not smaller than the object being examined. With a 5 MHz annular array transducer the beam is less than 1 mm in lateral resolution at the focal zone. Thus one has the technical ability to record small structures which was not possible only a few years ago.

Another development which has enhanced the practical examination of the coronary arteries is the ability to digitally record the ultrasonic examination [12]. By utilizing this approach one can illiminate that part of the examination when the artery is in view. One can now analyze just those few frames in which the artery is visualized. Such a review can be in greater detail and with greater convenience than can be accomplished with videotape recordings.

With the advent of annular array technology and the ability to digitally record and analyze the 2D images we have had renewed interest in the transthoracic visualization of the coronary arteries [13]. The interest is no longer limited to the left main coronary artery. Recently we have concentrated our efforts on visualizing the proximal left anterior descending artery [14]. This portion of the coronary tree is particularly important because of the high incidence of clinically important atherosclerotic plaque located in this area. In our experience it is unusual for a patient to have significant obstructive coronary artery disease and not have some ultrasonic evidence of disease within the proximal left anterior descending artery. Thus one can exclude the presence of significant obstructive coronary artery disease by finding a proximal left anterior descending artery which is essentially free of atherosclerosis.

We have found this application to be particularly valuable in assessing patients who present with large dilated left ventricles [15]. The differential diagnosis is an idiopathic dilated cardiomyopathy versus ischemic cardiomyopathy. Although the differential diagnosis can frequently be made on clinical grounds or on the findings within the two-dimensional echocardiogram, there are still patients in whom one resorts to cardiac catheterization and coronary angiography merely to make the differential diagnosis. In a recent study we were able to make this differentiation in a large percentage of patients. Hopefully one should be able to determine the etiology of the dilated malfunctioning left ventricle without having to resort to coronary angiography. In this particular study we were able to obtain clinically useful studies in 86% of our patients. In those patients with dilated cardiomyopathy our success rate was 95%. In the patients with coronary artery disease we were able to visualize the left anterior descending artery with a 75% incidence. The success rate of making the correct diagnosis was 90% in the patients with dilated cardiomyopathy and 80% in patients with coronary artery disease.

Conclusion

These newer developments in the ultrasonic visualization of the coronary arteries are indeed encouraging. The transthoracic approach is still one to be tried initially. Besides being truly noninvasive a major advantage of the transthoracic examination is the ability to move the transducer with ease and in multiple directions. Angulation of the ultrasonic beam is critical in looking at these small variable coronary arteries. The ability to move the transducer is clearly offset by the limitation of the ultrasonic window. The esophageal approach has a wider window but has greater limitations with regard to angulation of the transducer. Another advantage of the transthoracic approach is that the left anterior descending artery can be visualized in a large number of cases. The circumflex artery however is less accessible. As one might expect in the esophageal approach visualizing the coronary arteries is reversed. The circumflex artery is seen rather easily with the left anterior descending artery being more difficult.

It is highly unlikely that any ultrasonic technique will visualize the entire coronary tree. However there is every expectation that certain clinical subsets of patients will benefit from the ultrasonic visualization of the coronary arteries and that in these particular patients coronary angiography may be obviated. The ultrasonic visualization of the coronary arteries should be more sensitive than angiography in the detection of coronary atherosclerosis. On the other hand trying to quantitate coronary atherosclerotic disease is more challenging with ultrasound. Although transthoracic Doppler echocardiography has been used to examine the coronary arteries, this approach has many practical limitations. The experience with this examination is not nearly as extensive as with the two-dimensional approach. Further investigation will be necessary to know whether or not Doppler echocardiography with or without color will provide some of the missing information in the ultrasonic examination of the coronary arteries.

References

1. Weyman AE, Feigenbaum H, Dillon JD (1976) Noninvasive visualization of the left main coronary artery by cross-sectional echocardiography. *Circulation* 54: 169.
2. Rogers EW, Godley RW, Weyman AE (1980) Evaluation of left coronary artery anatomy in vitro using cross-sectional echocardiography. *Circulation* 62: 782.
3. Chandraratna PAN, Aronow SW (1980) Left main coronary arterial patency assessed with cross-sectional echocardiography. *Am J Cardiol* 46: 91.
4. Chen CC, Morganroth J, Ogawa S (1980) Detecting left main coronary artery disease by apical, cross-sectional echocardiography. *Circulation* 62: 288.
5. Rogers EW, Feigenbaum H, Weyman AE (1980) Possible detection of atherosclerotic coronary calcification by two-dimensional echocardiography. *Circulation* 62: 1046.
6. Friedman MJ, Sahn DJ, Goldman S (1982) High predictive accuracy for detection of left main coronary artery disease by antilog signal processing of two-dimensional echocardiographic images. *Am Heart J* 103: 194.

7. Rink LW, Feigenbaum H, Godley RW (1982) Echocardiographic detection of left main coronary artery obstruction. *Circulation* 65: 719.
8. Ronderos R, Salcedo EE, Kramer JR (1984) Value and limitations of two-dimensional echocardiography for the detection of left main coronary artery disease. *Cleveland Clin Q* 51: 7.
9. Block PJ, Popp RL (1984) Detecting and excluding significant left main coronary artery narrowing by echocardiography. *Am J Cardiol* 55: 937.
10. Ryan T, Armstrong WF, Feigenbaum H (1987) Annular array technology: Application to cardiac imaging. *Echocardiography* 4: 203.
11. Douglas PS, Fiolkoshi J, Berko B, Reichek N (1988) Echocardiographic visualization of coronary artery anatomy in the adult. *J Am Coll Cardiol* 11: 565.
12. Ryan T, Armstrong WF, Feigenbaum H (1986) Prospective evaluation of the left main coronary artery during digital two-dimensional echocardiography. *J Am Coll Cardiol* 7: 807.
13. Vasey CG, Ryan T, Armstrong WF (1986) Digital echocardiographic visualization of the left coronary arteries using an annular phased array system, (abstract). *J Am Coll Cardiol* 7: 147A.
14. Presti CF, Feigenbaum H, Armstrong WF (1987) Digital two-dimensional echocardiographic evaluation of the proximal left anterior descending coronary artery. *Am J Cardiol* 60: 1254.
15. Sawada SG, Feigenbaum H, Armstrong WF, Ryan T, Davis C (1988) Differentiation of coronary disease cardiomyopathy and idiopathic dilated cardiomyopathy by coronary ultrasound, (abstract). *Circulation* 78: II–418.

23. Evaluation of proximal left coronary artery anatomy and blood flow using digital transesophageal echocardiography

SABINO ILICETO, CATALDO MEMMOLA,
GIULIA DE MARTINO, VITO MARANGELLI,
CARLO CAIATI and PAOLO RIZZON

Introduction

Non-invasive evaluation of the proximal left coronary artery can be obtained by two-dimensional echocardiography [1–6]. Even if the feasibility of this kind of evaluation has been demonstrated, its clinical application has not yet obtained wide acceptance because of some difficulties that considerably hamper echocardiographic imaging of coronary arteries. First of all, reviewing and evaluation of real time 2D Echo images of the coronaries is troublesome because of the cyclic movement of the heart that does not allow continuous monitoring of a tubular structure as small as the coronary artery; furthermore, the quality of echocardiographic images is very often poor and, therefore, does not allow accurate definition of the coronary boundaries.

The first of the two above-mentioned problems has been overcome using digital reviewing systems that allow accurate reviewing of selected consecutive frames in a continuous loop format. The problem of the quality of echocardiographic imaging of the coronaries can theoretically be solved using transesophageal echocardiography [7], an emerging application of two-dimensional echocardiography that makes it possible to obtain high resolution real time echocardiographic images of cardiac and extra cardiac structures. Thus, to explore the potential of digital transesophageal echocardiography in evaluating coronary arteries we studied a series of consecutive patients undergoing coronary angiography. In the light of the excellent transmission of ultrasounds throughout cardiac structures, obtainable by means of transesophageal echocardiography, we also investigated the feasibility of analysing coronary artery blood flow using pulsed Doppler evaluation of blood flow in the left anterior descending artery.

Visualization of left coronary artery by transesophageal echocardiography

Coronary visualization by transesophageal echocardiography was attempted in 112 consecutive patients undergoing coronary angiography for diagnostic

S. Iliceto et al. (eds.), Ultrasound in Coronary Artery Disease, 269–276.
© 1991 *Kluwer Academic Publishers*.

purposes. Transesophageal echocardiography was performed 2–3 days before cardiac catheterization using a Hewlett Packard transesophageal probe (21362A) with a 5 MHz transducer connected up to Hewlett Packard 77020 echocardiographic equipment. All the patients were studied in the conscious state.

The transducer was inserted into the esophagus following the techniques and manoeuvres commonly used when carrying out a gastroscopy. After patient sedation, obtained by intravenous injection of small doses of Diazepam, the transducer was actually inserted with the patient in the left lateral decubitus.

Technique of visualization

In order to visualize the coronary arteries, the transducer must be placed at the level of the aortic root (Figure 1). The left main coronary artery usually appears emerging from the corresponding aortic sinus immediately above the aortic leaflets. The ostium of the left main coronary artery is imaged as an echo-free space that interrupts the continuity of the aortic wall borders. Once the ostium is visualized, slight upwards/downwards and leftwards/rightwards movements of the probe must be performed so as to image the left main coronary artery along its full length (Figure 2). This is usually successful in most patients without having to place the probe itself at an angle. On the other hand, in some cases it is necessary to push/pull the probe forwards or backwards in order to cut the left main coronary artery lengthwise. These procedures are necessary since the orientation of the left main coronary artery and its consequent relationships with the ultrasound exploring tomographic plane is extremely variable. The left main coronary artery bifurcation is usually visualized by just slightly moving the probe position and orientation from the position in which the left main coronary artery is imaged in its maximum length (downward direction of ultrasound beam obtained by means of down-

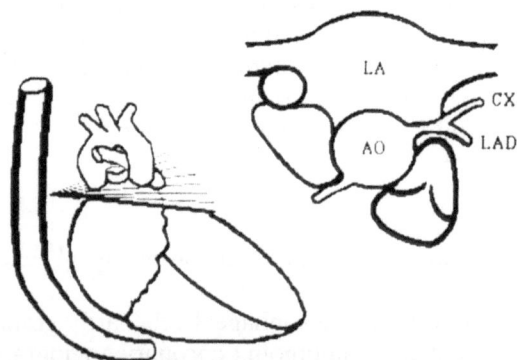

Figure 1. Relationship between the esophagus, left atrium (LA), aortic root (Ao), left main coronary, bifurcation, left anterior descending (LAD) and circumflex (CX).

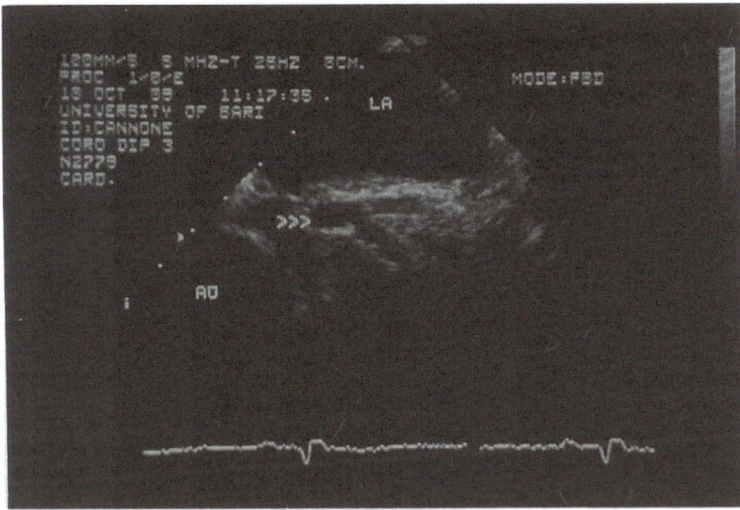

Figure 2. Transesophageal echocardiography visualization of the left main coronary artery (arrows), bifurcation and initial portion of the circumflex and left anterior descending artery. Ao = Aortic root, LA = left atrium.

ward angling of the transducer). A downward angulation of the ultrasound beam (transducer retroflection) is often necessary to visualize the left anterior descending artery along a reasonable length because of its typical longitudinal and downward direction (Figure 3). Finally, the circumflex artery (Figure 4) can be imaged by rotating leftwards and slightly pulling back the probe from

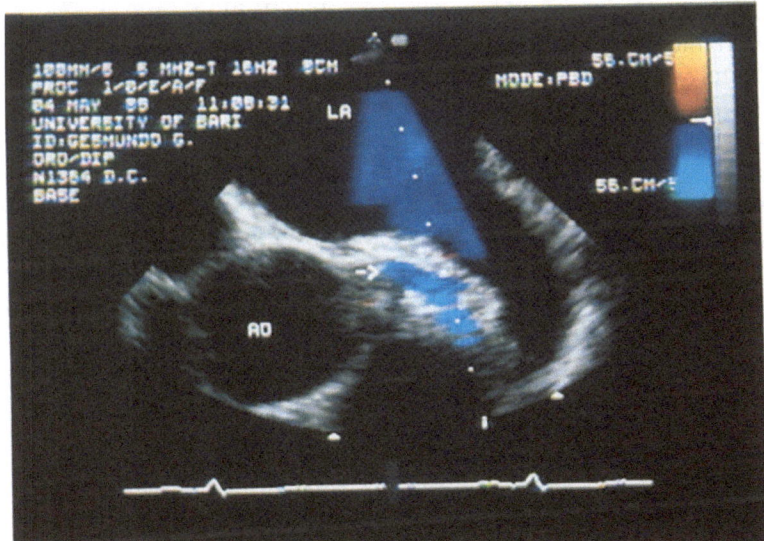

Figure 3. Visualization of the left anterior descending artery. Color Doppler mapping delineates the lumen in blue (flow away from the transducer). LA = left atrium, Ao = Aorta.

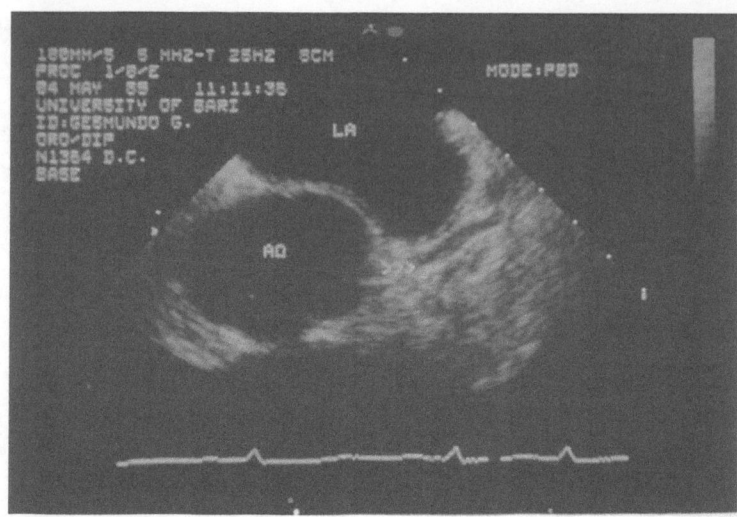

Figure 4. Visualization of the circumflex artery. The vessel is visualized as an echo-free tubular structure located behind the left atrium (LA). Ao = Aorta.

the position in which the ultrasound beam longitudinally intersects the left main coronary artery.

Digital reviewing of 2D echocardiographic images

Reviewing of 2D Echo images of coronary arteries is decidedly easier and more reliable if performed by means of a digital cine loop system. Acquisition of a variable number of video fields is automatically performed by means of the digital system.

Technique

Consecutive video fields have to be acquired every 17 msec; only consecutive frames clearly showing the lumen of the observed coronary arteries must be stored and then reviewed in a continuous cine loop format at a speed considerably higher than that of the acquisition phase. Frames in which the coronary vessel is not adequately visualized must be eliminated from the acquisition and, consequently, not included in the cine loop. Thus, the final number of frames usually included in the loop does not exceed 6–8. All the sequences can be permanently stored on a floppy disk.

Success rate in visualizing coronary segments and capability in identifying 'specific' coronary segments

Figure 5 summarizes the success rate of TEE in visualizing the left main coro-

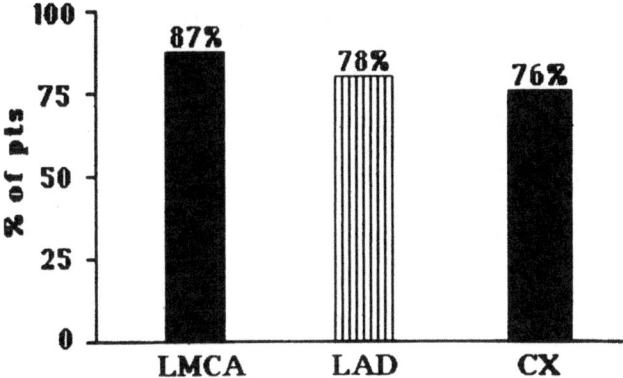

Figure 5. Success rate of transesophageal echocardiography in visualizing left coronary artery segments. LMCA = left main coronary artery, LAD = left anterior descending, CX = circumflex.

nary artery, left anterior descending and circumflex obtained in a consecutive series of 112 patients undergoing TEE for coronary visualization. According to the aspect of transesophageal echocardiographic images, 3 different 'coronary' patterns were identified:

– pattern A: patent coronary lumen;
– pattern B: presence of calcific plaques in the coronary walls though no narrowing;
– pattern C: calcific plaques and lumen narrowing (Figure 6).

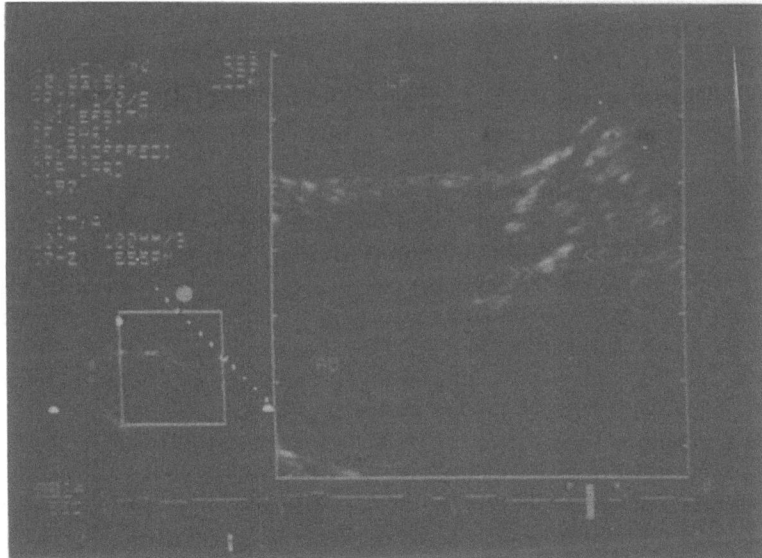

Figure 6. Severe stenosis of proximal part of the left anterior descending artery (LAD). The arrows indicate the presence of the calcific stenosis.

DETECTION OF CORONARY STENOSIS BY TEE

	TEE	n° pts	% Ang. sten.	
LMCA (98 pts)	Norm	70	0/70	(0%)
	Calc	24	0/24	(0%)
	Sten	4	4/4	(100%)
LAD (88 pts)	Norm	43	12/43	(27.9%)
	Calc	31	14/31	(45.1%)
	Sten	14	10/14	(71.4%)
CX (86 pts)	Norm	51	3/51	(5.8%)
	Calc	31	7/31	(22.5%)
	Sten	4	4/4	(100%)

Figure 7. Transesophageal echo (TEE) findings in a series of consecutive patients (pts) undergoing coronary angiography. The TEE findings are classified as: norm = normal vessel; calc = presence of non-stenotic calcific plaques on the coronary walls; sten = stenosis of the vessel; N° pts = number of patients with specific TEE findings; Ang. Sten = percentage of patients with significant stenosis documented by angiography.

Figure 7 summarizes the correlations found between these patterns and the presence of a coronary stenosis angiographically detected. Criterion A was highly predictive of patent lumen (especially if applied to the left main coronary artery and to the circumflex), while criterion C was highly predictive of significant coronary narrowing.

Pulsed Doppler evaluation of blood flow in the left anterior descending coronary artery

In those patients in whom the left anterior descending coronary artery (LAD) is clearly visualized during the transesophageal echocardiographic study, pulsed Doppler evaluation of blood flow in the visualized LAD can be attempted. First of all, it is necessary to image the LAD virtually parallel to the exploring ultrasound beam so that the angle between the coronary blood flow and the ultrasound beam directions is as close as possible to 0°. The sample volume, regulated at its minimum to facilitate its positioning within the vessel, has to be placed in the site in which the moving LAD reaches its diastolic position. In fact, because of the movement of the heart, the LAD also moves in space during each cardiac cycle. This movement is almost exclusively systolic in that throughout the whole of diastole the position of the LAD with respect to the transducer remains virtually constant. Therefore, the positioning of the sample volume is done after observing the systo-diastolic movement of the LAD and noting the position it reaches in diastole. The left panel in Figure 8 shows a typical example of flow velocity within the left anterior

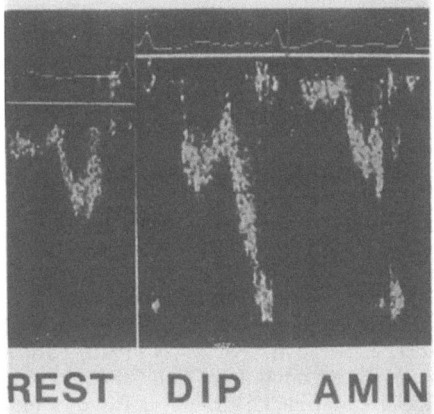

REST   DIP   AMIN

Figure 8. Doppler coronary blood flow velocity profile in a patient with normal coronary arteries (*left* panel). Coronary flow velocities (systolic and diastolic) increased markedly after dipyridamole (DIP) infusion (*middle* panel) and reverted to normal after aminophylline (AMIN) (*right* panel).

descending artery. Flow pattern is biphasic with a greater diastolic and a smaller systolic component. Several diastolic and systolic velocity parameters can be calculated.

We have studied a group of patients [8] who also underwent pulsed Doppler evaluation of coronary artery blood flow before and after a protocol specially designed to investigate the effects on coronary flow of vasoactive drugs. Doppler recordings were obtained before and after dipyridamole infusion (0.56 mg/kg in 4') and after aminophylline infusion. As expected, all velocity parameters increased during dipyridamole infusion and reverted to normal after aminophylline. Figure 8 shows an example of coronary blood flow before and after dipyridamole infusion.

The increase in coronary blood flow velocity was significantly greater in patients with a normal left anterior descending artery than in those with a significant stenosis on it and a consequently reduced coronary flow reserve [9].

Conclusion

Digital transesophageal echocardiography seems to be a useful tool for evaluating coronary anatomy. This approach also allows coronary blood flow to be explored, thus representing a potentially new approach for the evaluation of coronary blood flow reserve.

References

1. Presti CF, Feigenbaum H, Armstrong WF, Ryan T, Dillon JC (1987) Digital two-dimensional

echocardiographic imaging of the proximal left anterior descending coronary artery. *Am J Cardiol* 60: 1254–1259.

2. Rink LD, Feigenbaum H, Godley RW, Weyman AE, Dillon JC, Phillips JF, Marshall JE (1982) Echocardiographic detection of left main artery obstruction. *Circulation* 65: 719–724.

3. Rogers EW, Feigenbaum H, Weyman AE, Godley, Vakili ST (1980) Evaluation of left coronary artery anatomy in vitro by cross-sectional echocardiography. *Circulation* 62: 782–787.

4. Rogers EW, Feigenbaum H, Weyman AE, Godley, Johnston KW, Eggleton RC (1980) Possible detection of atherosclerotic coronary calcification by two-dimensional echocardiography. *Circulation* 62: 1046–1053.

5. Ryan T, Armstrong WF, Feigenbaum H (1986) Prospective evaluation of the left main coronary artery using digital two-dimensional echocardiography. *J Am Coll Cardiol* 7: 807–812.

6. Douglas PS, Fiolkoski J, Berko B, Reichek N (1988) Echocardiographic visualization of coronary artery anatomy in the adult. *J Am Coll Cardiol* 11: 565–571.

7. Iliceto S, Memmola C, De Martino G, Piccinni G, Rizzon P (1989) Visualization of the coronary artery during transesophageal echocardiography, in: Erbel R, Khanderia BJ, Brennecke R, Seward JB, Meyer J, Tajik AJ (eds), *Transesophageal Echocardiography*, pp 86–98. Springer, Berlin, New York.

8. Iliceto S, Memmola C, Marangelli V, Rizzon P (1989) Evaluation of coronary blood flow by transesophageal echo-Doppler. *Circulation* (suppl 2) 80 (4): 338.

9. Iliceto S, Marangelli V, Memmola C, De Martino G, D'Ambrosio G, Piccinni G, Rizzon P (1990) Assessment of coronary flow reserve by transesophageal echo-Doppler. *J Am Coll Cardiol* (abstract), (in press).

24. Intra-arterial ultrasonic imaging

N. BOM, W. J. GUSSENHOVEN, C. T. LANCÉE, C. J. SLAGER,
P. W. SERRUYS, H. TEN HOFF and JOS R. T. C. ROELANDT

Introduction

Present medical treatment for severe obstruction of the coronary disease is the surgical bypass procedure. Other and newer interventional techniques of a less traumatic nature are also being used to avoid surgery. Well-known is the balloon dilatation technique as described by Gruentzig et al. [1]. With this method the obstruction is stretched, not removed, by a balloon that is gradually inflated. Other methods, presently tested in research laboratories, include the abrasive tip method as suggested by Hansen [2], an atherectomy catheter tip method as suggested by Simpson [3] and various versions of laser energy. Laser angioplasty, which is the in situ ablation of arterial obstructions with laser radiation, has shown to work in animal models and early clinical trials. A problem, however, with this technique, is the possibility of thermal damage to adjacent or underlying normal tissue that also absorbs the radiation. Penetration of the normal arterial wall may occur particularly in strongly curved arteries and when eccentricity of obstructions with relation to the arterial wall exists. This requires high selectivity of the ablation method or a 'steering' capability.

Studies were published in which possibilities for differentiation between atheroma and normal tissue by flashlamp-excited laser at 465 nm have been described by Prince [4]. Although these studies are a step forward much work has to be done yet given the wide range of variations in tissue character of the arterial obstructions.

For optimal differentiation between the healthy and the diseased part of the artery angioscopy cannot be used since the viewing area only allows visualization of the innermost layer of the obstruction and also 'in depth' information is needed. As an attractive parameter Slager [5] studied the possibilities to differentiate using an electrical impedance measurement. On a series of 13 human aortic segments, freshly obtained at autopsy, the impedance was measured at 56 different atherosclerotic locations and at 11 normal areas. Histological examination was used to classify the tissues. The frequency distribution of the resistance at 100 kHz of different types of tissue

S. Iliceto et al. (eds.), Ultrasound in Coronary Artery Disease, 277–284.
© 1991 *Kluwer Academic Publishers*.

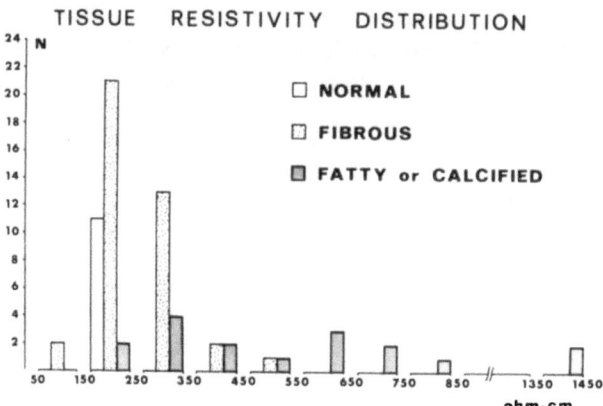

Figure 1. Resistance ranges for normal, fibrous and fatty or calcified area. The distribution over the resistance range is indicated for 69 measurements [5].

is shown in Figure 1. There exists, unfortunately, too much overlay. We must therefore conclude that the electrical impedance measurement also is not specific enough to guide an ablation method.

Ultrasound offers yet another possibility

If it would be possible to obtain cross-sectional images, then important diagnostic information would become available. It is with this in mind that a renewed activity in catheter tip echographic techniques has been stimulated to overcome the apparent limitations in present new interventional techniques.

Early intraluminal dimensional echo measurements

Already in 1960 Cieszynski [6] obtained echoes from within the heart with a single catheter-mounted transducer introduced via the jugular vein. It was a first feasibility test whereby the author obtained echoes from soft tissue in a medium filled up with blood in model experiments. He also carried out measurements in dogs where he obtained reflections from the inner walls of the left and the right side of the heart. Ten years later in a survey of diagnostic applications of ultrasound in cardiology Kossoff [7] illustrated an 8F catheter with a 2 mm diameter 8 MHz transducer used for measuring ventricular diameter and septal thickness. In 1968 Carleton [8] described a cylindrical nondirectional element which was used for the measurement of ventricular diameter.

Early intraluminal cross-sectional imaging

The idea to build a cross-sectional image by rotation of a single echo element

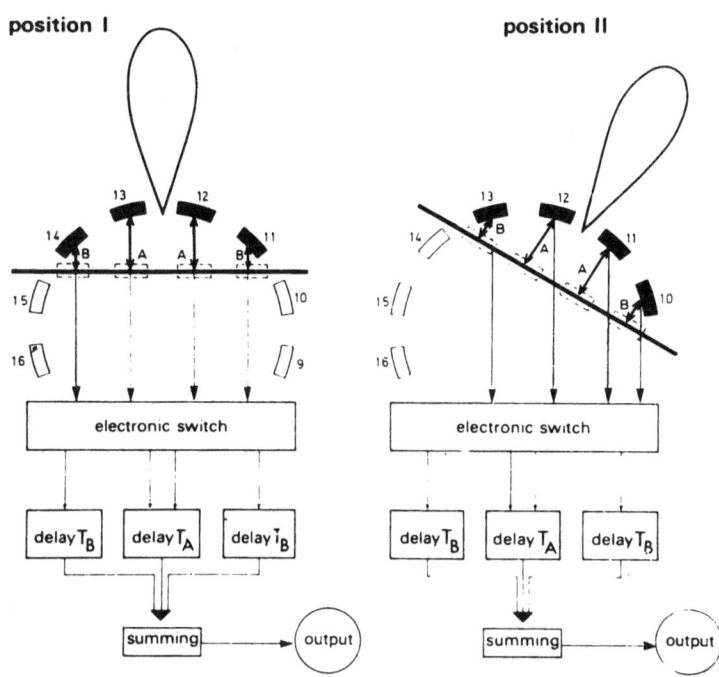

From: N. Bom et al. Ultrasonics 10:74, 1972

Figure 2. Principle of electronic phased array catheter tip for real-time imaging. In position I, elements 11, 12, 13 and 14 are delayed in reception by delay T_B, T_A, T_A and T_B, respectively. After summation, this creates the main beam axis as indicated. The same method can be used for adjacent subgroups as shown in position II.

and integration of the echoes into a cross-sectional image has appealed to many scientists. As early as 1955 Wild and Reid [9] suggested the use of a mechanically rotating element for rectal tumor location. Ebina in 1965 [10] suggested a similar transesophageal approach study of the heart and the vessels. In our laboratory we developed in 1971 the first real-time intra-cardiac scanner based on a 32 element's circular array and operating with a phasing technique. The principle of this method is shown in Figure 2. By introducing time delays in reception a subgroup of elements becomes vir-tually one larger element. This technique, combined with electronic switch-ing, allows the rapid rotational shift of the acoustic main beam. Integration of the echo data on a display allows high speed two-dimensional observation in a plane perpendicular to the catheter tip. With the technological capability at that time results were not sufficient to warrant continuation although real-time images of cardiac cross-sectional have been obtained in animal experi-ments.

Since the phased array approach was at that time too expensive and com-plicated to duplicate, it seemed that for the one-time use of disposable catheters required nowadays, a probably better way to follow would be the cheaper mechanically rotated beam approach. In recent years we have followed this direction.

Mechanically rotating catheters

In order to estimate the practical catheter diameter size it is necessary to have knowledge of the internal coronary artery diameter in normal adults. MacAlpin et al. [11] indicated that the lumen diameter of the right coronary artery ranges from 3.2 ± 0.6 mm (proximal) to 2.7 ± 0.7 mm (distal). The main left coronary artery lumen diameter was measured to be 4.0 ± 0.7 mm. For the left anterior descending artery a range was measured of 3.4 ± 0.5 mm (proximal) to 1.9 ± 0.3 mm (distal) and for the circumflex of 3.0 ± 0.7 (proximal). From this material it was concluded that in a first approach a 2 mm outer diameter catheter would be sufficiently small.

We studied a variety of 20 and 40 MHz mechanical single element catheter tip scanners based on 7F catheters. With rotational speed of 3000 rpm, intra-arterial images were obtained in vitro studies. Animal experiments showed real-time capabilities for observation of arterial wall motion. In Figure 3 three

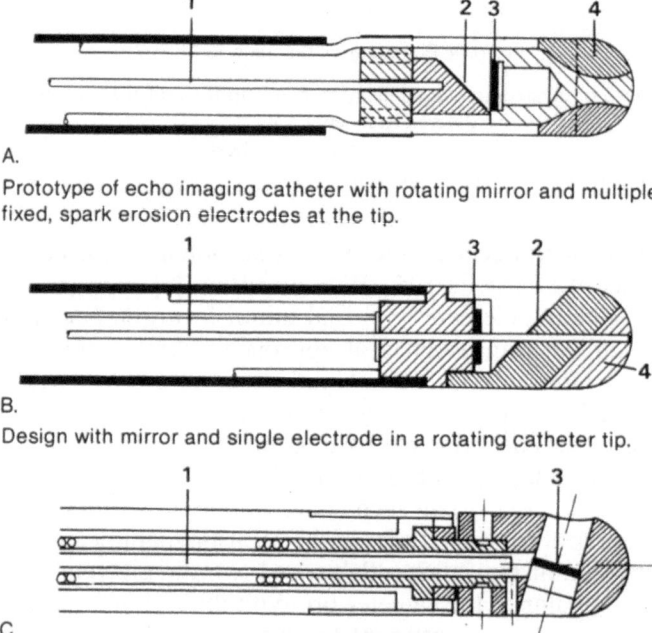

A.

Prototype of echo imaging catheter with rotating mirror and multiple, fixed, spark erosion electrodes at the tip.

B.

Design with mirror and single electrode in a rotating catheter tip.

C.

Design of the catheter tip as used for the cross-sectional arterial image as shown.

Figure 3. Schematic drawing of echo catheter prototypes, with spark erosion integration *(A, B)* and without *(C)*.

versions of the rotating catheter tip are shown. At first the catheter tip was – rather optimistically – already designed for integration with an ablation method. As reported by Slager et al. [5] spark erosion can be used to evaporate atherosclerotic plaques. The technique was studied in specimen of human aorta obtained at autopsy. As with many of the other techniques still some fundamental questions have to be solved.

In Figure 3 prototype A shows an early approach with driving shaft *1*, a rotating mirror *2*, the piezoelectric element *3* and the integration with the spark erosion electrodes *4*. For ablation, the spark erosion electrode was to be selected based on information obtained with echography. In prototype B, the catheter tip rotates and contains a mirror *2* and a spark erosion electrode. The advantage of this construction is the close proximity of the cross-sectional echo image and the ablation area. In a more recent design C, a slightly conical cross-section is obtained with a rotating tip construction without further integration with an ablation method (see also Figure 4).

One of our present designs has three characteristics. At the tip, it contains a small hole which allows a fluid drip. This can be used for local application of a therapeutic fluid, such as a thrombolyticum. In addition, the fluid serves to maintain the acoustic contact between the element within the dome and the obstruction area to be studied. The second and most important characteristic is the visualization method based on rotational motion of an acoustic element. This can be used for instant monitoring of therapeutic effects as well as for long term evaluation. The third characteristic is that the device includes the capability to assure the correct translation of echo information (beam position) obtained at the tip into correct visualization of this information (beam position) on the display. This part is based on an optical sensor which samples the tip position. Even if the tip does not move smoothly, the exact tip position is known and the echoes are displayed correctly.

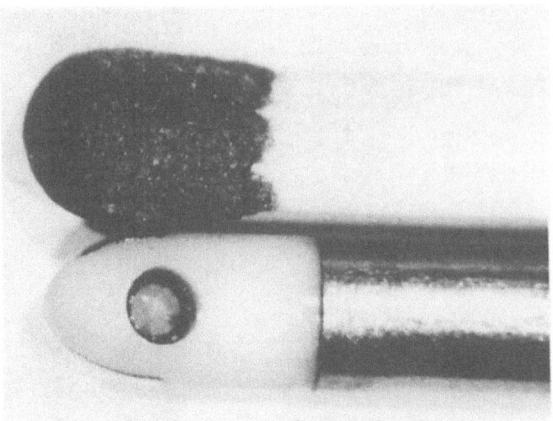

Figure 4. Early prototype of catheter tip of class C (see Figure 3).

Results and discussion

In vitro studies comparison was made between the echographic cross-section and the histology as obtained in the same cross-section. The arteries were fixed and stained for histologic study. Microscopic investigation showed two types of artery: a muscular and an elastin artery. Differences were apparent in particular when observing the media. The media of a muscular artery is composed of smooth muscle cells and practically devoid of elastin fibers. The media of an elastin artery consists mainly of densely packed concentrically arranged elastin fibers amidst smooth muscle cells. It is known that elastin fibers, when orderly arranged, are in part responsible for high echo density in echo images. Absence of elastin fibers will cause low echo density. The latter effect showed up in images of muscular arteries. Here the media could easily be recognized as an annular area with low echo intensity. It also appeared to be possible to measure the thickness of the plaque. There was a high correlation between measured plaque thickness in the echo image and the thickness measured in the histologic specimen when correction was made for shrinkage after dehydration during fixation. An example of an echo image and the corresponding histologic cross-section is shown in Figure 5. The arrow indicates the plaque area.

The need for better visualization of arterial obstructive lesions is a consequence of the rapid development of intervention radiology and cardiology and more particularly the newer methods for angioplasty (laser, atherectomy, abrasion, spark erosion, etc.) of stenosed arteries. Optical techniques such as angioscopy can visualize lumen morphology, but provide no information on the disease of the wall under the endothelial surface. Optical techniques are further hindered by the opacity of the blood requiring its complete replacement by a translucent liquid to allow structure visualization. This poses

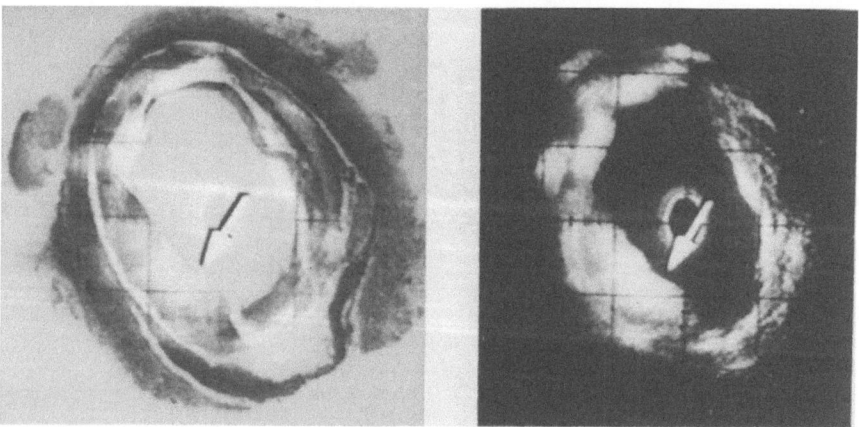

Figure 5. Histologic specimen of arterial cross-section *(left)* and the corresponding echo image *(right)* with indicated plaque (arrow).

serious limitations for the direct visualization of lesions both pre- and post-angioplasty especially in the coronary arteries.

An imaging method which could show lumen morphology and pathology within the vessel wall would have advantages for the diagnosis and treatment of arterial disease. Ultrasonic imaging offers this unique advantage, since it allows the operator to 'see' under the endothelial surface and to visualize the arterial wall components. In addition, the method has the potential for tissue characterization and this may provide further details of arterial wall pathology. The system described can be used for many clinical applications. It is particularly suited for instantaneous visual monitoring of therapeutic interventions, such as clotlyses with thrombolitica.

At the other end of the cardiac application spectrum, the system may be used to monitor valve area and commissural opening prior to and after valvular repair. The diagnosis and characterization of arterial atherosclerotic disease offers interesting experimental and clinical perspectives. Recent pathology studies have further elucidated the atherosclerotic disease process. In the earlier stages of the disease, coronary arteries enlarge as a result of a remodelling process in relation to plaque area and functionally important lumen stenosis may not develop until the lesion occupies 40 percent of the internal elastic lamina area. Thus, serious wall disease may be present despite a nearly normal lumen cross-sectional area on coronary arteriograms [12].

An intravascular imaging catheter as described here can be used to assess the degree and extent of atherosclerotic arterial disease prior to and after recanalization procedures. Equally important, however, is the functional significance of the stenosis. Doppler flow measurements prior to and after interventions at rest and following pharmacologically induced maximal vasodilatation can allow to assess the functional significance of the original and remaining stenosis [13]. The combination of measurement of arterial cross-sectional area by imaging and blood flow velocity would improve our understanding of coronary artery disease and further help to assess the results of intervention.

Conclusion

Intravascular real-time, high resolution ultrasonic imaging is an exciting new development. It produces cross-sectional images of the artery of interest and allows measurement of arterial lumen dimensions, wall thickness and extent of atherosclerotic disease. This unique diagnostic potential can be used to characterize and quantify the degree of atherosclerotic arterial disease, to grade the effects of pharmacological intervention and to guide angioplasty procedures and evaluate their effects.

Acknowledgements

These investigations are supported in part by the Netherlands Technology Foundation (STW).

Construction of our catheter prototype has been carried out by Produkt-centrum TNO and TPD-TNO, Delft, the Netherlands and the Central Research Workshop of the Erasmus University Rotterdam.

References

1. Gruentzig AR, Senning A, Siegenthaler WE (1979) Nonoperative dilatation of coronary artery stenosis: Percutaneous transluminal angioplasty. *N Engl J Med* 301: 61–68.
2. Hansen DD, Hall M, Intlekofer MJ, Auth D, Ritchie JL (1986) In vivo rotational angioplasty in atherosclerotic rabbits; comparison of angioscopy and angiography. *Circulation* 74 (suppl 2): 362 (abstract).
3. Simpson JB, Johnson DE, Brader LJ, Gifford HS, Thaplyal HV, Selmon MR (1986) Transluminal coronary atherectomy (TCA): Results in 21 human cadaver vascular segments. *Circulation* 74 (suppl 2): 202 (abstract).
4. Prince MR, Deutsch TF, Shapiro AH, Margolis RJ, Oseroff AR, Fallon JT, Parrish JA, Anderson RR (1986) Selective ablation of atheromas using a flashlamp-excited dye laser at 465 mm. *Proc Natl Acad* 83: 7064–7068.
5. Slager CJ, Essed CE, Schuurbiers JCH, Bom N, Serruys PW, Meester GT (1985) Vaporization of atherosclerotic plaques by spark erosion. *J Am Coll Cardiol* 5: 1382–1386.
6. Cieszynski T (1960) Intracardiac method for the investigation of structure of the heart with the aid of ultrasonics. *Arch Immun Ter Dow* 8: 551–557.
7. Kossoff G (1966) Diagnostic applications of ultrasound in cardiology. *Australas Radiol* X: 101–106.
8. Carleton RA, Clark JG (1968) Measurement of left ventricular diameter in the dog by cardiac catheterization. Validation and physiologic meaningfulness of an ultrasonic technique. *Circ Res* 22: 545–548.
9. Wild JJ, Reid JM (1950) Progress in techniques of soft tissue examination by 15 MC pulsed ultrasound, in: Kelly E (ed), *Ultrasound in Medicine and Biology*, p 30. Washington DC: American Institute of Biological Sciences.
10. Ebina T, Oka S, Tanaka M, Kosaka S, Kikuchi Y, Uchida R, Hagiwara Y (1964) The diagnostic application of ultrasound to the disease in mediastinal organs. Ultrasonotomography for the heart and great vessels. *Sci Rep Res Inst Tohoku Univ* 12: 199–212.
11. McAlpin RN, Abbasi AS, Grallman JA, Eber L (1973) Human coronary artery size during life. *Radiology* 108: 567–573.
12. Glagov S, Weisenberg E, Zarins CK et al. (1987) Compensatory enlargement of human atherosclerotic arteries. *N Engl J Med* 316: 1371–1375.
13. Serruys PW, Zijlstra F, Reiber JHC et al. (1988) Assessment of coronary flow reserve during angioplasty using a Doppler tip balloon catheter. Comparison with digital substraction cineangiography. *J Interven Cardiol* 19–33.

25. Intracoronary blood flow velocity, reactive hyperemia and coronary blood flow reserve during and following PTCA

PATRICK W. SERRUYS, FELIX ZIJLSTRA,
HANS H. C. REIBER, KEVIN BEATT, G. J. LAARMAN,
JOS R. T. C. ROELANDT and P. J. DE FEYTER

Introduction

Since the introduction of percutaneous transluminal coronary angioplasty (PTCA) in 1977 [1], the procedure has gained increasing importance in the treatment of coronary artery obstructions. So far, the immediate results of the procedure have been assessed by coronary angiography and the residual pressure gradient. However, the change in luminal size of an artery following the mechanical disruption of its internal wall cannot be assessed accurately from the detected angiographic contours [2, 3]. The measured residual pressure gradient may have short and long-term prognostic value, but it reflects only the hemodynamic state at rest [4–6] Recently the assessment of coronary flow reserve has been proposed as a better method to evaluate the functional results of dilatation of a coronary artery obstruction [7–10]. Papaverine is currently regarded as the vasodilator of choice for the induction of maximal hyperemia, as intracoronary administration results in an immediate, potent and short-lasting hyperemia [11, 12]. Intracoronary blood flow velocity measurements with a Doppler probe, and the radiographic assessment of myocardial perfusion with contrast media have previously been used to investigate regional coronary flow reserve [13–17]. In the present study we compared both techniques in the setting of PTCA, and compared the pharmacologically induced vasodilation after intracoronary papaverine with reactive hyperemia following transluminal occlusion.

Patients and methods. In the first study group twenty patients undergoing elective PTCA for angina pectoris were investigated (New York Heart Association functional class II to IV). Informed consent was obtained for the additional investigations. All patients were studied without premedication, but their medical treatment (nitrates, calcium antagonists and beta-blockers) was continued on the day of the procedure. Patients with left ventricular hypertrophy, valvular heart disease, angiographic evidence of collateral circulation, anemia, polycythemia or hypertension were excluded as these conditions may influence coronary flow reserve [18–20].

S. Iliceto et al. (eds.), Ultrasound in Coronary Artery Disease, 285–309.
© 1991 *Kluwer Academic Publishers.*

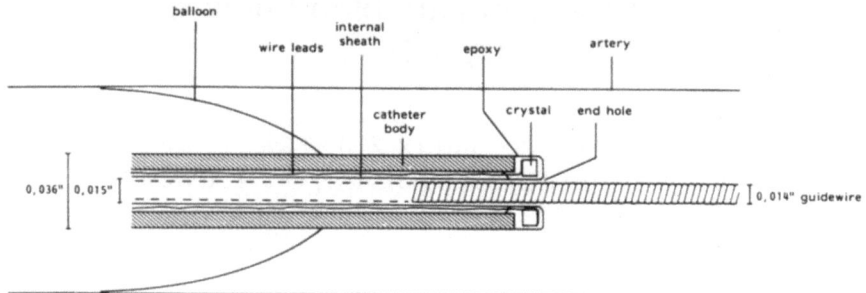

Figure 1. Schematic cross-sectional drawing of Doppler tip angioplasty catheter with inflated balloon in the artery.

Intracoronary blood flow velocity measurements

A 20 mega Hz ultrasonic crystal mounted on the tip of the angioplasty cathe-ter was used in all patients. The Doppler crystal has a 1.0 mm diameter annulus with a 0.5 mm central hole. Two leads are soldered to the crystal and pass through the catheter between the original 0.5 mm lumen and a thin-walled tube, which serves as a new 0.4 mm lumen (Figure 1). The leads exit near the proximal luer hub and are wired to a 2 pin plug for connection to the pulsed Doppler instrument. Blood flow velocity is measured from the cathe-ter tip transducer using a range-gated 20 MHz pulsed Doppler instrument. The master oscillator frequency of 20 MHz is pulsed at a frequency of 62.5 KHz. Each pulse is approximately 1 ms in width and therefore contains 20 cycles of the master oscillator frequency. The frequencies chosen allow velocities of up to 100 cm/s to be recorded at distances of up to 1 cm from the catheter tip. The sampling window is individually adjusted to obtain the optimal signal, which usually results in a sampling window of 1.8 mm (range: 1.5 to 2.2).

The output of the pulsed Doppler is displayed as a frequency shift (Δf, KHz) which can be related to blood flow velocity by the Doppler equation: $\Delta f = 2 F (V/c) \cos a$, where F is the ultrasonic frequency (20 MHz), V is the velocity within the sample volume, c is the speed of sound in blood (1500 m/s), and a is the angle between the velocity vector and the sound beam. Using an end-mounted crystal with the catheter parallel ($\pm 20°$) to the vessel axis (cos a equals $1 \pm 6\%$), the relation between the Doppler shift and velocity is approximately 3.75 cm/s per KHz [9]. Recently, Sibley et al. [17] validated cli-nically and experimentally the ability of a similar catheter with an end-moun-ted piezo-electric crystal to provide accurate continuous on-line measure-ment of coronary blood flow velocity and vasodilator reserve. In our labora-tory, we verified the accuracy of each velocity probe by correlating velocity recorded with the Doppler probe in a 9Fr femoral sheat with the volume flow measured by a timed collection of blood from the side branch of the same sheath. Graduated flow rates (range 12 to 165 ml/min) and the corresponding velocities (range 1.2 to 8.2 kHz) were obtained by incremental balloon inflation with the balloon positioned in the sheath. This simple model allows the assessment of the flow-velocity relation at different levels. As previously demonstrated, this relation is linear with correlation coefficients generally $\geqslant 0.95$, [21, 22, 23] but underestimates true volume flow for flows over 150 ml/min [17]. Flow rates of this magnitude, or velocities exceeding 7.5 kHz, were never encountered in this study population.

Protocol

After recording the baseline intracoronary blood velocity in the proximal segment, the balloon catheter (Schneider-Shiley dilatation catheter, Shiley Inc.) with a Doppler probe at the tip was advanced across the stenosis and 3 to 7 inflations with pressures up to 12 atmospheres were used to dilate the stenosis. Resting velocities before and after each balloon inflation and those during reactive hyperemia immediately after deflation were recorded with the Doppler probe situated across the stenotic lesion and expressed in kHz. A satisfactory functional result was considered to have been achieved if there was no further increase in peak velocity during reactive hyperemia. No additional dilatations were then performed and coronary angiography was repeated after removing the PTCA catheter. The balloon diameter size used in this study varied from 2.5 to 3.5 mm. The cross-sectional area of the catheter with the balloon deflated was 0.68 mm^2.

Quantitative analysis of the coronary artery

Coronary angiograms were performed in at least 2 orthogonal projections before and after PTCA and the same projections were repeated after the procedure (Figure 2). The determination of coronary arterial dimensions from 35 mm cinefilm was performed with the computer-based Cardiovascular Angiographic Analysis System (CAAS) [24–26]. In essence, boundaries of the relevant coronary artery segment are detected automatically from optically magnified and video digitized regions of interest of a selected single cineframe angiogram. The absolute diameter of the stenosis (in mm) is determined using the guiding catheter as a scaling device [24]. The detected contours of the arterial and catheter segments are corrected for pincushion distortion [25]. A computer-estimation of the original arterial dimension at the site of the obstruction is used to define the interpolated reference area or diameter [24–26]. The interpolated percentage area stenosis and the minimal luminal cross-sectional area (mm^2) are then calculated and averaged from at least 2, preferably orthogonal, projections.

In the second study group twenty-one patients undergoing elective PTCA for angina pectoris were studied. All patients had evidence of myocardial ischemia as indicated either by ECG changes at rest or during exercise thallium scintigraphy. Informed consent was obtained for the additional investi-

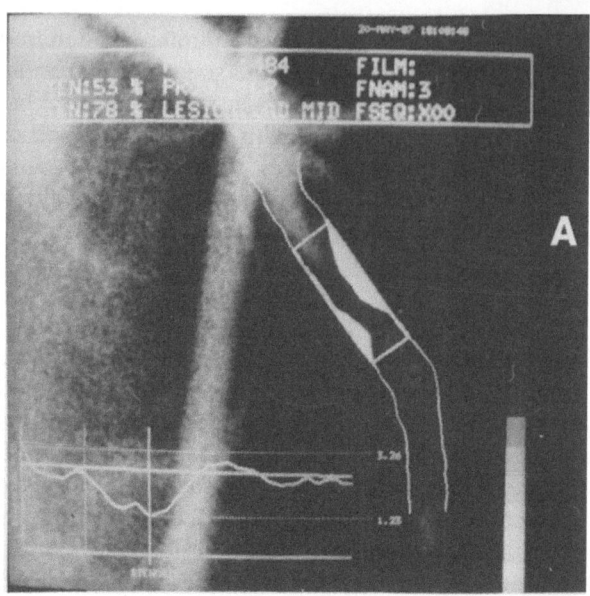

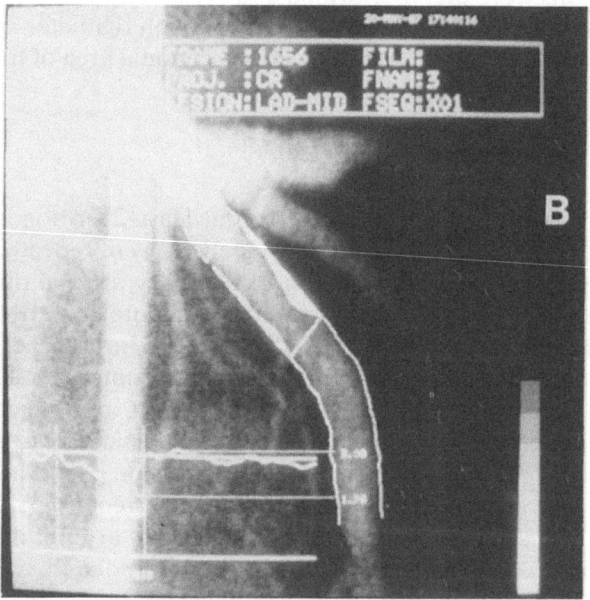

Figure 2. Angiograms of a left anterior descending coronary artery (cranial projection) before *(A)* and after *(B)* angioplasty with superimposition of the automated contours at the coronary artery segment of interest. Beneath this is shown the diameter function of the detected contours of the coronary artery. The minimal lumen diameter (vertical line) and the interpolated diameter function (horizontal line) from which the reference diameter is derived are shown.

gations. All patients were studied without premedication, but their medical treatment (nitrates, calcium antagonists and beta-blockers) was continued on the day of the procedure.

Protocol of the investigational procedure

– Coronary cineangiography was performed in at least two, preferably orthogonal projections for quantitative analysis of the coronary artery stenosis, after intracoronary administration of 2 or 3 mg intracoronary isosorbide dinitrate. The intracoronary administration of isosorbide dinitrate was repeated at regular intervals (20–30 min) to ensure constant and maximal epicardial coronary vasodilation during the entire procedure [27].

– Coronary flow reserve was measured by digital subtraction cineangiography.

– A long wire (length: 315 cm, diameter: 0.014 inch) was passed through the coronary artery stenosis.

– A balloon catheter with a Doppler probe at the tip [9] was advanced over the guide wire into the coronary artery to measure coronary blood flow velocity. The precise location of the tip of the balloon catheter with respect to the stenotic lesion – immediately proximal to the lesion and beyond any major side branches – was determined by injection of contrast medium. After recording the baseline intracoronary blood flow velocity, hyperemia was induced by injecting 12.5 mg papaverine through the guiding catheter. The ratio of peak mean intracoronary blood flow velocity to baseline was then determined as previously described by Wilson et al. [13]. This measurement was obtained in 14 patients (see Table 1).

– Thereafter the balloon was advanced across the stenosis and 3 to 7 inflations, lasting 40 to 80 s, and up to 12 atmospheres were used to dilate the stenosis until repeat cineangiography showed a good result (<50% diameter stenosis). The mean total inflation time was 162 s/patient (range: 120–352 s). Immediately following the final balloon inflation the reactive hyperemia was recorded as previously described [9].

– After subsidence of this reactive hyperemic response, the Doppler tip was pulled back into the proximal part of the coronary artery and the ratio of peak mean intracoronary blood flow velocity after 12.5 mg papaverine i.c. to baseline velocity was again determined. This measurement was obtained in 19 patients (see Table 1).

– After removal of the balloon catheter and the guide wire, coronary flow reserve was measured with digital subtraction cineangiography, at the same pacing rate and using the same radiographic and injection parameters as before PTCA.

– Coronary cineangiography was repeated post-PTCA in the same projections as used at the start of the procedure, for quantitative analysis of the coronary artery stenosis.

Coronary flow reserve measurements with digital subtraction cineangiography

The coronary flow reserve measurement from 35 mm cinefilm has been implemented on the CAAS [15]. The heart was atrially paced at a rate just above the spontaneous heart rate. An ECG-triggered injection into the coronary artery was made with Iopamidol at 37°C through a Medrad Mark IV® infusion pump. This nonionic contrast agent has a viscosity of 9.4 cP at 37°, and osmolarity of 0.796 osm.kg⁻¹ and an iodine content of 370 mg/ml. The angiogram was repeated 30 s after a bolus injection of 12.5 mg papaverine into the coronary artery by way of the guiding catheter [11, 12]. The injection rate of the contrast medium was judged to be adequate if back flow of contrast medium into the aorta occurred. When this was not observed on the hyperemic image, baseline and hyperemic image acquisition were repeated at a higher flow rate, necessitating flow rates of up to 6 ml/s in some patients. Five or six consecutive end-diastolic cineframes were – selected for analysis. Logarithmic nonmagnified mask-mode background subtraction was applied to the image subset to eliminate noncontrast medium densities [28]. The last end-diastolic frame prior to the administration of contrast was chosen as the mask. From the sequence of background subtracted images, a contrast arrival time image was determined using an empirically derived fixed density threshold [15]. Each pixel was labelled with the sequence number of the cardiac cycle numbered from the cycle in which the pixel intensity level first exceeded the threshold. In addition to the contrast arrival time image, a density image was computed, with the intensity of each pixel being representative of the maximal local contrast medium accumulation. The coronary flow reserve was defined as the ratio of the regional flow computed from a hyperemic image divided by the regional flow of the corresponding baseline image. Regional flow values were quantitatively determined using the following videodensitometric principle: regional blood flow (Q) = regional vascular volume/transit time [15]. Regional vascular volume was assessed from logarithmic mask-mode subtraction images, using the Lambert Beer relationship. Coronary flow reserve was then calculated as:

$$\text{CFR} = \frac{Qh}{Qb} = \frac{Dh}{Th} : \frac{Db}{Tb}$$

where D is the mean contrast density and T the mean appearance time at baseline (b) and hyperemia (h). Mean contrast medium appearance time and density were computed within a user-defined region of interest, which was chosen so that the epicardial coronary arteries visible on the angiogram, the coronary sinus, and the great cardiac vein were all excluded from the analysis [15]. Reproducibility data are shown in Table 2. Normal values for coronary

Table 1. Results of quantitative coronary angiography.

Pts	PTCA artery	Balloon size	Balloon inflation	Before PTCA MLCA (mm²)	Before PTCA DS (%)	Before PTCA AS (%)	After PTCA MLCA (mm²)	After PTCA DS (%)	After PTCA AS (%)	After PTCA RA (mm²)	After PTCA RD (mm)	Before PTCA cor. MLCA (mm²)	After PTCA cor. MLCA (mm²)
1	LAD	2.5	4	0.7	61	85	1.3	52	76	5.3	2.59	0.0	0.6
2	LC	2.5	5	0.9	56	80	1.4	48	73	5.4	2.61	0.2	0.7
3	LAD	2.5	4	0.4	66	88	1.4	43	67	4.6	2.30	0.0	0.7
4	LAD	2.5	5	1.3	53	77	1.2	49	73	5.4	2.61	0.6	0.5
5	LAD	3.0	5	0.7	66	88	1.2	48	73	4.7	2.64	0.0	0.5
6	LAD	3.0	4	0.7	55	77	2.0	32	54	4.3	2.16	0.0	1.3
7	LC	3.0	6	0.5	74	93	2.5	28	49	5.9	2.54	0.0	1.8
8	LAD	3.0	4	0.7	65	88	3.7	13	24	4.8	2.54	0.0	3.0
9	LAD	3.0	5	2.9	36	59	5.3	23	41	8.2	3.11	2.2	4.6
10	LAD	3.0	4	1.9	53	78	3.3	39	63	9.3	3.33	1.2	2.6
11	R	3.0	6	0.6	71	91	2.9	40	64	8.1	3.02	0.0	2.2
12	LAD	3.0	4	0.3	78	95	2.5	35	55	6.1	2.79	0.0	1.8
13	LAD	3.0	3	0.6	67	89	1.2	44	67	4.8	2.47	0.0	0.5
14	LAD	3.4	3	2.3	54	79	4.8	30	51	10.3	3.65	1.6	4.1
15	LAD	3.4	4	1.3	52	76	1.8	47	72	6.2	2.75	0.6	1.1
16	LAD	3.4	7	0.7	72	92	2.9	43	56	9.0	3.37	0.0	2.2
17	LC	3.4	4	3.3	48	72	4.1	34	51	9.7	3.57	2.6	3.4
18	LAD	3.4	4	1.6	47	72	3.5	30	32	7.4	2.96	0.9	2.8
19	LAD	3.4	4	0.3	74	93	3.0	18	40	4.9	2.51	0.0	2.3
20	LAD	3.4	4	0.9	63	86	3.5	22	57	6.4	2.81	0.2	2.8
Mean				1.1	60	83	2.7	36	57	6.5	2.85	0.5	2.0
± SD				±0.8	±11	±9	±1.2	±11	±15	±1.9	±0.41	±0.8	±1.2

AS = percentage area stenosis; cor. MLCA reduction due to the catheter across the lesion; DS = percentage diameter stenosis; LAD = left anterior descending coronary artery; LC = left circumflex coronary artery; MLCA = minimal luminal cross-sectional area; PTCA = percutaneous transluminal coronary angioplasty; RA = reference interpolated area; RD = reference interpolated diameter; SD = standard deviation.

flow reserve measured with this technique have previously been established [10, 15]. The coronary flow reserve of 12 angiographically normal coronary arteries was 5.0 ± 0.8. Therefore a flow reserve below 3.4 (2 SD below the mean) is taken to be abnormal.

Results

The first study group: Coronary blood flow velocity during PTCA as a guide line for assessment of the functional result

Clinical data (Table 1). The mean age of the 20 patients (14 men and 6 women) was 54 years (range 41–66). Eighteen patients had 1-vessel coronary narrowing and 2 patients 2-vessel narrowing. The investigated and dilated coronary artery was the left anterior descending artery in 16, the circumflex artery in 3 and the right coronary artery in 1 patient. All patients had normal systolic and diastolic wall motion and an ejection fraction of more than 55%. The mean number of balloon inflations were 4.4/patient (range 3 to 7). The PTCA was successful (diameter stenosis less than 50%) in all patients. Four patients had small localized superficial tear of the dilated coronary artery segment after the procedure.

Quantitative analysis of the coronary angiogram (Table 1). The minimal lumen cross-sectional area increased from 1.1 ± 0.8 to 2.7 ± 1.2 mm^2 (mean $\pm$ standard deviation) (Table 1). Percent of area stenosis decreased from $83 \pm 9\%$ to $57 \pm 15\%$. Percent of diameter stenosis decreased from $60 \pm 11\%$ to $36 \pm 11\%$. The actual minimal lumen cross-sectional area before and after dilatation with the catheter across the lesion was estimated after subtraction of the area (0.68 mm^2) of the PTCA catheter.

Intracoronary Doppler shift during percutaneous transluminal coronary angioplasty (Figures 3a–d). On average, 4 dilatations were performed per patient with sequential mean inflation times of 54, 60, 63 and 68 sec. The inflation pressure increased on average for the 4 inflations from 7.6 to 10.4, 11.4 and 12.0 atmospheres (Figure 3). Reactive hyperemia was maximal after 27 sec (range 21 to 33) s) after deflation. The time to subsidence of hyperemia was 56 sec (range 42 to 74).

After each of the first 3 dilatations, both resting and hyperemic velocities increased (Table 2). On average the velocities of the last 2 dilatations did not differ statistically, suggesting that the end result was already achieved by the third dilatation (Figure 4). However, 5 patients (1, 12, 16, 17 and 20) still had a substantial increase after the fourth dilatation and might have well benefited from additional dilatations.

The ratio of peak hyperemic velocity to resting velocity for each inflation are reported in Table 3. When calculating 'coronary flow reserve' using the

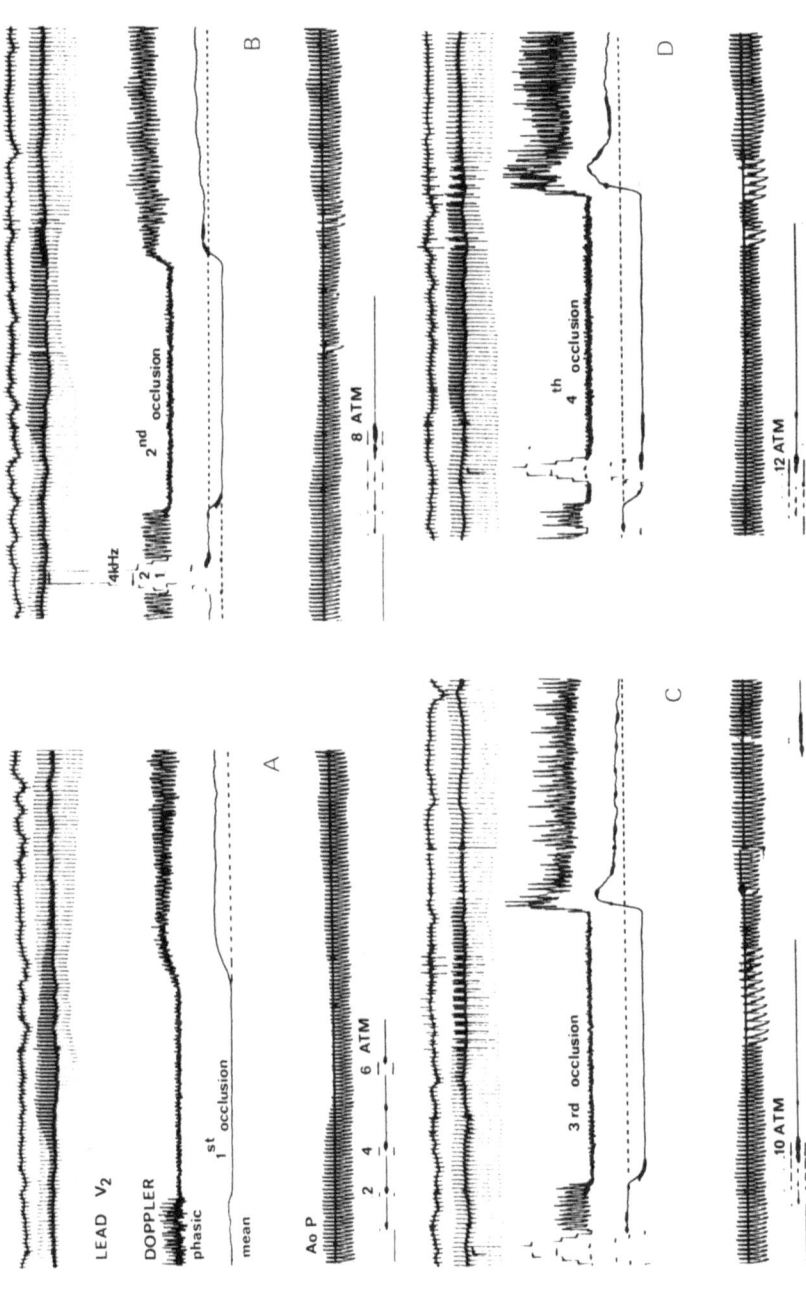

Figure 3. Examples of mean and phasic Doppler signals before, during and after balloon inflation. Reactive hyperemia occurs after balloon deflation. The precordial lead V shows ST-segment elevation (*A*) first transluminal occlusion using a balloon inflation pressure of 6 atmospheres (Atm). (*B*) second transluminal occlusion using a balloon inflation pressure of 8 Atm. (*C*) third transluminal occlusion during a balloon inflation pressure of 10 Atm. (*D*) fourth transluminal occlusion using a balloon inflation pressure of 12 Atm.

Table 2. Doppler shift (KHz) during four sequential dilations.

Pts	Vb				Vh				Va			
	D1	D2	D3	D4	D1	D2	D3	D4	D1	D2	D3	D4
Mean	0.37	0.78	1.03	1.06	1.15	1.35	1.72	1.73	0.59	0.93	0.95	0.99
± SE	±0.10	±0.19	±0.16	±0.16	±0.25	±0.18	±0.26	±0.21	±0.12	±0.15	±0.16	±0.13
		†		NS		*		NS		*		NS

Data are individual and mean ± standard error (SE).
D = dilatation; Va = resting velocity after dilatation; NS = difference not significanct; Vb = resting velocity before dilatation, Vh = peak reactive hyperemia.
Variance analysis plus paired t-test: * $p < 0.05$; † $p < 0.001$.

Table 3. Ratios of peak reactive hyperemia to resting velocity after each dilatation.

Pts	Dil 1		Dil 2		Dil 3		Dil 4	
	Vh/Vb	Vh/Va	Vh/Vb	Vh/Va	Vh/Vb	Vh/Va	Vh/Vb	Vh/Va
Mean	3.91	2.14	2.90	1.70	1.93	2.01	1.85	1.92
± SE	±0.65	±0.35	±0.63	±0.24	±0.17	±0.14	±0.24	±0.28

Data are individual and mean ± standard error (SE).
Abbreviations as in Table 2.

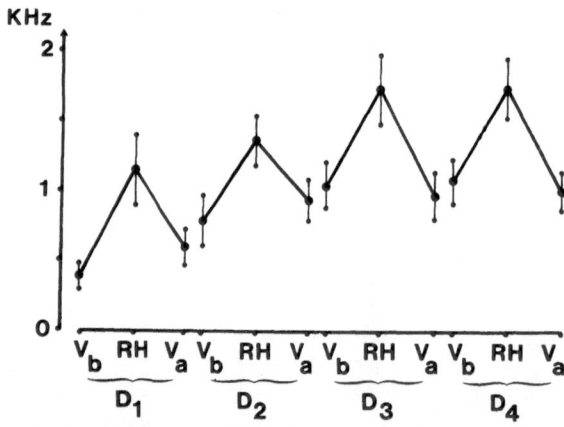

Figure 4. Doppler shift (kHz, mean ± standard error) during 4 sequential dilatations (D). Va = resting velocity after dilatation; Vb = resting velocity before dilatation; Vh = peak reactive hyperemia.

peak hyperemic velocity and the resting velocity recorded before the first 2 dilatations, we observed a paradoxical decrease of the ratio from 3.9 ± 0.6 to 1.9 ± 0.2. This is due to the major increase in resting velocity whose values were very low prior before the first inflation, with the catheter across the undilated lesion. When this ratio is based on the resting velocity recorded after dilatation, the coronary flow reserve differed little from 1 inflation to the next; values ranging between 1.7 and 2.1. This absence of change was confirmed statistically by variance analysis. In other words, this ratio does not seem to be an useful functional guideline for PTCA, whereas the peak hyperemic velocity following successive balloon deflations shows a gradual and significant increase, levelling off in the most patients after the third dilatation.

Second study group: A comparison of two methods to measure coronary flow reserve in the setting of coronary angioplasty: intracoronary blood flow velocity measurements with a Doppler catheter, and digital subtraction cineangiography

The clinical characteristics, results of the quantitative analysis of the coronary angiogram and the coronary flow reserve measurements are shown in Table 4. The mean age of the 21 patients was 57 years (range: 37–76), 17 were male. Eighteen patients had single vessel coronary artery disease and 3 patients two vessel disease. The investigated and dilated coronary artery was the left anterior descending artery in 14, the circumflex artery in 3 and the right coronary artery in 4 patients. In none of the patients a sidebranch was involved at the site of the lesion. The mean left ventricular ejection fraction was 67% and ranged from 38 to 81%. Patient 9 had sustained a myocardial infarction in the anterior wall resulting in a large akinetic segment and an ejection fraction of 38%. None of the other patients had clinical evidence for a myocardial infarction and all had normal wall motion and an ejection fraction of more than 55%. In two patients (patients 4 and 11) the coronary arteriogram showed grade III/IV collateral filling of the PTCA vessel [29]. Patient 12 (see Table 4) had long standing arterial hypertension with left ventricular hypertrophy. None of the other patients had electrocardiographic, echocardiographic or angiographic evidence of left ventricular hypertrophy. The mean number of balloon inflations was 4.3/patient and ranged from 3 to 7. The dilation was successful in all patients, and none of the patients had a CPK-rise after the procedure. Seven patients had a dissection of the dilated coronary artery segment after the procedure. Five dissections were small (patients 1, 7, 10, 11 and 20), two dissections were of moderate severity (patients 17, 18). None of the dissections had clinical repercussions. The hemodynamic data of the individual patients are shown in Table 4 and mean values ($\pm$ SD) of the heart rate and aortic pressure are given in Table 6. The cross-sectional area at the site of obstruction was 1.1 ± 0.6 mm^2 before, and 3.2 ± 1.1 mm^2 after PTCA. Percentage diameter stenosis was $58 \pm 9\%$ before, and $32 \pm 10\%$ after PTCA. Percentage area stenosis was $82 \pm 8\%$ before, and $52 \pm 14\%$ after PTCA. The interpolated reference area was 6.6 ± 1.6 mm^2 and ranged from

Table 4. Results of quantitative coronary angiography and coronary flow reserve measurements.

Pat.	F/M	Age	No of DV	Vessel	B/A	OA	AS	DS	HR1	Ao1	CFR DSC	HR2	Ao2	CFR DOP	RH
1	F	48	1	LAD	A	5.4	35	19	70	91	2.0	67	104	2.1	2.2
2	M	43	1	LAD	A	4.8	51	30	70	95	3.3	51	92	2.9	2.9
3	M	58	1	RCA	A	2.9	64	40	70	93	2.8	68	98	3.0	2.8
4	M	69	1	RCA	A	2.2	66	42	80	91	1.2	72	87	1.1	1.0
5	M	58	2	LAD	B	1.2	86	62	70	99	0.6	57	95	0.9	
					A	3.3	63	39	70	83	2.4	70	89	2.9	2.3
6	M	62	1	LAD	B	0.9	86	62	90	97	1.0	69	101	0.9	
					A	3.5	40	23	90	97	2.0	83	103	1.8	2.0
7	F	53	1	LAD	B	1.6	72	47	90	82	2.0	71	80	1.8	
					A	3.5	51	30	90	78	2.4	81	76	2.7	2.3
8	M	56	1	LAD	B	0.7	88	64	100	83	0.8	91	85	1.1	
					A	3.7	24	17	100	88	2.2	85	98	2.3	2.2
9	M	53	1	LAD	B	1.2	83	59	80	90	1.1	70	90	1.3	
					A	4.5	37	21	80	88	3.0	82	89	2.3	2.6
10	M	55	1	CX	A	2.5	49	28	80	96	1.7	70	97	1.9	1.7
11	M	53	1	CX	A	2.7	69	45	70	85	2.2	60	79	2.0	2.1
12	F	57	1	LAD	B	2.9	59	35	70	115	1.1	66	112	1.0	
					A	5.3	41	23	70	111	1.7	62	108	2.2	2.1
13	M	66	2	LAD	B	0.7	82	58	70	81	1.4	59	83	1.2	
					A	2.9	44	25	70	84	2.7	61	83	2.4	1.9
14	M	56	1	RCA	B	0.7	87	63	70	81	1.2	61	83	1.1	
15	M	67	2	CX	B	0.9	86	68	70	88	1.3	58	88	1.0	
					A	1.7	69	37	70	76	1.8	60	79	1.7	1.5
16	M	60	1	LAD	B	1.3	78	53	80	93	1.4	73	89	1.6	
17	M	56	1	LAD	B	0.8	86	62	70	91	1.1	61	96	2.5	
					A	2.7	61	37	70	92	1.0	57	99	1.4	1.3
18	M	37	1	LAD	A	1.8	70	45	70	87	1.1	63	89	1.1	1.0
19	M	49	1	RCA	B	1.4	84	60	80	95	1.3	73	99	1.4	
					A	2.5	73	48	80	86	1.6	76	83	1.7	1.3
20	F	76	1	LAD	B	1.1	75	50	80	91	1.3	63	90	1.4	
					A	2.8	36	20	80	82	2.3	81	80	2.5	1.5
21	M	58	1	LAD	B	0.6	90	69	70	80	1.0	65	82	1.2	
					A	2.2	64	40	70	75	2.2	63	76	2.3	1.6

Pat = patient, F = female, M = male, No of DV = number of diseased coronary arteries (diameter stenosis 50%), LAD = left anterior descending coronary artery, RCA = right coronary artery, CX = circumflex artery, B = before PTCA, A = after PTCA, OA = cross-sectional area at the site of obstruction (mm^2), AS = percentage area stenosis, DS = percentage diameter stenosis, HR = Heart rate in beats/min and Ao = mean aortic pressure (mmHg) 1 = immediately preceding CFR-DSC measurements.   2 = immediately preceding the CFR-DOP and RH measurements. CFR-DSC = coronary flow reserve measured with distal subtraction cineangiography, CFR-DOP = coronary flow reserve measured with Doppler.

Table 5. Reproducibility of the coronary flow reserve measurements.

		1°	2°	Difference ± SD	r	SEE
DSC	N = 13	2.1 ± 1.2	2.1 ± 1.2	−0.02 ± 0.26	0.98	0.26
DOP	N = 15	1.6 ± 1.3	1.6 ± 0.3	+0.03 ± 0.18	0.88	0.19

1° = first determination (mean ± SD), 2° = second determination (mean ± SD), DSC = digital subtraction cineangiography, analysis of repeated image acquisition taken 5 min apart, without change in patient position, pacing rate, contrast injection parameters or X-ray gantry settings, DOP = repeated intracoronary Doppler blood flow velocity measurements 5 min apart without change in patient – or Doppler catheter position.

Table 6. Hemodynamic data.

Heart rate (HR, beats/min) and mean aortic pressure (Ao, mmHg) immediately preceding the coronary flow reserve measurements with digital subtraction cineangiography (DSC-CFR) and coronary flow reserve and reactive hyperemia measurements with the Doppler catheter (DOP-CFR and DOP-RH).

	Before PTCA		After PTCA		
	DSC-CFR	DOP-CFR	DSC-CFR	DOP-CFR	DOP-HR
Hr	78 ± 10	67 ± 9	76 ± 9	69 ± 10	69 ± 10
Ao	90 ± 9	91 ± 9	88 ± 8	90 ± 10	90 ± 10

3.9 ± 9.8 mm^2. During the measurements with the Doppler catheter just proximal to the stenosis, the tip of the catheter (1.2 mm^2) occupied $18 \pm 5\%$ (range 12 to 31%) of the cross-sectional area of the coronary artery. The reactive hyperemia was measured with the balloon part of the Doppler catheter (0.65 mm^2) across the stenosis. In this situation the catheter occupied $20 \pm 5\%$, (range: 12–37%) of the luminal cross-sectional area at the site of the stenosis. This implies that coronary flow reserve assessed with both techniques after PTCA was measured in the presence of an area stenosis of $52 \pm 14\%$, whereas reactive hyperemia was assessed in the presence of a residual area stenosis of $62 \pm 16\%$. In 14 patients a coronary flow reserve measurement with the angiographic technique was also obtained in a myocardial region supplied by a coronary artery which was not dilated and which had no significant stenosis (<50% diameter stenosis). The mean coronary flow reserve of these vessels was 3.4 ± 0.8 before PTCA and 3.3 ± 0.9 after PTCA. The relationship between coronary flow reserve measured with digital subtraction cineangiography (CFR-DSC) and the cross-sectional area at the site of obstruction (OA) is shown in Figure 5. Patients 1, 4, 7, 9, 10, 11, 12, 17, 18 and 20 had conditions associated with a reduced coronary flow reserve, in addition to the presence of a coronary stenosis. In these patients only a weak relationship was found between these two parameters: CFR-DSC = 0.27 OA + 0.9, (r = 0.55, SEE = 0.57). In the other patients in whom the epicardial

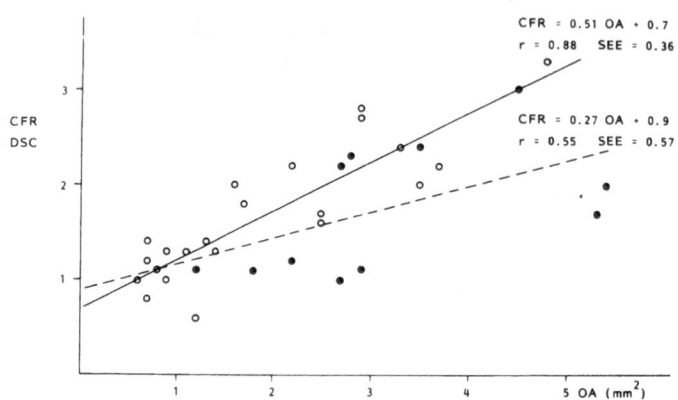

Figure 5. Relationship between coronary flow reserve measured with digital subtraction cinean-giography (CFR-DSC) and cross-sectional area at the site of obstruction (OA). The open symbols are the patients with any of the following characteristics: Left ventricular hypertrophy, hypertension, previous myocardial infarction, collaterals or dissection after PTCA. The closed symbols are the patients without any of the above listed characteristics.

narrowing was the sole factor determining the coronary flow reserve, a good relationship was found between these two parameters: CFR-DSC = 0.51 OA + 0.7, (r = 0.88, SEE = 0.36).

The relationship between coronary flow reserve measured with Doppler (CFR-DOP) and the cross-sectional area at the site of obstruction (OA) is shown in Figure 6. The resting Doppler-shift before PTCA was 1.4 ± 0.7 kHz and after PTCA 1.5 ± 0.7 kHz. In the patients with conditions associated with a reduced coronary flow reserve aside from the presence of a coronary stenosis the relationship between these two parameters was weak: CFR-DOP = 0.27 OA + 1.0 (r = 0.59, SEE = 0.50). In the other patients a reasonably

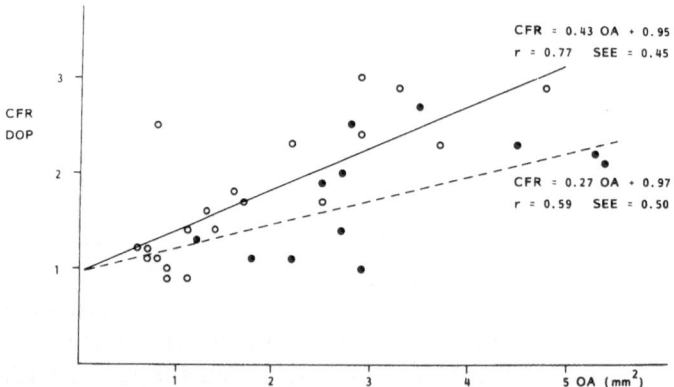

Figure 6. Relationship between coronary flow reserve measured with the Doppler probe (CFR-DOP) and cross-sectional area at the site of obstruction (OA). See for explanation of symbols Figure 1.

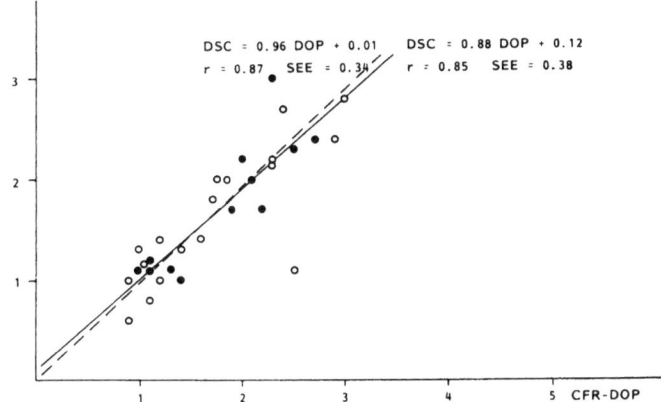

Figure 7. Relationship between coronary flow reserve measured with digital subtraction cinean-giography (CFR-DSC) and coronary flow reserve measured with the Doppler probe (CFR-DOP). See for explanation of symbols Figure 1.

good relationship was found between these two parameters: CFR-DOP = 0.43 OA + 1.0 (r = 0.77, SEE = 0.45).

The relationship between the coronary flow reserve measured with the angiographic technique and the coronary flow reserve measured with Doppler probe is shown in Figure 7. There is a good relationship between the measurements made with these two techniques, irrespective of whether the flow reserve is limited solely by the severity of the coronary stenosis (CFR-DSC = 0.88 CFR-DOP + 0.12, r = 0.85, SEE = 0.38) or whether there are additional patient characteristics present such as previous infarction, hypertrophy, collaterals or dissection after PTCA (CFR-DSC = 0.96 CFR-DOP + 0.01, r = 0.87, SEE = 0.34).

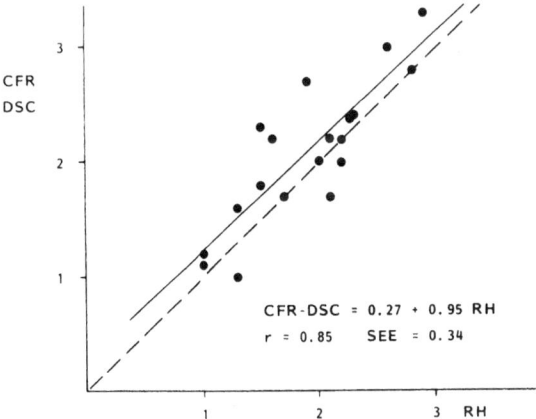

Figure 8. Relationship between coronary flow reserve measured with digital subtraction cinean-giography (CFR-DSC) and the reactive hyperemia recorded with the Doppler probe across the dilated lesion after the final balloon inflation (RH).

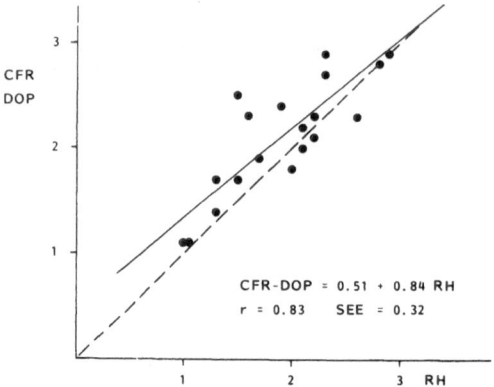

Figure 9. Relationship between coronary flow reserve measured with the Doppler probe (CFR-DOP) proximal to the dilated lesion and the reactive hyperemia recorded with the Doppler probe across the dilated lesion after the final balloon inflation (RH).

The relationships between the reactive hyperemia (RH) recorded after the final balloon inflation with the angioplasty catheter still across the lesion, and coronary flow reserve measured with the angiographic technique (CFR-DSC $= 0.27 + 0.95$ RH, $r = 0.85$, SEE $= 0.34$) and with the Doppler catheter (CFR-DOP $= 0.51 + 0.84$ RH, $r = 0.83$, SEE $= 0.32$) are shown in Figures 8 and 9, respectively. As expected the mean reactive hyperemia was somewhat lower than the coronary flow reserves measured with the angiographic technique or with the Doppler probe located proximal to the dilated stenosis. Reactive hyperemia was 1.9 ± 0.6, coronary flow reserve measured with the angiographic technique 2.1 ± 0.6 and coronary flow reserve measured with the Doppler catheter 2.1 ± 0.6.

Discussion

Intracoronary blood flow velocity: An on line assessment of the functional result of the dilatation?

We measured the changes of the intracoronary blood flow velocity during PTCA by means of a Doppler tip balloon catheter. Our original purpose was to use this information as an 'on-line' assessment of the functional result of the dilatation, with the PTCA catheter still across the stenosis. The technical innovation of this catheter is the combination of a diagnostic and therapeutic tool. Although the catheter is a prototype of first generation, it provides an unique opportunity to assess the reactive hyperemia in awake human beings.

The poststenotic velocities recorded with the catheter across the lesion are low when compared with the previously published data that document values recorded proximal to the stenotic lesion [13, 18]. Recently it has been suggested [30] that the 'zero crossing' method underestimates post-stenotic velocity possibly because of disturbance of laminar flow and this may also explain the discrepancy between our results and those previously published. The routine calibration of each Doppler probe by the timed blood volume collection from the femoral sheath (cross-sectional area: 6.9 mm^2) makes it unlikely that the intracoronary flow velocities recorded in this study with an end-mounted Doppler catheter are in error. The duration of the hyperemia observed in all patients was longer than that in the previously reported [10, 18, 31, 32]. However, in contrast to our results, previous results were obtained after occlusion of normal arteries and after a shorter occlusion time (20 s maximal). Marcus et al. [32] have demonstrated that the duration of the hyperemic response increased progressively with increasing duration of occlusion.

Peak reactive hyperemia a useful functional guide line during the procedure

Intracoronary blood flow velocity measurements with a Doppler probe have previously been used to investigate regional coronary flow reserve, assessing the maximal reactive hyperemia induced by pharmacological vasodilation of ischemia [5–9]. However, because coronary flow reserve is a ratio between maximal and resting coronary blood flow, any increase in resting flow results in a decrease of this ratio. This phenomenon was observed after the first 2 dilatations when the resting velocity preceding the inflation was used as the denominator of the ratio (peak hyperemic velocity/resting velocity). If the resting velocity after the deflation was used as denominator, the ratio remained unchanged during 4 dilatations; this alternative is therefore useless as a functional guide-line during the procedure. Because peak hyperemic velocity shows a gradual increase with successive dilatations which presumably reflects progressive enlargement of the lumen stenosis we attempted to correlate the cross-sectional area of the stenotic lesion 'corrected' for the presence of the catheter across the stenosis, with the absolute value of the peak velocity during reactive hyperemia. Despite an orderly ranking of the 2 parameters no close correlation (r = 0.41) could be established. Ideally cross-sectional areas measured after each stepwise enlargement of the lumen by the gradual inflation of the balloon should have been correlated with the peak hyperemic velocity after the transluminal occlusion. Unfortunately, the poor quality of the coronary angiography performed with the PTCA catheter in the guiding catheter precludes quantitative analysis.

In the setting of PTCA, the absence of precise mathematical relation between the peak hyperemic velocity measured after the last inflation and the post-PTCA 'corrected' minimal lumen cross-sectional area is not so surprising. First, the changes in luminal size of an artery following the mechanical disruption of its internal wall may be difficult to assess by angiographic means [2, 3]. The irregular shape with internal tears that fill with contrast medium to a variable extent will result in some overestimation of the true functional luminal size immediately following PTCA. Second, the extent of coronary atherosclerosis may be difficult to delineate angiographically.

McPherson et al. [33] have documented substantial intimal atherosclerosis resulting in diffuse obstructive disease and involving the entire length of an epicardial artery, is often present, even when angiograms reveal only discrete lesions. As a consequence relative measurements of stenosis severity are an inadequate approach to assessing the severity of coronary obstructions. In addition, the calculated cross-sectional area of the stenotic lesion after the subtraction of the cross-sectional areas of the catheter (mean 2.0 ± 1.2 mm^2, range: $0.5–4.6$ mm^2) clearly suggests that the catheter is not only impeding the flow through the stenotic lesion, even after dilatation, but might unpredictably disturb the velocity profile in the post-stenotic segment [34]. Further miniaturization of the catheter may improve this major draw-back. For all these reasons, the measurement of the peak velocity with this proto-type catheter of first generation does not permit, on-line, and accurate prediction of the morphological change of the stenotic lesion. However, during sequential dilatations the plateau observed in the peak hyperemic and resting velocity signals still provides valuable information which indicates that no further improvement in flow velocity can be expected from additional dilatations.

The purpose of the investigation in the second study group was twofold: firstly, to compare in the setting of an angioplasty procedure two different techniques of assessing regional coronary blood flow; secondly, to compare the pharmacologically induced vasodilation after intracoronary papaverine with reactive hyperemia following transluminal occlusion.

Rationale for comparison of the two techniques to measure coronary flow reserve

Extensive validation studies with the Doppler technique have been performed in which the measured changes in velocity have been compared with changes in perfusion measured with timed-venous coronary sinus collection [13, 32], labelled microspheres [35], and electromagnetic flow probes [32]. These studies indicate that under a great variety of conditions, changes in coronary blood flow velocity measured by the Doppler technique accurately reflect changes in flow [36]. Recently, small sized Doppler catheters have been developed and validated. They are able to make selective measurements of flow velocity in the major proximal coronary arteries [9, 13, 17], without causing coronary obstruction [36]. For instance, in this report the cross-sectional area of the Doppler balloon catheter was only $18 \pm 5\%$ of the cross-sectional area of the coronary artery in the segment proximal to the stenosis. However, two important limitations of the Doppler technique are, firstly: it measures flow velocity rather than volume flow – which may lead to inaccurate values for flow reserve if significant change occurs in cross-sectional areas between baseline and hyperemia [18] – and secondly: subselective coronary cannulation increases the risk during cardiac catheterization [13, 36]. Therefore less invasive approaches to determine the regional coronary flow reserve are urgently needed.

Selective coronary angiography is the standard means for obtaining anatomical information and is the most important tool for clinical decision making used by the clinician caring for patients with coronary artery disease. Recently, several attempts have been made to measure coronary blood flow parameters during cardiac catheterization using recent developments in radiographic technology [16]. However, radiographic contrast media cannot be used to measure coronary blood flow by the traditional methodological approaches [16]; an essential prerequisite of indicator-dilution (Stewart-Hamilton), inert substance washout (Kety-Schmidt), or firstpass distribution (Sapirstein) techniques is that the indicator substance does not affect the regional flow being measured [8]. Unfortunately, all radiographic media have substantial vascular effects [37], although nonionic media may disturb blood flow less than ionic agents [16]. Using ECG-gated power injection of a contrast agent at a rate that is presumed to be sufficiently rapid to achieve complete replacement of blood with contrast, Hodgson et al. [38] developed a mask mode subtraction technique that determines myocardial time-density curves before and during maximal hyperemia before the vascular effects of the contrast medium disturb the ratio between resting and hyperemic coronary blood flow. Since some of this techniques fundamental assumptions may not be met under clinical conditions, validation studies are of special interest [39]. In this study we found a reasonable good correlation between radiographically determined coronary flow reserve and the coronary flow velocity reserve measured with a Doppler probe, despite the fact that the two approaches have methodologically nothing in common and that their respective regions of interest (myocardium for the radiographic technique and intracoronary lumen for the Doppler technique) are basically different.

Maximal coronary blood flow after pharmacological vasodilation versus reactive hyperemia induced by coronary occlusion

In the animal laboratory it has been shown that pharmacologically induced vasodilation after intracoronary administration of papaverine is of the same magnitude as the reactive hyperemia after a 15 s occlusion of the coronary artery [40]. There is some question as to whether the same quantity of flow reserve that can be recruited pharmacologically, can be recruited during ischemia [39]. In this study, we found that reactive hyperemia in patients without hypertrophy, infarction, hypertension, collaterals or dissection was 2.1 ± 0.6 (range 1.3 to 2.9), whereas coronary flow reserves in these patients both with the Doppler probe and the radiographic technique were 2.3 ± 0.6 (range 1.6 to 3.3) after PTCA. The cross-sectional area at the site of obstruction averaged 3.05 mm^2 in these patients. Since the balloon catheter was still across the lesion the functional lumen averaged 2.4 mm^2 (see Table 1). In a previous study from this laboratory we established the relationship between cross-sectional area at the site of obstruction and the measured coronary flow reserve in a patient population with single vessel coronary disease and the absence of other factors that might reduce flow reserve such as hypertrophy, infarction, hypertension, collaterals or dissection [15]. This relationship is shown in Figure 10. A coronary artery with an obstruction area of 2.4 mm^2 would be expected to have a vascular reserve of 2.2 with confidence limits extending from 1.3 to 3.0, which corresponds almost exactly to the range found in this study. Therefore, we feel that our data support the conclusion that the coronary vasodilation after an optimal dose of intracoronary papaverine [11] is equipotent to the reactive hyperemia following a transluminal occlusion of more than 40 s in patients with significant coronary artery disease.

Limitations

When comparing these three measures of the functional capacity of a coronary artery one has to bear in mind the potential sources of data scatter. Fortunately, the radiographic technique as well as the Doppler technique have a good reproducibility (see 'Methods'). Coronary flow reserve and reactive hyperemia are both ratios between maximal coronary blood flow and resting flow. Resting coronary blood flow is mainly determined by aortic pressure and heart rate and coronary blood flow during maximal vasodilation is linearly related to the prevailing perfusion pressure [7, 8]. These two hemodynamic parameters change little between the measurements of flow reserve and reactive hyperemia [see Table 1 and 3), although they certainly contribute to the scatter of the data (see Figures 3, 4 and 5).

Several studies have shown that in selected patients a close relationship exists between quantitatively determined stenosis geometry and measured coronary flow reserve [15, 41]. However, coronary flow reserve can be influenced by many factors other than epicardial coronary stenosis, such as myocardial hypertrophy, tachycardia, hypertension, prior myocardial infarction, collaterals, dissection after PTCA [42, 43], changes in coronary vasomotor tone and changes in ventricular end-diastolic and intrathoracic pressures [7, 8]. Therefore, in order to relate the measured coronary flow reserve to quantitatively determined stenosis geometry, we have carefully divided our study population into a group of patients (A) with one or more of the above mentioned characteristics and a group of patients (B) without any of these characteristics (see Figures 1 and 2). We tried to prevent changes in vasomotor tone which is relevant to both techniques [24] by inducing a constant maximal epicardial coronary vasodilation with repeated intracoronary administration of isosorbide dinitrate [27]. In accordance with previous reports [15, 41] we found a good correlation between cross-sectional area at the site of obstruction and measured coronary flow reserve in group B, in contrast to a poor correlation between these two parameters in group A.

Coronary flow reserve immediately after PTCA

Several authors [10, 42] have shown that the coronary flow reserve of the myocardial region supplied by the dilated vessel increases substantially after PTCA, but is not restored to normal values. The measurements obtained in the present study with two independant techniques confirm this fact. We also measured the coronary flow reserve of an adjacent myocardial region supplied by a not significantly diseased coronary artery, by the radiographic technique and found a marked difference in vasodilator response. For ethical reasons we did not obtain this measurement with the Doppler catheter as we felt that introduction of the Doppler probe into a second coronary artery might introduce additional risks to the investigational part of the procedure. Nevertheless, the results of the radiographic technique indicate that the abnormal vasodilatory response is restricted to the myocardium supplied by the dilated coronary artery. There are several potential explanations for this phenomenon.

– Since coronary flow reserve is a ratio between resting flow and maximal coronary blood flow, any increase in resting flow results in a decrease of this ratio. Neither of the techniques we used, provided us with absolute measurements of volume flow. Therefore, we cannot make a definite conclusion regarding resting coronary volume flow after the PTCA. However, the resting Doppler shift was virtually the same before and after the PTCA procedure, 1.4 ± 0.7 kHz and 1.5 ± 0.7 kHz, respectively. Furthermore, several authors using the thermodilution technique in the coronary sinus or the great cardiac vein have reported comparable resting volume flows before and after PTCA [44–46].

– Metabolic, humoral or myogenic factors could potentially play a role in the limited restoration of coronary flow reserve after PTCA. However, the metabolic derangements due to the PTCA seem quickly reversible [44, 47, 48]. Although humoral factors may play a role in a specific subgroup of patients with complicated PTCA, sofar no evidence has been presented that implicates that humoral factors are important in this regard in the majority of patients [49]. The chronic reduction in perfusion pressure distal to the stenotic lesion may induce alterations in the complex mechanism of autoregulation and a prolonged period of time may be needed before these abnormalities subside [50].

– Finally, the impaired coronary flow reserve could be directly related to the residual stenosis [10]. Cross-sectional area measured immediately after PTCA generally increases about threefold due to the procedure but remains grossly abnormal [10, 51]. The relationship between cross-sectional area at the site of obstruction and coronary flow reserve as found in a previous study from our laboratory [15], is shown in Figure 10 with the 95% confidence intervals. The data of the present study for patients fulfilling the same exclu-

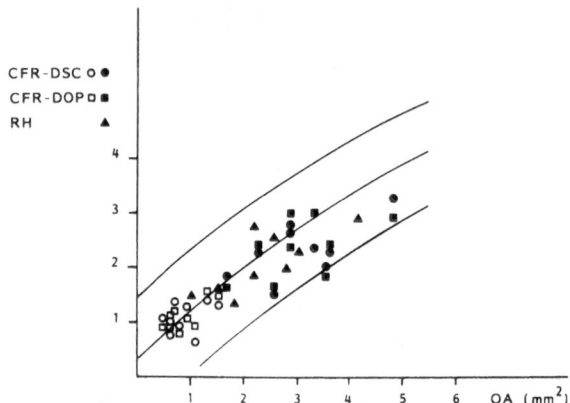

Figure 10. Relationship between flow reserve and cross-sectional area at the site of obstruction (OA) as described in a previous report of our laboratory [16]. The lines indicate the best fit curve and the 95% confidence limits. The data of the present study are superimposed. The open symbols are the measurements obtained before PTCA. The closed symbols are the measurements obtained after PTCA. CFR-DSC = coronary flow reserve measured with digital subtraction cineangiography, CFR-DOP = coronary flow reserve measured with the Doppler probe, RH = reactive hyperemia recorded following the final balloon inflation.

sion criteria (group B) are superimposed: coronary flow reserve measured with both techniques and the reactive hyperemia following the final balloon inflation with residual obstruction area corrected for the presence of the Doppler balloon catheter. The large majority of measurements fall within the 95% confidence limits of this relation, suggesting that the persisting reduction in cross-sectional area perse constitutes a sufficient explanation for the limited restoration of coronary flow reserve, although it does not exclude other contributing pathophysiological mechanisms.

Acknowledgements

Kevin Beatt is recipient of the Joint Fellowship from the British and Netherlands Heart Foundations.

We gratefully acknowledge to Anja van Huuksloot en Claudia Sprenger de Rover for their secretarial assistance.

References

1. Grüntzig AR, Senning A, Siegenthaler WE (1979) Nonoperative dilatation of coronary artery stenosis: percutaneous transluminal angioplasty. *N Engl J Med* 301: 61–68.
2. Block PC, Myler RK, Stertzer S, Fallon JT (1981) Morphology after transluminal angioplasty in human beings. *N Engl J Med* 305: 382–385.
3. Serruys PW, Reiber JHC, Wijns W, Brand M van den, Kooyman CJ, Katen HJ ten, Hugen-

holtz PG (1984) Assessment of percutaneous transluminal coronary angioplasty by quantitative coronary angiography: Diameter versus densitometric area measurements. *Am J
Cardiol* 54: 482–488.

4. Leimgruber PP, Roubin GS, Hollman J, Cotsonis GA, Meier B, Douglas JS, King SB,
Gruentzig AR (1986) Restenosis after successful coronary angioplasty in patients with
single-vessel disease. *Circulation* 73: 710–717.

5. Serruys PW, Wijns W, Reiber JHC, Feyter P de, Brand M van den, Piscione F, Hugenholtz
PG (1985) Values and limitations of transstenotic pressure gradients measured during percutaneous coronary angioplasty. *Herz* 6: 337–342.

6. Redd DCB, Roubin GS, Leimgruber PP, Abi-Mansour P, Douglas JS, King SB (1987) The
transstenotic pressure gradient trend as a predictor of acute complications after percutaneous transluminal coronary angioplasty. *Circulation* 76: 792–801.

7. Hoffman JIE (1984) Maximal coronary flow and the concept of vascular reserve. *Circulation* 70: 153–159.

8. Klocke FJ (1983) Measurements of coronary blood flow and degree of stenosis: Current
clinical implications and continuing uncertainties. *J Am Coll Cardiol*: 31–41.

9. Serruys PW, Juillière Y, Zijlstra F, Beatt KJ, Feyter PJ de, Suryapranata H, Brand M vd,
Roelandt J (1988) Coronary Blood Flow velocity during PTCA: A guide-line for assessment of functional results. *Am J Cardiol* 61: 253–259.

10. Zijlstra F, Reiber JC, Juillière Y, Serruys PW (1988) Normalization of coronary flow
reserve by percutaneous transluminal coronary angioplasty. *Am J Cardiol* 61: 55–60.

11. Wilson RF, White CW (1986) Intracoronary papaverine: An ideal coronary vasodilator for
studies of the coronary circulation in conscious humans. *Circulation* 73: 444–451.

12. Zijlstra F, Serruys PW, Hugenholtz PG (1986) Papaverine: The ideal coronary vasodilator
for investigating coronary flow reserve: A study of timing, magnitude, reproducibility and
safety of the coronary hyperemic response after intracoronary papaverine. *Cath Cardiovasc
Diagn* 12: 298–303.

13. Wilson RF, Laughlin DE, Ackell PH, Chilian WM, Holida MD, Hartley CJ, Armstrong
ML, Marcus ML, White CW (1985) Transluminal subselective measurement of coronary
artery blood flow velocity and vasodilator reserve in man. *Circulation* 72: 82–92.

14. Bates ER, Aueron FM, Le Grand V, Le Free MT, Mancini GBJ, Hodgson JM, Vogel RA
(1985) Comparative long-term effects of coronary artery bypass graft surgery and percutaneous transluminal coronary angioplasty on regional coronary flow reserve. *Circulation*
72: 833–839.

15. Zijlstra F, van Ommeren J, Reiber JHC, Serruys PW (1987) Does quantitative assessment
of coronary artery dimensions predict the physiological significance of a coronary stenosis?
Circulation 75: 1154–1161.

16. Vogel RA (1985)The radiographic assessment of coronary blood flow parameters. *Circulation* 72: 460–465.

17. Sibley DH, Millar HD, Hartley CJ, Whitlow PL (1986) Subselective measurement of coronary blood flow velocity using a steerable Doppler catheter. *JACC* 8: 1332–1340.

18. Marcus ML (1983) Physiological effects of a coronary stenosis, in: *The Coronary Circulation in Health and Disease*, pp 242–269. New York: Mc Graw-Hill.

19. Marcus ML (1983) Effects of cardiac hypertrophy on the coronary circulation, in: *The
Coronary Circulation in Health and Disease*, pp 285–306. New York: Mc Graw-Hill.

20. Marcus ML, Doty DB, Hiratzka LP, Whight CB, Eastham CL (1985) Decrease coronary
reserve: A mechanism for angina pectoris in patients with aortic stenosis and normal coronary arteries. *N Engl J Ned* 307: 1362–1366.

21. Cole JS, Hartley CJ (1977) The pulsed Doppler coronary artery catheter. Preliminary
report of a new technique for measuring rapid changes in coronary artery flow velocity in
man. *Circulation* 56: 18–25.

22. Hartley CJ, Cole JS (1974) An ultrasonic pulsed Doppler system for measuring blood flow
in small vessels. *J Appl Physiol* 37: 626–629.

23. Wilson RF, Laughlin DE, Ackell PH, Chilian WM, Holida MD, Hartley CJ, Armstrong

ML, Marcus ML, White CW (1985) Transluminal subelective measurement of coronary artery blood flow velocity and vasodilator reserve in man. *Circulation* 72: 82–92.

24. Reiber JHC, Serruys PW, Kooyman CJ, Wijns W, Slager CJ, Gerbrand JJ, Schuurbiers JCH, Boer A den, Hugenholtz PG (1985) Assessment of short-, medium-, and long-term variations in arterial dimensions from computer-assisted quantification of coronary cineangiograms. *Circulation* 71: 280–288.

25. Reiber JHC, Kooijman CJ, Slager CJ, Gerbrands JJ, Schuurbiers JHC, Boer A den, Wijns W, Serruys PW, Hugenholtz PG (1984) Coronary artery dimensions from cineangiograms; methodology and vasodilation of a computer-assisted analysis procedure. *IEEE Trans Med Imaging* MI-3: 131–141.

26. Reiber JHC, Kooijman CJ, Boer A den, Serruys PW (1985) Assessment of dimensions and image quality of coronary contrast catheters from cineangiograms. *Cath Cardiovasc Diagn* 11: 521–531.

27. Zijlstra F, Reiber JHC, Serruys PW (1988) Does intracoronary papaverine dilate epicardial coronary arteries? Implications for the assessment of coronary flow reserve. *Cath Cardiovasc Diagn* 14: 1–6.

28. Werf T van der, Heethaar RM, Stegehuis H, Meyler FL (1984) The concept of apparent cardiac arrest as a prerequisite for coronary digital subtraction angiography. *J Am Coll Cardiol* 4: 239–244.

29. Rentrop KP, Cohen M, Blanke H, Philips RA (1985) Changes in collateral channel filling immediately after controlled coronary artery occlusion by an angioplasty balloon in human subjects. *J Am Coll Cardiol* 5: 587–592.

30. Kajiva F, Ogasawara Y, Tsuyioka K, Nakai M, Coto M, Wada Y, Tadaoka S, Matsuoka S, Mito K, Fuwruara T (1986) Evaluation of human coronary blood flow with an 80 channel transform methods during cardiac surgery. *Circulation* 74 (suppl 3): 53–60.

31. Sibley D, Bulle T, Baxley W, Dean L, Whitlow P (1986) Continuous on-line assessment of coronary angioplasty with a Doppler tipped balloon dilatation catheter (abstracts). *Circulation* 74 (suppl 2): 459.

32. Marcus M, Wright C, Doty D, Eastham C, Laughlin D, Krumm P, Fastenow C, Brody M (1981) Measurements of coronary velocity and reactive hyperemia in the coronary circulation of humans. *Circ Res* 877–897.

33. Mc Pherson DD, Hiratzka LF, Lamberth WC, Brandt B, Hunt M, Kieso RA, Marcus ML, Kerber RF (1987) Delineation of the extent of coronary atherosclerosis by high-frequency epicardial echocardiography. *N Engl Med* 316: 304–309.

34. Kilpatrick D, Webber SB (1986) Intravascular blood velocity in simulated coronary artery stenoses. *Cathet Cardiovasc Diagn* 12: 317–3.

35. Wangler RD, Peters KG, Laughlin DE, Tomanek RJ, Marcus ML (1981) A method for continuously assessing coronary velocity in the rat. *Am J Physiol* 10: H816–H820.

36. Marcus ML, Wilson RF, White CW (1987) Methods of measurements of myocardial blood flow in patients: A critical review. *Circulation* 76: 245–253.

37. Hodgson JM, Mancini GBJ, LeGrand V, Vogel RA (1985) Characterization of changes in coronary blood flow during the first six sec after intracoronary contrast injection. *Invest Radiol* 20: 246–252.

38. Hodgson JM, LeGrand V, Bates ER, Mancini GBJ, Aueron FM, O'Neill WW, Simon SB, Beauman GJ, LeFree MT, Vogel RA (1985) Validation in dogs of a rapid angiographic technique to measure relative coronary blood flow during routine cardiac catheterization. *Am J Cardiol* 55: 188–193.

39. Klocke FJ (1987) Measurements of coronary flow reserve: Defining pathophysiology versus making decisions about patient care. *Circulation* 76: 1183–1189.

40. Bookstein JJ, Higgins CB (1977) Comparative efficacy of coronary vasodilatory methods. *Investigate Radiology* 12: 121–127.

41. Wilson RF, Marcus ML, White CW (1987) Prediction of the physiologic significance of coronary arterial lesions by quantitative lesion geometry in patients with limited coronary artery disease. *Circulation* 75: 723–732.

42. Hodgson JM, Riley RS, Most AS, Williams DO (1987) Assessment of coronary flow reserve using digital angiography before and after successful percutaneous transluminal coronary angioplasty. *Am J Cardiol* 60: 61–65.
43. Bates ER, Mc Gillem MJ, Beats TF, DeBoe SF, Mickelson JK, Mancini GBJ, Vogel RA (1987) Effect of angioplasty induced endothelial denudation compared with medial injury on regional coronary blood flow. *Circulation* 76: 710–716.
44. Serruys PW, Wijns W, Brand M van den, Mey S, Slager C, Schuurbiers JCH, Hugenholtz PG, Brower RW (1984) Left ventricular performance, regional blood flow, wall motion, and lactate metabolism during transluminal angioplasty. *Circulation* 70: 25–36.
45. Feldman RL, Conti R, Pepine CJ (1983) Regional coronary venous flow responses to transient coronary artery occlusion in human beings. *J Am Coll Cardiol* 2: 1–10.
46. Rothman MT, Baim DS, Simpson JB, Harrison DC (1982) Coronary hemodynamics during percutaneous transluminal coronary angioplasty. *Am J Cardiol* 49: 1615–1622.
47. Serruys PW, Piscione F, Wijns W, Harmsen E, Brand M van den, Feyter P de, Hugenholtz PG, Jong JW de (1986) Myocardial release of hypoxanthine and lactate during percutaneous transluminal coronary angioplasty: A quickly reversible phenomenon, but for how long', in: Serruys PW, *Transluminal Coronary Angioplasty: An Investigational Tool and a Non-operative Treatment of Acute Myocardial Ischemia*, p 75. (Doctoral thesis, Erasmus University, The Netherlands).
48. Webb SC, Rickards AF, Poole-Wilson PA (1983) Coronary sinus potassium concentration recorded during coronary angioplasty. *Br Heart J* 50: 146–152.
49. Peterson MB, Machay V, Block PC, Palacios I, Philbin D, Watkins WD (1986) Thromboxane release during percutaneous transluminal coronary angioplasty. *Am Heart J*: 111–119.
50. Wilson RF, Aylward PE, Leimbach WH, Talman CL, White CW (1986) Coronary flow reserve late after PTCA. Do the early alterations persist? (abstracts). *J Am Coll Cardiol* 7: 212A (suppl).
51. Johnson MR, Brayden GP, Ericksen EE, Collins SM, Skaton DJ, Harrison DG, Marcus ML, White CW (1986) Changes in cross-sectional area of the coronary lumen in the six months after angioplasty: A quantitative analysis of the variable response to percutaneous transluminal angioplasty. *Circulation* 73: 467–475.

26. Long term result of revascularization after angioplasty
Should we 'randomize'?

P. W. SERRUYS, B. J. MEESTER and P. J. DE FEYTER

Introduction: Now and then

Last year, on both sides of the Atlantic, we celebrated the tenth anniversary of the first coronary angioplasty performed in Zürich by Andreas Grüntzig. It is common place to say that many things have changed over the last ten years. Indeed, if we analyze the baseline data of the PTCA registry of the National Heart Lung and Blood Institute [1] and if we compare the patients enrolled between 1978 and 1982 with those treated in 1985–1986, then it becomes apparent that new PTCA cases have significantly higher incidence of previous CABG and previous MI than the early registry cases, 13% versus 9% and 37% versus 21%. (Table 1). The percentage of patients with multivessel disease has increased from 25% to 53% and are now more common than the single vessel disease. A much higher proportion of the current cohort have multiple lesion attempted, 40% versus 9% in the early registry. Despite generally sicker patients and more ambitious procedures, the rates of major inhospital events have decreased for the new registry cohort. The incidence of elective CABG has dropped dramatically from 20.7% to 2.2%. Similarly, the incidence of emergency CABG in the new cohort is 3.4% compared to 5.8%. The incidence of dissection and non fatal MI, as well as the death rate are almost identical for the old and new cohort. Complementing these lower rates of events and complications there are much higher rates of angiographic and overall success. In the new cohort, at least one dilatation per patient was successful in 91% of the cases compared to 68% in the earlier cases. Eighty-two percent of the new cohort had all attempted lesions successfully dilated compared to 65% of earlier PTCA cases. The overall success rate when all lesions are attempted is up significantly from 61% to 78% for new registry patients and the success per lesion has increased from 67% to 88%.

Acute closure and death: A predictable procedural event?

With current techniques, acute closure occurs in only 4% of the attempts, but

S. Iliceto et al. (eds.), Ultrasound in Coronary Artery Disease, 311–321.
© 1991 *Kluwer Academic Publishers.*

Table 1. 'Then and now': NHLBI PTCA registry: Baseline data and results (first PTCA without AMI), (Detre et al. 1988) [1].

	Old cohort		New cohort
	1978–82		1985–86
	n = 1155		n = 1857
	%		%
Prior CABG	9	**	13
Prior MI	21	***	37
Single VD	75	***	46
Multiple VD	25	***	53
Left main	2		2
Multiple attempts	9	***	40
Spasm	5	***	1.3
Dissection	5	ns	4.6
Elective CABG	20.7	***	2.2
Emergency CABG	5.8	**	3.4
Non fatal MI	4.9	ns	4.5
Death	1.2	ns	1.1
Success (⩾ 20%) by patients:			
At least one dilatation	68	***	91
No death, MI or CABG	63	***	85
All lesions attempted	65	***	82
No death, MI or CABG	61	***	78
Success by lesion	67	***	88
	(n = 1263)		(n = 2959)

*** < 0.001   ** < 0.01

it is still the major cause of morbidity and mortality. To determine predictors of acute coronary closure, the Emory group compared 140 procedures complicated by acute closure with 311 successful attempts all taken from a study population of more than 5000 procedures [2]. Sixteen clinical, 35 angiographic and 7 procedural variables were analyzed. Multivariate analysis found 7 independent preprocedural factors related to closure. These seven factors are:

- Lesion length ⩾ 2 luminal diameters
- Female gender
- Bend point ⩾ 45 degrees
- Branch point
- Thrombus
- Other stenoses ⩾ 50% in same vessel
- Multivessel disease

The importance of the presence of multiple preprocedural risk factors is demonstrated by the finding that, in this study sample, containing a 33% mix of patients with acute closure, the risk of closure on average was 14% in the

Table 2. Effects of presence of multiple pre-procedural risk factors on risk of closure (Ellis et al.) [2].

Risk factors	Sample containing a 33% mix of patients with acute closure	'Estimated' risk
None	14%	1.4%
One risk factor	26%	5%
Two risk factors	35%	14%
Three risk factors	58%	12%
Four risk factors	100%	30%

presence of no risk factors, 26% with one risk factor, 35% with two risk factors, 58% with 3 risk factors and 100% with four risk factors. Since by definition the incidence of closure in this study population was artificially elevated to 33%, the absolute risk associated with the presence of one or more of these morphological factors cannot be easily transferred to the general population of PTCA candidates. The study, however emphasizes the additive effect of these identified risk factors on acute closure associated with PTCA (Table 2).

Cardiac death as a consequence of acute vessel closure after coronary angioplasty occurred in thirteen of 294 closures from 8207 consecutive procedures performed at Emory and at the San Francisco Heart Institute since 1981 [3]. Multivariate analysis found collaterals originating from beyond the site dilated, female gender and multivessel disease to be independent predictors of death. (Thus, cardiac death after elective PTCA is very rare in experienced centers and occurs most often in females with large amounts of potentially ischemic myocardium). As the apparent indications for coronary angioplasty expand, it would seem prudent to proceed very carefully when dealing with such high risk patients.

Restenosis: The Achille's heel of angioplasty

When the patient has passed the test of the procedure, what can he expect for the future? Between 1980–1985, the French PTCA Registry has collected more than 5000 patients [4]. Just before discharge, 2373 patients underwent an exercise test: a maximal negative exercise test was obtained in 63% of patients with single vessel disease and 47% of patients with multiple vessel disease. In both groups 22% and 26%, respectively had submaximal negative tests – the patients being unable to reach the maximal age predicted heart rate. Before discharge, 15% of patients with single vessel disease and 27% of patients with multiple vessel disease still had a positive exercise test. Six months after the procedure, 1881 patients had a complete clinical and angiographic examination; seventy-one percent of patients with single vessel disease remained symptom free versus 65% of patients with multiple vessel disease. One thousand, three hundred, eleven patients underwent ECG exercise

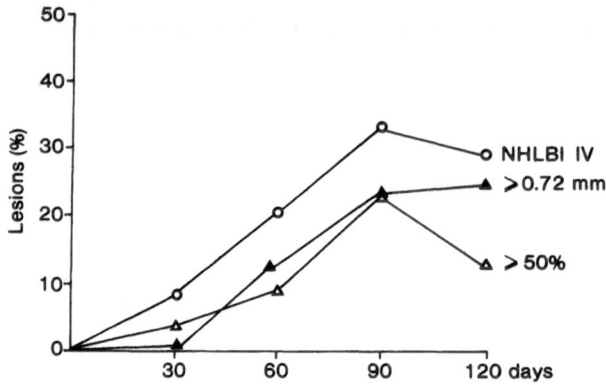

Figure 1. Percentages of lesions that fulfilled the various restenosis criteria at 30, 60, 90 and 120 days [5].

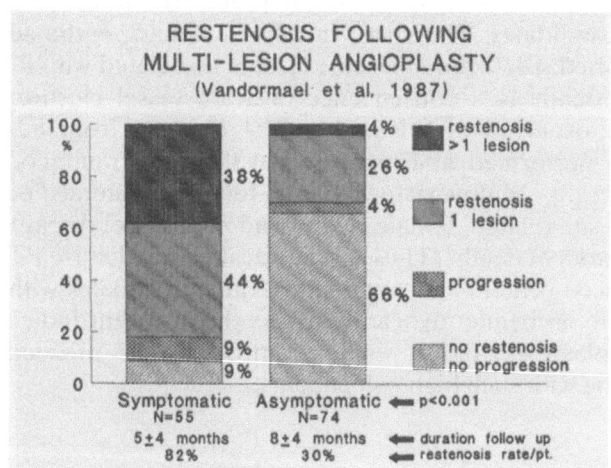

Figure 2. Restenosis following multi-lesion angioplasty, adapted from Vandormael et al. 1987 [6].

Table 3. Restenosis after successful multilesion/multivessel PTCA.

Author	Yr	N PT	FU Angiography (%)	Restenosis PT/ Lesion	F-U MTH (%)
Mata [12]	85	61	97	34/23	6
Roubin [13]	86	411	64	45/38	7
Van Dormael [6]	87	209	62	52/29	7
Myler [14]	87	286	57	32/n.a.	6
Finci [15]	87	85	91	51/31	12

test. Among the patients with single vessel disease, 71% had a negative test as opposed to 60% of patients with multivessel disease. This left 40% in the multivessel group and 29% in the single vessel with positive exercise test. Restenosis, defined as a 50% loss of the initial gain achieved at PTCA was observed in 31% of patients with single vessel disease versus 34% of patients with multiple vessel disease. We have prospectively studied the incidence of restenosis using the four NHLBI and more than 50% diameter criteria, as well as a criteria based upon a decrease of more than .72 mm in luminal lumen diameter [5]. Patients were recatheterized at either 30, 60, 90, and 120 days following successful PTCA. A wide variation in the incidence of restenosis was found dependent upon the criterion applied. But the important point is that the incidence of restenosis proved to be progressive to at least the third or the fourth month (Figure 1). The problem is even more complex in patients with multivessel dilatation. Restenosis rates reported after multilesion and multivessel angioplasty vary from 26 to 50%, with one study reporting a restenosis rate of 68% after multivessel angioplasty (Table 3).

Determination of the restenosis rate after multilesion angioplasty has been recently published by the group of St. Louis [6], (Figure 2). Of 209 patients who underwent successful multilesion angioplasty, 55 symptomatic and 74 asymptomatic patients were restudied at an average of 7 months after dilatation. In this study, restenosis was defined as a diameter stenosis greater than 50%. The restenosis rate was 82% in the symptomatic patients and 30% in the asymptomatic patients. In the symptomatic patients, restenosis occurred at more than one dilatation site in 38% and at one dilatation site in 44% of patients, in 9% of the patients, progression of coronary artery was observed. In the asymptomatic patients, silent restenosis occurred at more than one site in 4% and at one dilatation site in 26% of patients. In other words, 66% of these asymptomatic patients had neither restenosis nor progression of their disease. The likelihood of a restenosis in a patient who undergoes multiple dilatations is greater than that reported after single lesion angioplasty. However, this should not be a deterrent in recommending multilesion coronary angioplasty, because the procedure provides important symptomatic relief to the majority of patients. Furthermore, recurrent narrowings are usually amenable to a second dilatation attempt, if clinically indicated.

At long term, what can we expect from coronary angioplasty?

The Registry data center in Pittsburg has continued the follow-up of the first 1000 patients in whom the PTCA was classified as initially successful. We believe that this original cohort of patients with successful PTCA will remain a good predictor of long-term results in patients who are currently successfully dilated. Figure 3 shows the event and symptom status after a mean follow-up of 4.9 years in the first one-thousand patients who underwent an initially successful PTCA. Looking at the freedom of events, we see that 95% of the patients were alive. Eighty-six percent were alive and had no MI at follow-

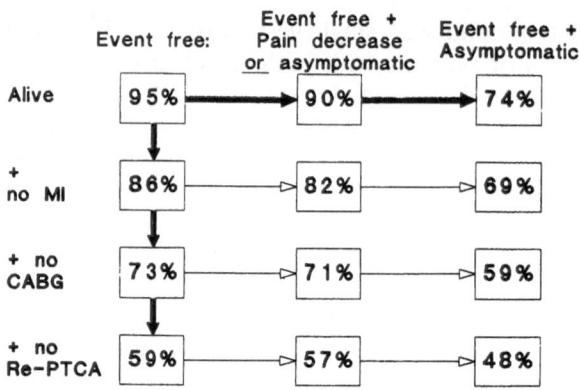

Figure 3. Event and symptom status after a mean follow-up of 4.9 years in the first one thousand patients of the NHLBI registry in whom the PTCA was classified as initially successful.

up. Seventy-three percent were alive and had neither MI nor bypass surgery at follow-up.

Finally, at five years 59% of the patients were free of all events: death, MI, CABG and repeat PTCA. Fifty-seven percent among this one thousand patients were event free, asymptomatic or had their symptoms improved. Fourty-eight percent were event free and asymptomatic. With the adjunction of a second PTCA, 59% were asymptomatic at 5 years. Almost two thirds remain plain free, without having undergone a MI or a coronary bypass surgery. To date the longest reported follow-up concerns the first 133 patients successfully treated by Andreas Grüntzig between September 1977 and October 1980 [7]. These patients have now been followed for five to eight years. In the follow-up period, five of the 133 patients died of cardiac disease that is to say 4% of the population (Table 4). Early recurrence within 6 months was demonstrated in 31%, late recurrence was observed in 5%. –

Table 4. Long-term follow-up (5 to 8 years); the Zurich experience (sept '77–oct '80), (Gruentzig et al. 1987), [7].

	n	%
Primary success	133	100
Death (cardiac)	5	4
Early recurrence (6 mths)	38	31
Late recurrence (2–7 yrs)	5	5
Progression (other vessel)	10	7
re-PTCA	27	20
CABG	19	14
Long-term success (with re PTCA)	98	74
Asymptomatic	89	67

Progression of coronary artery disease occurred in 10 patients, that is to say 7%. Over the mean follow-up period of six years 20% of the patients had a second angioplasty and 14% had bypass grafting for the original lesions. However, the important fact is that 74% of these patients, originally candidates for surgery have been successfully treated without surgery and 67% were asymptomatic at the last follow-up study. It would be difficult to match these patients with a control group in whom medical therapy or coronary bypass surgery was the primary treatment. However, the fact that there were five death from cardiac disease among the 169 original patients followed for six years makes the series at least comparable to other surgically or medically treated series of symptomatic patient with coronary artery disease.

PTCA for unstable angina and multivessel disease: two unsettled issues. Two subsets of patients merit further comment: the first one is characterized by its clinical syndrome: they have unstable angina, the second by its anatomy: they have a multivessel disease.

At the thoraxcenter, we have compared the long term follow-up of patients undergoing PTCA for stable and unstable angina [8]. The median follow-up of these patients was 3.1 years, ranging from 18 months to 7 years. The indication for PTCA was stable angina in 530 pts and unstable in 366 pts. In terms of mortality, there was no significant difference between the two groups, 3.4% versus 5.2%. In the unstable group the incidence of acute non fatal myocardial infarction was significantly higher: 8.3 versus 14.2% and the difference in non fatal myocardial infarction at follow-up was entirely explained by a higher incidence of infarction in the first 24 hrs after PTCA. (The influence of PTCA on the increased risk of non fatal myocardial infarction in unstable AP is difficult to determine, but these figures seem comparable for medical or surgical outcome). At follow-up, an increased rate of CABG was noticed in the unstable group 20.8% versus 14.7%. There was no difference in the need for repeat PTCA in the two groups and 68% of the stable and 61% of the unstable were event free at follow-up.

Relevant clinical, electrocardiographic, angiographic and angioplasty related variables were analysed to identify predictors for unfavorable outcome PTCA for unstable angina:

– Procedure related major complications,
– procedure related myocardial infarct,
– coronary events at one year and
– angiographic restenosis [9].

Multivariate stepwise logistic regression analysis showed that variables with an increased risk for major complication were ST elevation, persistent negative T wave and diameter stenosis ≥65%. Multivessel disease, and total occlusion of coronary events at one year were predictive, whereas ST-segment elevation paradoxically predicted a favorable outcome. As far as restenosis is concerned: presence of angiographically visible collaterals to the dilated vessel, transient ST segment depression during an ischemic attack, multivessel

Table 5. Factors predictive for unfavourable PTCA for unstable angina (De Feyter et al. 1987), [9].

	%
− Procedure related major complication:	
ST-segment elevation odds natio	3.7
persistent negative T-wave	3.7
% stenosis > 65%	3.3
− Procedure related myocardial infarct:	
St-segment elevation	3.3
Persistent negative T-wave	3.3
− Coronary events at 1 year	
ST-segment elevation: *negative*	0.4
Multivessel disease	3.7
Total occlusion	2.8
− Restenosis	
ST depression	2.0
Collaterals	2.2
Multivessel disease	1.9
LAD lesion	1.9

Multivariate logistic regression analysis.

disease, LAD stenosis were predictive of restenosis (Table 5). Thus the initial success rate of PTCA in patients with unstable angina is 90%, but the hazards of dilatation in these patients clearly exceeds that of patients with stable angina. However, after an initially successful procedure the prognosis is excellent with a low death rate and a low rate of myocardial infarction. The angiographic restenosis rate at 6 months hovers around the 30% and therefore appears comparable to those obtained in patients with stable angina.

What about multilesion PTCA?

Geoffrey Hartzler and his group have extended the follow-up period of the first 500 multilesion angioplasty patients treated at the mid America heart institute (personal communication). Successful dilatation was achieved in 92% of the attempted stenoses. The procedural mortality amounts to 1.2% and it should be noted that approximately 17% of these patients did undergo repeat PTCA within the first twelve months following their initial procedure, while 27% underwent re-PTCA at last follow-up. A 97.2% late follow-up was achieved in these patients at a mean time of 37 months. Actuarial survival at one year was 94%, at two years 91%, at three years 90%, and at four years 88%. Freedom of bypass surgery at twelve months, was 89% and, at five years 79%. In other words, 21% of the angioplasty patients required late revascularization because of progression of the disease, restenosis or inadequate initial revascularization.

Table 6. Extent of PTCA revascularization and late outcome in patients with 2 or 3 vessel disease (fu: 12–36 mths), (Van Dormael et al. 1987), [10].

n = 222	2 VD		3 VD	
	CRV	IRV	CRV	IRV
Event free %	71	63	70	55
Angina class > II	18	20	9	18
CABG	8	9	9	9
MI	1	3	9	9
Death	2	5	4	9

Abbreviations: VD = Vessel Disease; CRV = Complete Revascularization; IRV = Incomplete Revascularization [10].

Does the extent of PTCA revascularization influence the late outcome in patients with two or three vessel disease?

Another crucial question remains whether the extent of PTCA revascularization influences late outcome in patients with two and three vessel disease. The group of St. Louis has addressed this question [10]. Twohundred and two patients eligible for one year follow-up were contacted. The average FU was 27 months. A comparison of the cardiac event rate in patients with complete revascularization to those with incomplete revascularization in 2 or 3 VD revealed no significant difference, (71–70% in the patients with 2 and 3 VD and complete revascularization versus 63% and 55% with incomplete revascularization) (Table 6). However, a trend towards an increased risk of MI and death exists in the patients with incomplete revascularization. It is therefore still unclear whether angioplasty should best be limited to patients in whom all proximal severe stenoses are amenable to dilatation, so that revascularization is completed.

From the beginning, Andreas Grüntzig appreciated the difference in outcome between dilatation in single vessel disease and dilatation in multivessel disease [7]. A large number of patients, 71, in his original series had multivessel disease, allowing comparison of patients with multivessel and single vessel disease over a long follow-up period. It must be emphasized that in these patients with multivessel disease the artery considered to be responsible for the patient's symptoms was the only one dilated. Between these 2 groups, there were important differences. The group with multivessel disease had a lower primary success rate, a higher rate of death from cardiac disease, a lower longterm success rate without bypass surgery, a higher percentage of patients with a positive exercise stress test and fewer asymptomatic patients (Table 7). This difference in outcome between patients with single vessel and multivessel disease is not to be overlooked since many centers are accepting more patients with multivessel disease for angioplasty. From the beginning, in

Table 7. Long-term follow-up (5 to 8 years) the Zürich experience (Sept. 77–Oct 80), (Grüntzig et al. 1987), [7].

Patients	SVD 98	MVD 71
Primary success	83%	73%
Death (non cardiac)	3%	8%
Long-term success without CABG in patients with primary success	77%	60%
Positive exercise test	3%	23%
Class I at follow-up	77%	60%

1978 Andreas Grüntzig told us that 'randomized trials were clearly needed if we were to evaluate the efficacy of this new technique as compared with current and surgical treatment' [11]. Now in 1988 he would tell us: 'Patients with single vessel disease treated with angioplasty seem to have passed the test of time; however, patients with the more complex multivessel disease present more difficult problems in the follow-up period. Randomized trials now underway will help to determine the value of angioplasty in patients with multivessel disease'.

References

1. Detre K, Holubkov R, Kelsey S, Cowley M, Kent K, Williams D, Myler R, Faxon D, Holmes D Jr, Bourassa M (1988) Percutaneous transluminal coronary angioplasty in 1985–1986 and 1977–1981. The National Heart, Lung and Blood Institute Registry. *N Engl J Med* 318 (5): 265–270.
2. Ellis SG, Roubin GS, King III SB, Doublas JS Jr, Weintraub WS, Thomas RG, Cox WR (1988) Angiographic and clinical predictors of acute closure after native vessel coronary angioplasty. *Circulation* 77: 372–379.
3. Ellis SG, Roubin GS, King III SB, Douglas JS Jr, Shaw RE, Stertzer SH, Myler RK (1988) In-Hospital Cardiac Mortality After Acute Closure After Coronary Angioplasty: Analysis of Risk Factors from 8,207 Procedures. *J Am Coll Cardiol* 11 (2): 211–216.
4. Bertrand ME, Marco J, Cherrier F, Schmiff R, Gaspard Ph, Puel J, Valeix B, Bory M, Crochet H, Berland R, Machecourt J, Foucault JP, Bassand JP, Bourdonnec CL, Quirck A, Jault F. (1986) French percutaneous transluminal coronary angioplasty (PTCA) registry: Four years experience. *J Am Coll Cardiol* 7 (2): 21A.
5. Serruys PW, Luijten HE, Beatt KJ, Geuskens R, Feyter PJ de, Brand M van den, Reiber JHC, Katen HJ ten, Es GA van, Hugenholtz PG (1988) Incidence of restenosis after successful coronary angioplasty: A time-related phenomenon. *Circulation* 77: 361–371.
6. Vandormael MG, Deligonul U, Kern MJ, Harper M, Presant S, Gibson P, Galan K, Chaitman BR (1987) Multilesion coronary angioplasty: Clinical and angiographic follow-up. *J Am Coll Cardiol* 10 (2): 246–252.
7. Gruentzig AR, King SB, Schlumpf M, Siegenthaler W (1987) Long-term follow-up after percutaneous transluminal coronary angioplasty. The early Zurich experience. *N Engl J Med* 316 (18): 1127–1132.
8. Kamp O, Serruys PW, Feyter PJ de, Brand M van den, Suryapranata H, Domburg R van

(1987) Medium and long term follow-up (F/U) after PTCA for stable and unstable angina (AP). *Eur Heart J* (8) 3: 1029.

9. Feyter PJ de, Suryapranata H, Serruys PW, Beatt K, van Domburg R, Brand M van den, Tijssen JJ, Azar AJ, Hugenholtz PG (1988) Coronary Angioplasty for Unstable Angina: Immediate and Late Results in 200 Consecutive Patients With Identification of Risk Factors for Unfavorable Early and Late Outcome. *J Am Coll Cardiol* 12 (2): 324–333.

10. Deligonul U, Vandormael MG, Kern MJ, Zelman R, Galan K, Chaitman BR (1988) Coronary Angioplasty. A Therapeutic Option for Symptomatic Patients with Two and Three Vessel Coronary Disease. *J Am Coll Cardiol* 11 (6): 1173–1179.

11. Grüntzig AR (1978) Transluminal dilatation of coronary artery stenosis. *Lancet* 1: 263.

12. Mata LA, Bosch X, David PR, Rapold HJ, Corcos T, Bourassa MG (1985) Clinical and Angiographic Assessment 6 Months After Double Vessel Percutaneous Coronary Angioplasty. *J Am Coll Cardiol* 6 (6): 1239–1244.

13. Roubin G, Redd D, Leimgruber P, Abi-Mansour P, Tate J, Gruentzig A (1986) Restenosis after multi-lesion and multi-vessel coronary angioplasty (PTCA). *J Am Coll Cardiol* 7 (2): 22A.

14. Myler, RK, Topol EJ, Shaw RE, Stertzer SH, Clark DA, Fishman J, Murphy MC (1987) Multiple vessel coronary angioplasty: Classification, results, and patterns of restenosis in 494 consecutive patients. *Cathet Cardiovasc Diagn* 13 (1): 1–15.

15. Finci L, Meier B, Bruyne B De, Steffenino G, Divernois J, Rutishauser W (1987) Angiographic Follow-up after multivessel percutaneous transluminal coronary angioplasty. *Am J Cardiol* 60 (7): 467–470.

PART FOUR

Myocardial perfusion

27. Pathophysiology of the coronary circulation
Role of myocardial contrast echocardiography and relation with other techniques

DAVID D. McPHERSON

Introduction

Two-dimensional ultrasound imaging is an excellent means of identifying anatomical cardiac structure and determining myocardial function. However, until recently, cardiovascular ultrasound offered no means of evaluating myocardial perfusion other than assessment of the end result of ischemia and infarction-ie wall motion abnormalities. Two ultrasound techniques are now available for assessing coronary perfusion in vivo: contrast-enhanced echocardiography and Doppler ultrasonic flow devices.

Contrast-enhanced echocardiography consists of vascular injection of an ultrasound contrast agent that results in an altered acoustic appearance of the myocardium being perfused. Ultrasound contrast agents include agitated saline, renograffin, and gelatin or albumin encoated microbubbles. The injectate, number of microbubbles per unit injectate, and source of injection are important variables. Agents now available can be injected peripherally and give ultrasound myocardial signals proportional to bubble concentration. Tissue characterization techniques can identify regional contrast variability in the myocardium and the ultrasonic backscatter may correlate with contrast determined myocardial perfusion. Tissue characterization techniques include pixel brightness, and if the contrast material is not so large that it becomes trapped within the myocardium the T1/2 (contrast decay) within the myocardium. If the contrast decay is prolonged then significant stenosis proximal to the myocardial perfusion field exists. Recent data has shown that although significant baseline regional variation in contrast-enhanced echocardiographic images occurs unrelated to anatomic distribution of the contrast, this variability is attributable to factors intrinsic to the ultrasound imaging techniques and that methods are available to compensate for this variability. As well, risk area measurements demonstrated that risk area measurement by ultrasound contrast techniques is not affected by varying contrast injections, injection rates, or vasodilation. However, peak gray level intensity is variable among contrast agents and may result in variability of time-activity curve analysis. Others have demonstrated that contrast estimated infarct size corre-

S. Iliceto et al. (eds.), Ultrasound in Coronary Artery Disease, 325–349.
© 1991 *Kluwer Academic Publishers.*

lates well with pathologic infarct mass although contrast ultrasound tends to overestimate infarct size. Problems with ultrasound contrast assessment of myocardial perfusion include image blooming, regional gray scale variability, alterations in image information due to depth of field and tissue attenuation.

Other direct methods are available to determine myocardial blood flow. These are nuclear imaging techniques and ultrafast cine tomography. Both techniques are hampered by inability to assess regional blood flow to small areas.

New Doppler ultrasound techniques have been recently developed to measure epicardial coronary arterial velocity and reactive hyperemia. These techniques directly assess flow velocity in epicardial coronary arteries from which regional myocardial perfusion can be extrapolated. They involve the use of 20 MHz doppler ultrasound probes applied to the epicardial coronary arteries using a small suction cup in patients undergoing open heart surgery or intracoronary insertion of coronary doppler flow catheters in the cardiac catheterization laboratory. These probes measure mean coronary velocity in the artery evaluated. A new generation of epicardial probes are being evaluated that can measure absolute coronary flow by integration of the coronary velocity across the arterial lumen. Using doppler flow probes, changes in mean coronary velocity have been shown to closely correlate with changes in coronary flow. A coronary reactive hyperemic response can be demonstrated by the use of transient epicardial coronary arterial occlusion (intraoperatively), or intravenous injection of an arterial vasodilator (catheterization laboratory). The reactive hyperemic response describes the ability of the artery to vasodilate in response to physiologic or pharmacologic vasodilator stimuli. These doppler techniques with reactive hyperemia can be used to identify a physiologically significant coronary stenosis, diffuse coronary atherosclerosis in the presence of minimal luminal irregularities or abnormalities of myocardial perfusion-function relationships including those due to left ventricular hypertrophy.

In summary these exciting new ultrasound techniques can directly (contrast enhanced echocardiography) and indirectly (doppler ultrasound) evaluate regional myocardial blood flow.

The determination of a myocardial perfusion field is most commonly done using coronary arteriography. Coronary arteriography provides information concerning arterial caliber, and indirectly estimates the size of the myocardial perfusion field due to vessel size and distal arborization. As this technique provides little direct information concerning the actual size of a coronary perfusion field, two other techniques were subsequently developed. The first was the use of exercise stress or dipyridamole followed by thallium scanning to visualize the resultant myocardial perfusion defect [1]. The second was the use of an intracoronary injection of radioactive particles at the time of coronary arteriography [2]. These two techniques are hampered by visualization only of ischemic myocardium [1] or the identification of the risk area only at the time of cardiac catheterization and only with a limited number of observations due to available isotopes [2].

Until recently, cardiovascular ultrasound was only able to evaluate the end result of ischemia and infarction-i.e. left ventricular wall motion abnormalities. However, the development of two new ultrasound techniques, myocardial contrast echocardiography [3] and doppler ultrasonic flow devices [4], have allowed clinicians and physiologists to better assess coronary and myocardial perfusion.

This chapter will review our experiences and literature to date concerning both myocardial contrast echocardiography and doppler ultrasonic flow devices and briefly discuss two other methods available to determine myocardial blood flow.

Myocardial contrast echocardiography

This technique consists of injection of ultrasonic contrast agents either intravenous or intraarterially. The resultant acoustic agents (most commonly microbubbles) are strong discrete echo reflectors. They reflect ultrasound proportional to the concentration within the blood stream. The presence of an air-liquid interface in the microbubble creates an altered physical state that results in a large acoustic mismatch. This in turn results in a near perfect reflectant surface. Here the reflected ultrasound energy is near total, with little energy being transmitted and the majority of the sound energy being scattered or reflected. It is this air-liquid interface within the microbubble that permits the marked reflection of echo contrast agents.

With the development of agents that generate high concentrations of microbubbles in the left sided cardiac chambers and the arterial system, the rapid development of myocardial contrast ultrasonic imaging has become possible.

Ultrasound contrast agents

Early work involving ultrasound contrast agents included the use of hand agitated saline and various mixtures of indocyanin green dye/saline mixtures. Reflectivity of ultrasonic contrast agents is due to the concentration of microbubbles and not their actual size. The size of the microbubbles is less than 1/2 the wavelength of sound emitted from standard imaging transducers (approximately 300 microns per 1/2 wavelength in soft tissue using a 2.5 MHz transducer). Therefore, reflectivity of ultrasonic contrast agents is due to the concentrations of microbubbles and not their actual size. New agents were then developed that could generate large numbers of microbubbles. Agents tested included indocyanin green dye/saline mixtures (this caused a reduction of liquid surface tension and an increased generation of microbubbles); lipid emulsions (stabilization of microbubbles) [5] and the use of highly viscous agents such as sodium diatrizoate (Renograffin) [6, 7], dextrose, or sorbitol [7]. Other techniques for increasing the concentration of microbubbles included using gelatin encapsulated microspheres [8–10], albumin microspheres [11–13], or the use of polysaccharide solutions [14–16]. Some researchers even used injectable substances that form gaseous bubbles in vivo as a source of microbubbles for ultrasound contrast visualization; these have included sodium bicarbonate and ascorbic acid that produce carbon dioxide [17]; and dilute hydrogen peroxide to produce oxygen microbubbles [18, 19].

Of all of the possible combinations, two agents have been shown to be relatively stable, potentially providing large concentrations of microbubbles after transpulmonary flow into the coronary circulation and myocardium. These are agitated or sonicated sodium diatrizoate [7] and sonicated albumin microbubbles [7, 11–13, 20]. As Renograffin has a relative short 1/2 life and has well described hemodynamic effects [21] efforts were made to develop new contrast agents that could accurately reflect tissue blood flow without altering tissue dynamics. The agent that seems most appropriate at the present time is sonicated solutions of human albumin. These solutions and their microbubbles are relatively free of hemodynamic side effects and relatively stable, enabling their passage through the pulmonary vascular circulation in quantities sufficient to opacify the left ventricular cavity and subsequently the myocardium.

Protocols and methods for injection of contrast agents

The initial studies for evaluation of myocardial contrast agents required direct aortic root injection or direct intracoronary injection. These techniques were required to achieve sufficient contrast intensity such that perfusion could be demonstrated. Early difficulties arose when trying to demonstrate myocardial contrast after intravenous injection of the contrast agents. After peripheral intravenous injection there are several factors that result in failure of most microbubbles to pass through the pulmonary capillary bed. These include large bubble size that allowed bubbles to be trapped within the pulmonary circulation [22], and altered surface tension of the microbubbles in transpulmonary passage that caused a natural decay of the microbubbles prior to passing into the pulmonary venous circulation [23]. Subsequently newer agents including gelatin-encapsulated microspheres and polysaccharide solutions were identified to produce smaller more stable agents [9, 15, 16]. However the ability of these new agents to cross the pulmonary circulation unaltered has yet to be demonstrated. Other methods included injection of agents into a wedged venous catheter directly into the pulmonary venous circulation, allowing direct passage into the left sided chambers and coronary arteries [24–26]. However, with this technique, the amount of contrast produced is insufficient for myocardial blood flow analysis.

Two agents have been developed that seem to be relatively unaltered after transpulmonary passage. The first is sonicated diatrizoate which produces microbubbles in the range of 10–16 microns [7]. The other is the use of a chilled 5% albumin solution which is sonicated for 40 sec [27]. This produces a supernatent with a mean microbubble size of 2.8 microns and a concentration of 64 million bubbles per cubic centimeter. The foamy layer has a mean microbubble size of 5.8 microns with a concentration of 8 millions bubbles per cubic centimeter. The echo reflectivity (microbubble stability) of the sonicated solution has been demonstrated for up to 48 h. Therefore, myocardial contrast is now possible using injection of intravenous agents that are relatively stable.

Methods to detect ultrasound contrast and relation to myocardial blood flow

The ideal microbubble would be proportional in the myocardium to the blood volume; cause neither vasodilation nor vasoconstriction; and have flow velocity and transit similar to that of red blood cells. Although there are no ideal myocardial contrast agents available, most agents do have flow characteristics that are proportional to that of blood.

There are a number of parameters that can be evaluated when studying the properties of ultrasonic contrast agents in the myocardium. These include the peak intensity of the contrast agent, the change of intensity from base line, the time to peak intensity of the contrast agent, the slope of the initial appearance of the contrast agent, and the disappearance (or wash-out of total area under the curve) of the contrast agent. These parameters are most easily derived using myocardial tissue characterization techniques on digitized video images. These techniques consist primarily of gray level analysis of regions of interest.

With regard to identification of myocardial contrast intensity and flow, there should be a linear relationship between the contrast concentration (i.e. the bubble number) and the image intensity. However all commercially available echocardiographic instructments greatly modify the signal, even at the time of registration of the signal by the transducer. This equipment generated non-linearity of the signal is especially important at higher image intensity levels. The extent of non-linearity between the actual recorded image and the image presented on the screen varies significantly among different equipment types and must be considered when comparing results of myocardial blood flow from different laboratories. A further compounding factor when comparing ultrasound contrast intensity and myocardial blood flow is the position-dependent varibility of gray levels in the scanning sector [28, 29]. As well as the varibility between lateral and axial resolution, regions of the myocardium that lie in the direct anterior/posterior plane to the transducer have much greater backscatter than those oriented more parallel to the beam. This later phenomenon, accentuated by contrast enhancement, results in substantial geometry-dependent variability of the image with and without the contrast. Although this phenomenon may not greatly complicate the determination of risk area, it may be an important factor in determination of image intensity for quantitative flow determination and relation to myocardial blood flow.

With regard to individual agents, Kemper and his colleagues used hydrogen peroxide and found a correlation between the ultrasound contrast intensity of the myocardium and normal myocardial blood flow [30]. Armstrong and co-workers were able to correlate peak image intensity, intensity change, and the slope of the initial appearance of contrast agent (using an injection of agitiated Renograffin and saline into the aortic root) with coronary arterial blood flow determined using electromagnetic flow meters [31]. Wash-out time was of no use in evaluating myocardial blood flow, most likely due to the size of the renograffin microbubbles being greater than red blood cells resulting in a longer wash-out period. These investigators were also able to evaluate hyperemia and demonstrated that the absolute intensity and the shortened time of initial appearance of contrast agents in the myocardium identified the reactive hyperemic response. They found that peak contrast correlated poorly with the hyperemic ratio. If smaller microbubbles are used which pass freely through the coronary circulation, the wash-out half time seems to be proportional to the level of coronary blood flow [32, 33]. With these smaller microbubbles, Ten Cate and others demonstrated that wash-out half time can accurately discriminate between resting or normal flow, hyperemic flow, and flow reduction [32]. These indices seem to be able to detect 30% or greater flow reduction within the myocardium.

Two groups of investigators have evaluated the ability of agents to differentiate between flow in the endocardium and flow the epicardium. Feinstein et al. used sonicated human albumin [34] and Lim et al. renograffin-76 (meglumine diatrizoate) [35]. In a pacing model of left ventricular ischemia, Lim demonstrated that contrast echocardiography could distinguish decreased subendocardial flow compared to epicardial flow.

In summary it can be shown that multiple parameters can be evaluated that have some relation to myocardial blood flow. These parameters include myocardial contrast intensity, peak intensity, slope of initial appearance, washout half-time for total myocardial flow and flow in the epicardium verses the endocardium. Each ultrasonic agent is different and different parameters must be individually evaluated when assessing myocardial blood flow.

Methods to detect ultrasound contrast and relation to risk area

Early work done by investigators at Cedars Sinai Hospital using myocardial contrast echo techniques found that non-perfused myocardial risk areas could be identified and that quantitation of these nonperfused regions was highly reproducible [7]. The methods of analyzing contrast echocardiograms for evaluation of myocardium perfusion and risk area have varied from laboratory to laboratory, with most investigators using standard unmodified ultrasound equipment, and simple planimetery of risk region verses the total myocardial area. Other techniques have included the assessment of the circumferential extent of the perfusion defect (rather than detailed planimetery) [29].

A potential problem in risk area determination research is the site of contrast agent injection. Although for most clinical studies ultrasound contrast is injected proximal to the site of the coronary occlusion, in animal studies the site of agent injection varies and therefore determination of risk area is altered. When ultrasound contrast is injected distal to the coronary arterial occlusion the estimated perfusion area is overestimated than when compared to estimation following injection proximal to the occlusion. This phenomenon is presumed to be due to the presence of collateral flow and secondary to 'blooming' and relatively poor lateral resolution of the echocardiographic equipment [36]. It seems, therefore, that in the experimental setting, if ultrasound agents are to correlate closely with risk area regions, they must be injected proximal to the coronary stenosis.

Armstrong and his group in Indiana evaluated the percent myocardium at risk using contrast echo techniques (by planmetery of the region at risk versus the total myocardial area) and found that there was high intra and inter reproducibility observer variability for one slice correlations between the extent of myocardium identified to be at risk during ultrasound contrast and the anatomic extent of infarction [18]. They found that myocardial contrast imaging techniques using one slice comparisons tended to overestimate small infarct areas and underestimate high infarct areas.

Taylor et al. from the group at the University of Iowa used ultrasound contrast on single slice echocardiograms and compared two methods of regional analysis to autoradiograms of the coronary perfusion field. A circumferential method (tracing the outer ventricular wall boundary including regions which may not have a full contrast effect) showed better correlation with the coronary arterial perfusion field than tracing only those areas that were fully opacified by contrast echocardiography [29]. Taylor felt that this variability was due primarily to regional variability and acoustic shadowing. However they determined that difficulties with using the total circumferential method of tracing the perfusion area would occur in patients who had chronic coronary occlusions and collateralization or in patients with differing endocardial/epicardial anatomic distribution of coronary flow. They concluded that in patients having chronic coronary arterial disease and collateralization, a circumferential method may not be a reproducible estimator of myocardial area at risk. Figure 1 illustrates the tracing method for evaluating myocardial area at risk using either the circumferential technique or the exact measurement technique. Figure 2 illustrates the correlation between angiographic and the two echocardiographic measurement techniques.

Armstrong and co-workers went on to evaluate other methods which may better handle 'acoustic contrast drop out' for measurement of myocardial risk area. They developed digital imaging techniques with digital subtraction of averaged pre and post contrast echocardiograms [37]. Figure 3 illustrates the creation of a digital subtraction image. This image is produced by averaging

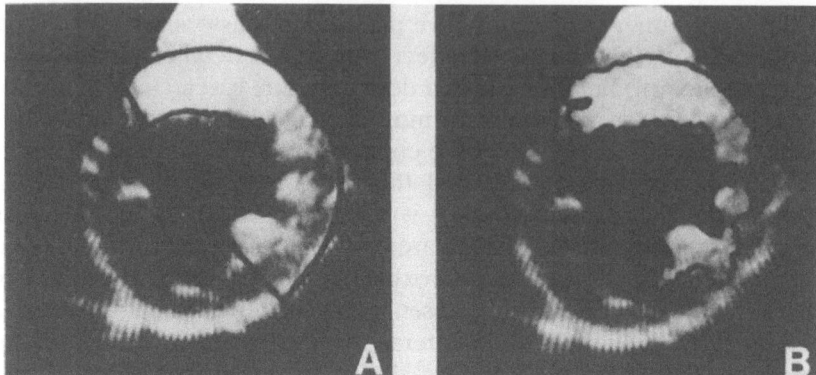

Figure 1. 'Circumferential' *(A)* and 'exact' *(B)* methods of measuring the echocardiographic perfusion bed. The left anterior descending artery perfusion bed is outlined by the criteria of each method. By the circumferential method, there are subepicardial areas that fail to opacify but are nonetheless included in the perfusion bed measurement because subendocardial contrast enhancement is seen. In the exact method the non-enhanced areas are excluded in the measurement of the perfusion bed.

(Reprinted with permission from the American College of Cardiology and Taylor A et al., *J Am Coll Cardiol* 1985, 6: 834.)

three end-diastolic fields. Figure 4 compares the risk region analysis using digital subtraction imaging and contrast echocardiography with the pathologic correlation of infarct size. These investigators found that digital subtraction techniques to evaluate myocardial risk area and subsequent plainmetery of the region at risk versus the total myocardial area correlated well with resultant infarct size for single myocardial slices ($r = 0.97$). Reproducibility

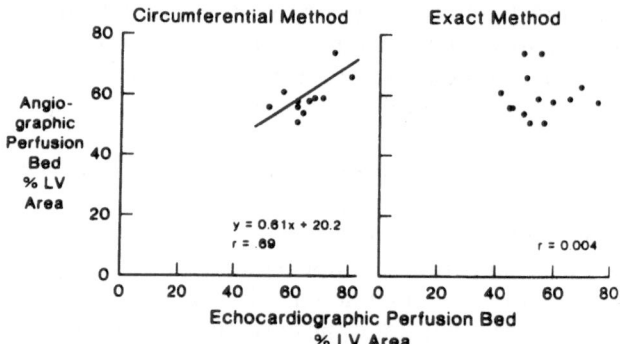

Figure 2. Correlations between angiographic and echocardiographic left anterior descending perfusion bed contrast enhancement measurement methods. There is a significant correlation only between the circumferential echocardiographic measurement method and angiography. LV = left ventricle.

(Reprinted with permission from the American College of Cardiology and Taylor A et al., *J Am Cardiol* 1985, 6: 836.)

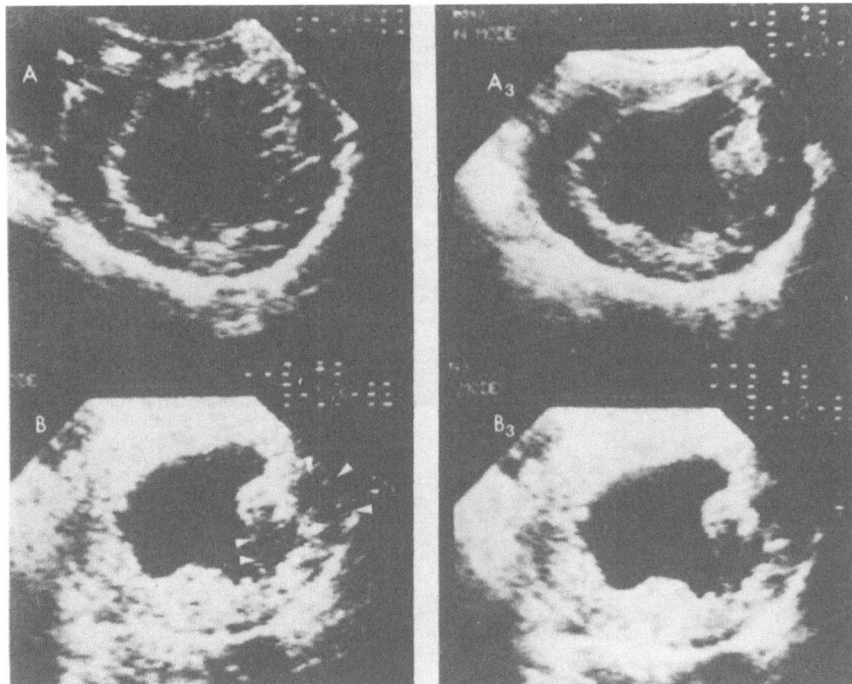

Figure 3. This figure illustrates the creation of a digital subtraction image. *(A)* a single echo-cardiographic field before injection of contrast medium. *(A₃)* the image produced by averaging three end-diastolic frames. *(B)* the post-contrast image showing an ischemic myocardium that is not contrast enhanced (demonstrated by arrowheads). *(B₃)* the image produced by averaging three post-contrast end-diastolic frames. There has been substantial smoothing of the image and the non-perfused area of the myocardium is again apparent.

(Reprinted with permission from the American College of Cardiology and Armstrong A et al., *J Am Coll Cardiol* 1984, 4: 141–148.)

data was very good. This correlation between anatomic and contrast evaluated risk area was better than their previous methods of contrast analysis. For clinical purposes, this technique of digital subtraction estimation of risk area would be applicable to patients including those with chronic coronary arterial disease and coronary collateral formation. Digital processing and subtraction techniques may also allow the use of reduced contrast loads.

Vandenberg and others from Iowa have assessed the effect of micro-bubble size and concentration, injection rate and role of intracoronary vaso-dilation on the determination of myocardial risk area and peak gray level by contrast echocardiography [38]. He evaluated diatrizoate meglumine/ diatrizoate sodium (MD-76), either hand agitated or sonicated, hand agitated MD-76 with saline, and sonicated 70% sorbitol. At a slow intracoronary injection rate of 13cc/sec, the average background-subtracted peak gray level intensity was higher with hand agitated MD-76 than with other agents. How-

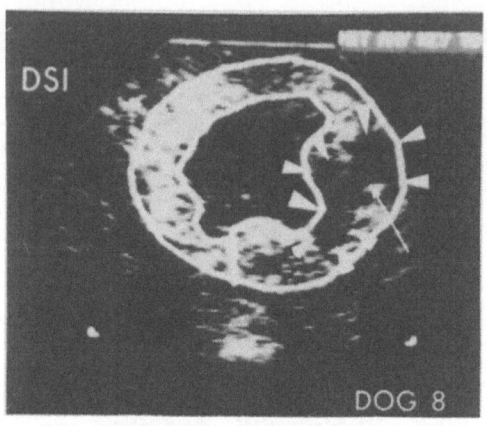

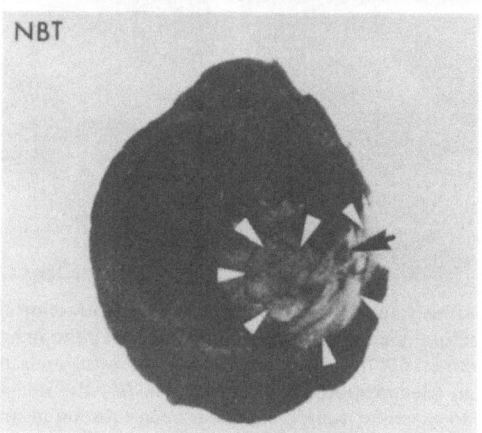

Figure 4. The upper panel illustrates a digital subtraction image (DSR) created by subtracting the averaged pre-contrast image in Figure 3 from the averaged post-contrast image. The epicardial and endocardial borders of the averaged pre-contrast images have been superimposed to assist in the delineation of the non-perfused region. There appears to be an island of perfused myocardium (white area) within the non-perfused region. The lower panel is a photograph of the corresponding anatomic specimen stained with nitroblue tetrazolium (NBT). The pale area with the white arrowheads represents recent myocardial infarction. There is a very good prediction of location and infarct size by digital subtraction contrast echocardiography.

(Reprinted with permission from the American College of Cardiology and Armstrong A et al., *J Am Coll Cardiol* 1984, 4: 141–148.)

ever at higher injection rates, 38cc/sec there were no differences in peak gray level intensity. Perfusion area determination by planimetry was unaffected by the contrast agent used, the injection rate, or by intracoronary administration of adenosine. His conclusions were that risk area measurement by the ultrasound contrast technique was not affected by varying contrast agents, injection rates or vasodilation. However peak gray level intensity was variable among contrast agents and this may result in variability of the time-activity curve analysis.

ECHOCARDIOGRAPHY IN CORONARY ARTERY DISEASE

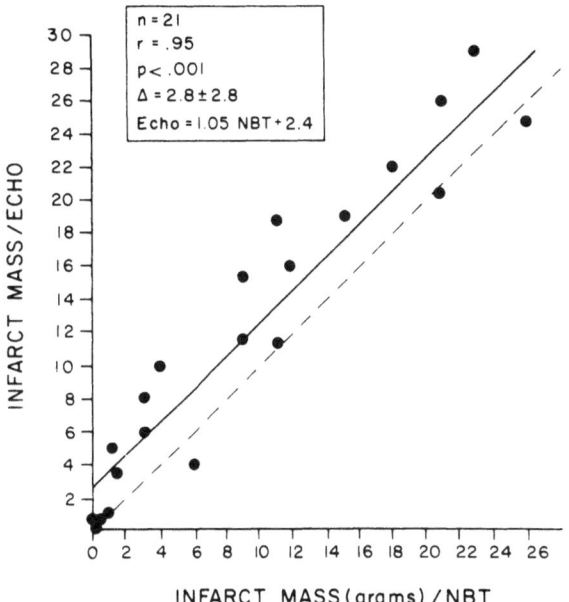

Figure 5. This figure illustrates the comparison of the results obtained between anatomic infarct mass and mass of non-perfused myocardium predicted by contrast echo in closed-chest dogs using digital subtraction techniques on contrast enhanced images.

(Reprinted with permission from Armstrong A et al., 'Assessment of myocardial perfusion,' Chapter 19, in: Kerber RE (ed), *Echocardiography and Coronary Artery Disease.* Futura Publishing Company, Mount Kisco, NY, 1988.)

Numerous studied have demonstrated the ability of contrast echo to predict total myocardial infarct size in a closed-chest model [39–40]. Armstrong and co-workers using digital subtraction techniques on contrast enhanced images evaluated total left ventricular risk area and compared it to the pathologic extent of myocardial infarction as determined by nitroblue tetrazolium staining (Figure 5) [39]. They found an excellent correlation between these two methods. These results have been confirmed by other investigators using similar methods [40, 41]. Kemper and colleagues [41] extended the study of Armstrong to demonstrate that the extent of the contrast deficit during reperfusion correlated with the resultant infarct size present within the region of risk. These studies demonstrate the ability of contrast echo to predict total myocardial infarct size in a closed-chest model.

As well, contrast determined myocardial area at risk demonstrated early after total coronary occlusion has been shown to be a stable marker of the area of non-perfused myocardium in the absence of reperfusion [42].

Although most of the risk area studies have not separated transmural from non-transmural myocardial infarction, Kemper and colleagues specifically addressed this [43]. They found that the delayed appearance of contrast to a risk area or that the non-transmural contrast effect was a marker of non-transmural myocardial infarction.

It seems therefore, that ultrasound contrast demonstrates consistent and good correlations with risk area following infarction and reperfusion, irrespective of the circumferential extent or transmural extent of infarction.

Adverse effects

In addition to the well described toxicities of agents containing sodium diatrizoate (Renograffin) [21] and other viscous radioplaque contrast agents, two major sources of potential toxicities are present in all ultrasound contrast agents. One is associated with the carrier solution, the second is associated with microbubbles themselves that are produced or contained within the solution.

With respect to microbubble size, not only the initial size but coalescence of microbubbles spontaneously increases microbubble size and may cause microbubble obstruction. Microbubble agents range in size from 3+/−2 microns for sonicated albumin [27] to > 50 microns for hydrogen peroxide [44]. Hydrogen peroxide also tends to increase in size over time. Hand agitation produces variably sized microbubbles whereas sonication produces more uniform sized smaller microbubbles.

The hemodynamic and pathological effects of hand agitated Renograffin solutions were investigated by Gillam, Levine [45, 46] in an animal model. They found transient hypotension and increased left ventricular end diastolic pressure as well as reduced myocardial motion during the myocardial contrast effect. This reduced motion was transient and there was no associated tissue damage noted in the myocardium, brain, or kidney at pathologic analysis. They also demonstrated that abnormal wall motion after injection of agitated Renograffin was due to the microbubbles themselves and not to the carrier solution [46].

Sonicated solutions of contrast agents do not however, seem to cause the same abnormalities in ventricular wall motion that hand agitated solutions produce [46, 47]. Sonicated solutions produce smaller, more uniform sized microbubbles than hand agitation produces and this may explain the differing toxicities between the two methods. Using sonicated solutions investigators have demonstrated no major adverse effects on the myocardium [48].

A less harmful effect of ultrasound contrast agents is that to some degree, these agents all produce a hyperemic effect in the coronary circulation and this may complicate the correlation of myocardial perfusion with the myocardial contrast effect.

Although more recent preparations (primarily sonicated human albumin [27, 47, 48] have been shown to produce less toxic effects, these agents cannot be considered totally inert. Immunologic effects of large concentrations of these newer agents also requires evaluation.

Applicability

Animal experimentation
The majority of studies performed to date have determined the accuracy of myocardial contrast echocardiography. These techniques can now be used in the experimental setting as valid methods to identify myocardial risk area and myocardial perfusion. Armstrong et al. have used myocardial contrast echocardiography as a marker of non perfused myocardium in an effort to evaluate the systolic behavior of infarcted myocardium [49]. Others have used risk area techniques to demonstrate the effect of systolic lengthening of an infarct segment and tethering on wall motion analysis [50]; to determine the region of non-perfused myocardium and assess its behavior under varying loading conditions [51]; and to evaluate the behavior of the border zone in an animal model of myocardial infarction [52]. Vasey and co-workers have also examined contrast risk area in an animal model to assess pharmacologic infarct size modification using metoprolol [53].

Experimental models using myocardial contrast coronary arterial perfusion have been slower to develop due to the more complicated methodology required. Feinstein and co-workers have recently shown that sonicated albumin microbubbles possess the appropriate characteristics required to adequately determine coronary perfusion [27]. Sonicated albumin microbubbles cause essentially no reactive hyperemia, no change in the aortic pressure, no change in left ventricular pressure or change in wall thickness. The contrast effect produced by these agent is excellent, and the wash out of the contrast effect is rapid, indicating a physiological transit through the myocardial vasculature. With sonicated human albumin and newer contrast agents we will be able to accurately determine myocardial perfusion during animal experimentation.

Clinical uses
Although myocardial contrast ultrasound techniques are in preliminary phases with respect to visualization of myocardial risk area in patients, some studies have been done demonstrating the efficacy for identification of myocardial perfusion.

The most extensively used methods for evaluating myocardial contrast clinically are that of intracoronary or aortic root injection. Feinstein and colleagues from the University of Chicago have demonstrated the feasibility of intracoronary injection in conjunction with coronary angiography and outlined the distribution of the major coronary arteries [54]. Moore and his colleagues from the University of Virginia have demonstrated the relative safety of myocardial contrast perfusion in conjunction with cardiac catheterization and have demonstrated the perfusion beds of the left and right coronary arteries [55]. In a study of normal patients they evaluated the effect of sonicated Renograffin on left ventricular hemodynamics and electrocardiographic abnormalities and found that abnormalities with sonicated Renograffin were no different than derangements found following the injection of the carrier solution alone (nonagitated Renograffin). Armstrong has been able to demonstrate in patients undergoing cardiac catheterization that intracoronary contrast injection easily demonstrates perfusion defects associated with coronary arterial obstructions and that these defects are similar to that demonstrated in animal experiments [56].

Of great interest is the assessment of regional myocardial blood flow before and after interventions designed to relieve coronary obstructions (angioplasty and thrombolysis). Both the investigators at the University of Chicago and those at the University of Indiana used myocardial contrast echocardiography and demonstrated serial changes in contrast appearance before and after balloon dilation of the coronary artery [57, 58]. Mindich and Goldman have used this technique at the time of coronary artery bypass surgery and feel that echocardiography may be a means of identifying the most significant coronary occlusions at operation prior to cardiac bypass [59].

In summary ultrasound contrast of the myocardium seems to have similar applications in the clinical arena as in the animal lab, that of identifying myocardial risk area and identifying changes in myocardial perfusion.

Future applications

The most exciting development in contrast evaluation of myocardial perfusion will be the generation of appropriate microbubbles which will cross the transpulmonary circulation relatively unaltered and can be detected within the myocardium. With sonicated human albumin its seems possible that this goal will be achieved.

Once we can demonstrate that ultrasound contrast is an effective technique for assessing myocardial perfusion, then online evaluation of myocardial perfusion in myocardial ischemia, infarction and in procedures which tend to increase myocardial perfusion (angioplasty and thrombolysis) will become possible. Ultrasonic myocardial contrast determination is a well documented technique for quantitation of nonperfused myocardium in the experimental laboratory and is now starting to show potential for general clinical use.

Other techniques for evaluation of myocardial perfusion

Radioactive tracers have been used for some time to assess myocardial perfusion. The most commonly used tracer, thallium, with exercise stress or stress following the injection of dipyridamole can give a relative estimation of variable perfusion to one area of the myocardium verses another. The sensitivity and specificity of thallium stress testing has been recently reported to be lower than previously thought. Specificity is reported to be 60–70% in symptomatic patients [60, 61] and in symptomatic patients with coronary disease specificity is 50–60% and sensitivity is 70–80% [62]. In addition to a reasonably low sensitivity and specificity for detecting ischemic coronary disease, localization of involved vessels is poor with thallium imaging. Single photon emission computed tomography is better at localizing the involved artery but both thallium and single photon emission computed tomography cannot quantitate the severity of a coronary stenosis. Both these techniques suffer from decreased radionuclide uptake during maximal perfusion and therefore do not accurately represent maximal regional blood flow.

Positron emission tomography (PET) is a radionuclide technique using a radioactive tracer (such as ^{13}N) to visualize perfusion and subsequent washout of the tracer in a perfusion field. This technique reconstructs the cardiac silhouette in multiple sections and allows better quantitation of regions of normal and abnormal flow in the myocardium. With the use of exercise and/or dipyridamole stress, PET can identify areas of decreased perfusion, ischemia, and collateral flow. PET by being similar to other nuclear imaging techniques is limited by falling extraction of the radiotracer at high flows. However the sensitivity and specificity of PET for determining ischemic disease is high and Gould and others feel that PET is the best noninvasive method for identifying and assessing the severity of coronary arterial stenosis [63].

Another non ultrasound technique for evaluating regional myocardial perfusion is ultrafast computerized tomography (cine CT). Using this technique, tomographic images of the myocardium are obtained that have a resolution of 0.7 to 2.0 mm in the X-Y plane and 3.0 to 10.0 mm in the Z plane [64]. Temporal resolution of this imaging modality is 17 frames per sec. in the cine mode and image density resolution permits separation of approximately 2,000 gray levels. This technique has the potential to evaluate regional myocardial perfusion. Rumberger and others in an animal model evaluated cine CT and found that regional flow and changes of flow reserve could be evaluated [65]. The correlation between CT measurements of perfusion with radio-labelled microspheres showed a modest correlation ($r = 0.70$). At least three problems were evident in this approach to accurately estimating myocardial perfusion from cine CT image data. First, if the contrast agent was injected intravenously, the contrast density in the cardiac chambers far exceeds the density of the contrast in the left ventricular wall. The intense contrast in the cardiac chambers causes beam hardening and scatter, and subsequently distorts contrast clearance curves obtained from the left ventricular wall. A second problem is that coronary transit time in animal preparations is much shorter than previously assumed and the width of the bolus injection is generally longer than coronary transit time. This problem confounds approaches to measuring myocardial perfusion using classical indicator dilution principles. The third problem is that when intense pharmacologic coronary dilation is performed, the vascular volume of the vessels that perfuse the left ventricular wall increase substantially. This increase in vascular volume alters the total contrast density in the left ventricular wall and distorts the contrast clearance curves. It is difficult to carefully account for all three factors and each one can seriously impair the accuracy of measurements of myocardial perfusion using cine CT image data. Wang and others from the Mayo recently presented preliminary data identifying a new algorithm that tries to deal with each of these three confounding factors [66]. They feel that this new algorithm may allow accurate evaluation of regional myocardial perfusion using cine CT image data.

Therefore these new non ultrasound imaging modalities, that of PET scanning and that of cine CT imaging may in the future allow precise calculation of regional myocardial perfusion. At the present time technical problems prevent them from being routinely employed in the clinical arena.

Doppler flow probes for functional assessment of regional myocardial perfusion

The physiological assessment of myocardial blood flow has clinical importance. Specifically this is the functional ability of coronary arteries to increase blood supply during physiologic stress. Contrast ultrasound techniques, positron emission tomography and cine CT can all to some degree assess changes in regional coronary flow however these techniques evaluate flow to the myocardium only and do not directly assess coronary arterial blood flow.

The concept of coronary flow reserve was first proposed by Gould fifteen years ago and has developed into an accepted descripter of stenosis severity [67]. Flow reserve evaluates the change between resting and maximal coronary flow and therefore identifies the ability to increase myocardial perfusion under stress. Although noninvasive perfusion imaging was initially used to evaluate coronary flow reserve, newer and more effective doppler flow probes have now become available to evaluate coronary arterial perfusion and changes in perfusion [4]. These doppler flow probes can be used during cardiac surgery intraoperatively, or intravascularly in the cardiac catheterization laboratory. Figure 6 is an illustration and a schematic of the suction doppler flow probe for intraoperative evaluation of physiologic coronary arterial flow. Figure 7 is an illustration and schematic of the intracoronary doppler flow probe for arterial flow determination at the time of cardiac catheterization.

Doppler methods for assessment of the physiologic significance of coronary atherosclerosis

Both the intraoperative and the intracoronary techniques utilize similar principles for measurement of coronary arterial flow. Both instruments have 20 MHz side mounted ultrasonic crystals. These crystals are placed at a 45° angle with respect to the blood flow and measure mean flow velocity in the artery evaluated. Both techniques utilize physiologic or pharmacologic stress to assess the ability of the artery to increase flow in response to ischemia. In

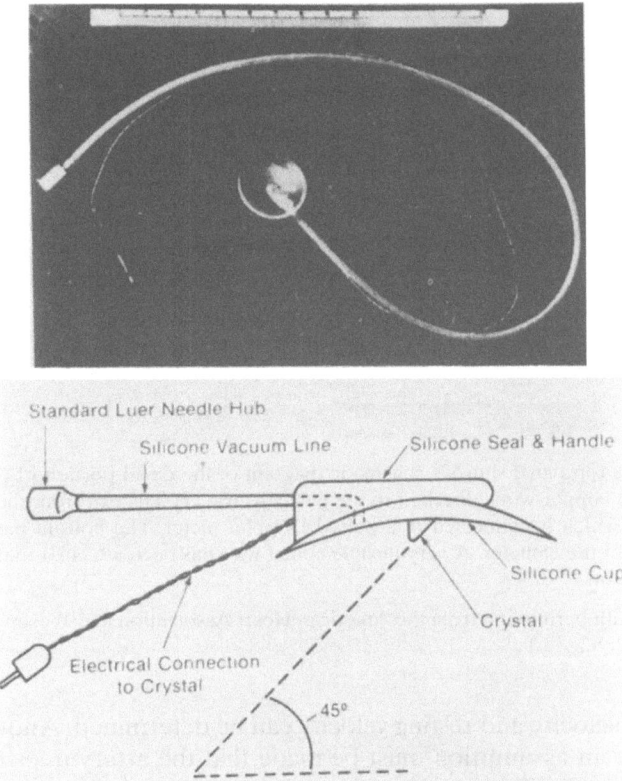

Figure 6. The top panel illustrates the suction Doppler probe utilized to perform intraoperative studies. The bottom panel shows a diagram of the critical components of the suction doppler probe.

(Reprinted with permission from Marcus ML, *Methods of measuring coronary blood flow,* Chapter 2, in: *The Coronary Circulation in Health and Disease.* McGraw-Hill, New York, 1983, 25–62.)

the operating room the probe is attached to a suction tip which is placed directly over the epicardial coronary artery to be evaluated [4]. This probe requires no traumatic dissection for accurate measurements of flow velocity. Changes in flow velocity have been shown to correlate with changes in volume flow. An adequate reactive hyperemic response occurs following 20 sec of transient coronary arterial occlusion and this correlates with maximum vasodilation and flow increase (Figure 8). With this transient coronary arterial occlusion, control and maximum blood flow (the reactive hyperemic response) can safely be determined in individual coronary arteries. Marcus and others have shown that sex and age do not interfere with the quantitative characteristics of the coronary reactive hyperemic response [68]. A disadvantage of doppler flow assessment is that mean velocity rather than absolute coronary flow is measured and therefore only relative changes between

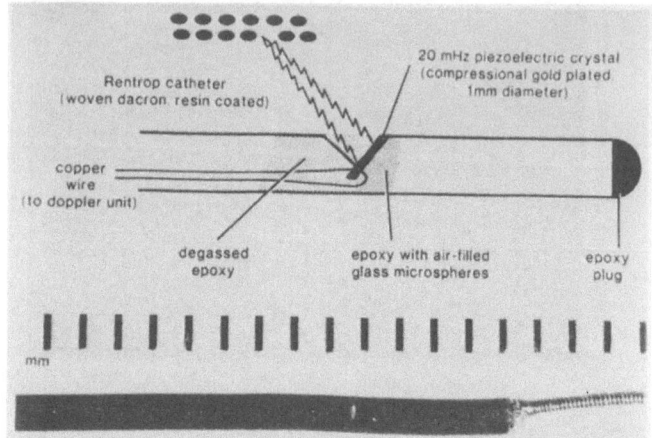

Figure 7. The top panel shows a schematic diagram of the distal portion of coronary Doppler catheter. The copper wires attached to the piezoelectric crystals exit from the proximal end of the catheter which is connected to a pulsed Doppler meter. The bottom panel illustrates the distal 3 CM of the catheter. A very flexible coiled wire has been attached to the tip to enhance safety in humans.

(Reprinted with permission from the American Heart Association and Wilson RF et al. *Circulation* 1985, 72: 82–92.)

maximum velocity and resting velocity can be determined. Another disadvantage is that an assumption must be made that the artery does not change its shape or size significantly throughout the reactive hyperemic response and in animal studies this has been shown to be true [69].

In the cardiac catheterization laboratory, intracoronary doppler flow probes utilize similar principles [70]. These flow probes are directly placed into the coronary arterial bed at the time of catheterization. Resting velocity

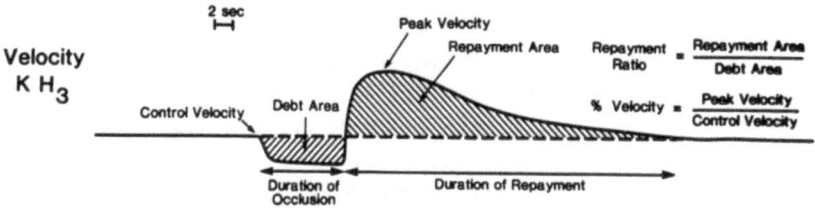

Figure 8. This figure illustrates diagrammatically the intraoperative assessment of the reactive hyperemic response using the coronary doppler suction flow probe. After control velocity has been determined a transient coronary occlusion is imposed. After release of the occlusion coronary flow velocity rises to a peak and subsequently returns to normal. The ratio of peak to resting velocity indicates the reactive hyperemic response (see text for the details).

(Reprinted with permission from Marcus ML, *Metabolic regulation of coronary blood flow*, Chapter 3, in: *'The Coronary Circulation in Health and Disease'.* McGraw-Hill, New York, 1983, 65–92.)

measurements are then obtained. Subsequently, vasodilators consisting of Renograffin (meglumine diatrizoate), dipyridamole, or papavarine are given. Changes in velocity after maximum vasodilation correspond to changes in flow. Papavarine and dipyridamole have been shown to cause maximum changes in subselective assessment of coronary vasodilator reserve. Disadvantages of the intracoronary doppler flow probe are primarily that the maximal stimulus to vasodilation that is present in the operating room (i.e. transient ischemia) is not present in the cardiac catheterization laboratory. Therefore peak to resting velocity ratios (the reactive hyperemic response) are lower using the intracoronary doppler flow catheter than using the intraoperative doppler flow probe.

Peak to resting flow ratios can also be influenced by situations which increase coronary flow (severe anemia, coronary collaterals supplying the artery being interrogated, increases in myocardial oxygen consumption secondary to hypertension, tachycardia) or situations which decrease coronary flow (severe polycythemia, marked hypothermia, decreased arterial perfusion pressure, significant ventricular hypertrophy or infarction in the perfusion field being studied). However in the vast majority of patients the peak to resting velocity ratio either intraoperatively or at the time of cardiac catheterization can be used as an accurate indicator of the physiologic ability of the artery to increase flow to meet demands.

Doppler coronary flow studies assessing the physiologic significance of coronary disease

Using the intraoperative coronary doppler device with transient coronary arterial occlusion, Marcus and others studied the relationship between visual estimates of percent diameter stenosis from the coronary angiogram and the coronary vasodilator capability [71]. Figure 9 illustrates their results. Patients with normal arteries had normal coronary dilator responses; patients with very severe coronary obstruction (>90% diameter coronary stenosis) had severely depressed coronary dilator responses; however patients with percent stenosis between 10% and 90% had extremely variable coronary dilator responses in individual arteries. Their conclusions were that these data strongly support the concept that percent stenosis is not a clinically useful approach to predicting the physiologic significance of a coronary obstruction. As percent stenosis was felt to be a poor indicator of the severity of coronary arterial lesions, a second study comparing percent area stenosis measured using quantitative coronary angiography to coronary vasodilator reserve assessment using doppler reactive hyperemia was undertaken [72]. These investigators again found that there was a very poor relationship between percent coronary area stenosis and physiologic coronary vasodilator reserve.

As the residual lumen area does not take into account variability of coronary atherosclerosis and wall thickening, we undertook a study to compare the physiologic reactive hyperemic response with measurements of coronary

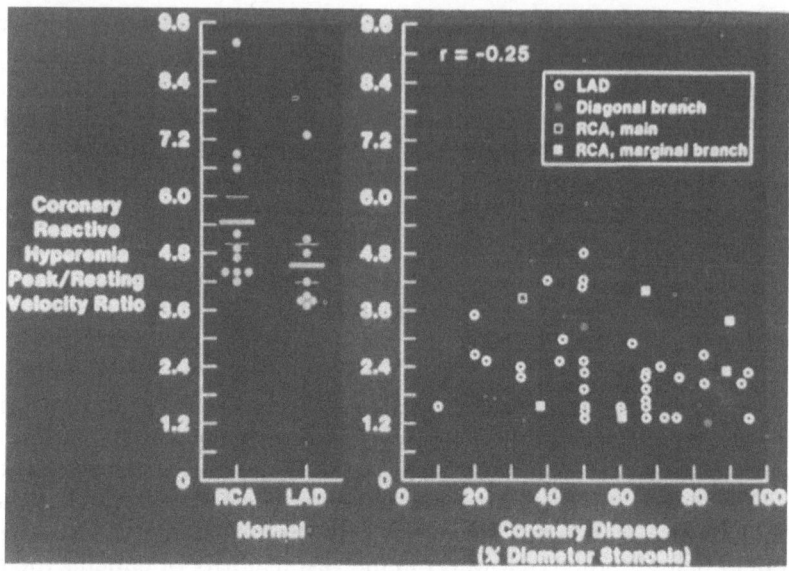

Figure 9. This figure illustrates the coronary reactive hyperemic responses in patients with angiographically normal coronary arteries perfusing a normal ventricle *(left panel)* and angiographically diseased coronary arteries perfusing a normal ventricle *(right panel)*. Peak to resting velocity ratio was measured following a 20 sec coronary occlusion. These studies were performed at the time of open heart surgery prior to insertion of cardiopulmonary bypass. The peak to resting velocity ratio was greater than 3.6 in all normal arteries studied. In patients with coronary obstructive lesions there was a very poor relationship between the percent diameter stenosis and the reactive hyperemic response. LAD = left anterior descending coronary artery. RCA = right coronary artery.

(Reprinted with permission the New England Journal and from CW White et al., *N Engl J Med* 1984, 310: 819–824.)

arterial wall and lumen using high frequency epicardial echocardiography probes at the time of cardiac surgery [73]. Figure 10 illustrates our results. There was a poor correlation between percent residual luminal area with reactive hyperemia. There was a better correlation between luminal diameter/ wall thickness ratios with the reactive hyperemic response. These data indicate that another factor which may be a major determinant of the physiologic vasodilator ability of the coronary artery is the extent of atherosclerosis within the arterial bed.

Using the intracoronary doppler flow catheter, Wilson and others demonstrated that dipyridamole infusion provides an adequate vasodilator response and should be able to predict the functional significance of atherosclerosis at the time of cardiac catheterization [10]. Their group performed other studies including the effect of coronary angioplasty on coronary flow reserve at the time of cardiac catheterization [74]. They demonstrated that in 1/2 of the patients there was a transient reduction in coronary flow reserve immediately after angioplasty. This reduction later normalizes. Their conclusions were that

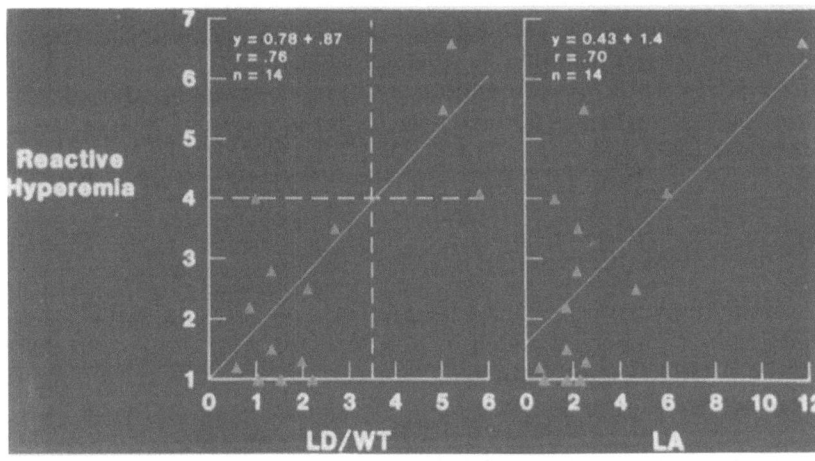

Figure 10. This figure illustrates our data comparing the doppler reactive hyperemic response and lesion characteristics assessed by high frequency epicardial echocardiography in patients with coronary arterial disease. The left panel compares the luminal diameter/wall thickness ratios at the site of a coronary lesion to the reactive hyperemic response. The right panel compares minimal luminal area at the site of the lesion to the reactive hyperemic response. Note that the correlation is better when wall thickness is taken into account (Reference 73).

coronary flow reserve measurement immediately after angioplasty may not reflect the eventual success of the procedure to relieve the physiologic obstruction to coronary flow.

Doppler assessment of coronary reactive hyperemia is very useful in many circumstances. Patients who have minimal luminal irregularities but may have significant functional coronary arterial disease can be identified using this technique. In addition patients who have left ventricular hypertrophy with minimal lesions may have very little vasodilator response and small alterations in coronary flow reserve due to atherosclerosis may cause profound effects on the ability of the perfusion bed to achieve adequate blood supply during periods of stress. Although limitations have been cited, the reactive hyperemic techniques as they presently exist can provide physiologic assessment of myocardial perfusion in many patients.

Future applications of vascular doppler techniques

New doppler flow measuring devices are being developed. These devices evaluate doppler velocity over multiple gates across the coronary arterial lumen. The integration of this velocity gives an absolute measure of coronary blood flow. This may allow, intraoperatively or at the time of cardiac catheterization, absolute blood flow measurements in the coronary arteries. The doppler assessment of coronary flow in addition to evaluating the vasodilator and functional ability of the vascular bed to increase flow, will allow the determination of benefits derived from techniques used to increase myocardial perfusion (thrombolytic therapy, angioplasty etc.). In addition to providing clinically useful information, these techniques can be used to validate other indirect methods of myocardial perfusion (nuclear angiographic techniques, cine CT, PET, myocardial contrast echocardiography) for accurate assessment of coronary flow.

Summary

The evaluation of myocardial blood flow is an important field in cardiac diagnosis. It is important to identify non perfused areas of myocardium which would indicate recent or chronic infarction, and to identify the ability of areas of the myocardium to increase flow in response to stress (ischemia). Myocardial contrast echocardiography is a technique that has been developed to specifically evaluate myocardial perfusion. At the present time sonicated human albumin remains the agent of choice for adequate visualization of myocardial perfusion. Soon this agent will be available for routine use. No complicated image processing techniques are required to determine areas of no flow. Simple and more complicated image processing techniques will be required to determine areas of decreased perfusion. The ability of the myocardium to increase flow to areas under stress will require even more complicated image processing modalities. In all, myocardial contrast echocardiography remains a technique that has some immediate clinical use. With the development of simple and complicated image processing techniques contrast echocardiography may gain more widespread use for evaluating regional myocardial perfusion.

At present the addition of intracoronary doppler flow devices and epicardial coronary doppler flow devices gives us the ability to assess changes in myocardial perfusion. This includes the physiologic ability of the distal vascular bed to increase blood flow under stress. These doppler techniques combined with regional wall motion analysis or analysis of myocardial perfusion with contrast echocardiography give important clinical and pathophysiologic information. They are important clinical tools which all clinical echocardiographers should be familiar.

References

1. Bergen HJ, Zaret BL (1981) Nuclear cardiology. *N Engl J Med* 305: 799–807.
2. Adelstein SJ, Maseri A (1977) Radioindicators for the study of the heart: Principles and applications. *Prog Cardiovascular Dis* 20: 3–17.
3. Kaul S, Pandian NG, Okade RD, Pohost GM, Weyman AE (1984) Contrast echocardiography in acute myocardial ischemia. I. In vivo determination of total left ventricular 'area at risk'. *J Am Coll Cardiol* 4: 1272–1282.
4. Marcus M, Wright C, Doty D, Eastham C, Laughlin D, Krumm P, Fastenau C, Brody M (1981) easurements of coronary velocity and reactive hyperemia in the coronary circulation of humans. *Circ Res* 49: 877–891.

5. Valdes-Cruz LM, Sahn DJ, Horowitz S, Mesel E, Fischer DC, Banner W, Vargas Barron J, Golberg SJ, Allen HD (1982) Left ventricular opacification by intravenous injection of safe echo contrast agents: Comparative studies in animals and initial human trails. *Circulation* 66: II–28.

6. Tei C, Sakanaki I, Shah PM, Meerbaum S, Shimoura K, Kondo S, Corday E (1983) Myocardial contrast echocardiography: A reproducible technique of myocardial opacification for identifying regional perfusion deficits. *Circulation* 67: 585–593.

7. Feinstein SB, Ten Cate FJ, Zwehl W, Ongk, Maurer G, Tei C, Shah PM, Meerbaum S, Corday E (1984) Two-dimensional contrast echocardiography. I. In vitro development and quantitative analysis of echo contrast agents. *J Am Coll Cardiol* 3: 14–20.

8. Carroll BA, Turner RJ, Tickner EG, Boyle D, Young S (1980) Gelatin encapsulated microbubbles as ultrasonic contrast agents. *Invest Radiol* 15: 260–266.

9. Meltzer RS, Klig V, Teichholtz LE (1985) Generating precision microbubbles for use as an echocardiographic contrast agent. *J Am Coll Cardiol* 5: 978–982.

10. Armstrong WF, Mueller TM, Kinney EL, Tickner EG, Dillon JC, Feigenbaum H (1982) Assessment of myocardial perfusion abnormalities with contrast-enhanced two-dimensional echocardiography. *Circulation* 66: 166–173.

11. Bommer WJ, Mason DT, DeMaria AN (1979) Studies in contrast echocardiography: Development of new agents with superior reproducibility and transmission through lungs. *Circulation* 60: II–17.

12. Feinstein SB, Keller MW, Dick CD, Keller MW, Dick C, Bridenshine TR, Wissler R (1987) Successful transpulmonary contrast echocardiography in monkeys. *J Am Coll Cardiol* 9: 111 A.

13. Keller MW, Feinstein SB (1986) Successful transpulmonary Contrast echocardiography for quantitation of myocardial perfusion. *Clin Res* 313A.

14. Schartl M, Fritzsch Th, Friedmann W, Lange L (1984) Quantitative myocardial perfusion studies with a new safe echo contrast agent. *J Am Coll Cardiol* 3: 563.

15. Smith MD, Kwan OL, Reiser HJ DeMaria AN (1984) Superior intensity and reproducibility of SHU-454, a new right heart contrast agent. *J Am Coll Cardiol* 3: 992–998.

16. Smith M, Kwan OL, Nissen S, Elion J, Rovai D, DeMaria A (1985) Left heart opacification after peripheral venous injection pulmonary transmission of ZK 44012, a new echo contrast agent. *Circulation* 72: III–57.

17. Jiang L, Pu Sy, Yang MZ, Chen HZ (1984) Left heart contrast echocardiography using a carbon dioxide producing agent. *Circulation* 70: II–5.

18. Armstrong WF, West SR, Mueller TM, Dillon JC, Feigenbaum H (1983) Assessment of location and size of myocardial infarction with contrast-enchanced echocardiography. *J Am Coll Cardiol* 2: 63–69.

19. Kemper AJ, O'Boyle JE, Sharma S, Cohen CA, Kloner RA, Kituri S, Parisi A (1983) Hydrogen peroxide contrast-enchanced two-dimensional echocardiography real-time in vivo delineation of regional myocardial perfusion. *Circulation* 68: 603–611.

20. Keller MW, Feinstein SB, Briller RA (1986) Automated production and analysis of echo contrast agents. *J Ultrasound Med* 5: 493.

21. Friesinger GC, Schaffer J, Criley JM, Gaertner RA, Ross RS (1965) Hemodynamic consequences of the injection of radioplaque material. *Circulation* 31: 730–740.

22. Feinstein SB, Shah PM, Bing RH, Meerbaum S, Corday E, Bing-Lo C, Santillano G, Fujibayashi Y (1984) Microbubble dynamics visualized in the intact pulmonary capillary circulation. *J Am Coll Cardiol* 3: 595–600.

23. Meltzer RS, Tickner EG, Popp RL (1980) Why do the lungs clear ultrasonic contrast? *Ultrasound Med Biol* 6: 263–269.

24. Meltzer RS, Serruys PW, McGhie J, Verbaan N, Roelandt J (1980) Pulmonary wedge injection yielding left sided echocardiographic contrast. *Br Heart J* 44: 390–394.

25. Ten Cate FJ, Feinstein J, Zwehl W, Meerbaum S, Fishbein M, Shah PM, Corday E (1984) Two-dimensional Contrast echocardiography. I Transpulmonary Studies. *J Am Coll Cardiol* 3: 21–27.

26. Xin Fang W, Jia-en W, Lin-Shen C et al. (1985) Left-sided heart contrast echocardiography by pulmonary wedge injection of hydrogen peroxide. *Chin Med J* 98: 121.

27. Keller MW, Feinstein SB (1988) New developments in contrast echocardiography, in: Kerber RE (ed), *Echocardiography in Coronary Artery Disease*, Chapter 20. Futura Publishing, Mount Kisco, NY.

28. Zwehl W, Areeda J, Schwartz G, Feinstein S, Ong K, Meerbaum S (1984) Physical factors influencing quantitation of two-dimensional contrast echo amplitudes. *J Am Coll Cardiol* 4: 157–164.

29. Taylor A, Collins SM, Skorton DJ, Keiso RA, Melton J, Kerber RE (1985) Artifactual regional gray level variability in contrast enhanced two-dimensional echocardiographic images: Effect on measurement of the coronary perfusion bed. *J Am Coll Cardiol* 6: 831–838.

30. Kemper AJ, Force T, Kloner R, Gilfoil M, Perkins L, Hale S, Aiker K, Parisi AF (1985) Contrast echocardiographic estimation of regional myocardial blood flow after acute coronary occlusion. *Circulation* 72: 1115–1124.

31. Gage S, Vasey G, Dillen JC, Feigenbaum H (1980) Reactive hyperemia: Evaluation with myocardial contrast echocardiography. *J Am Coll Cardiol* 7: 189A.

32. Ten Cate FJ, Drury JK, Meerbaum S, Noordsy J, Feinstein S, Shah PM, Corday E (1984) Myocardial contrast two-dimensional echocardiography: Experimental examination at different coronary flow levels. *J Am Coll Cardiol* 3: 1219–1226.

33. Tei C, Kondo S, Meerbaum S, Ong K, Maurer G, Wood F, Kamaki TS, Shimaura K, Corday E, Shah PM (1984) Correlation of myocardial echo contrast disappearance rate ('washout') and severity of experimental coronary stenosis. *J Am Coll Cardiol* 3: 39–46.

34. Feinstein SB, Lang R, Geiser E, Powsner S, Neuman A, Borrow KM (1986) A new method for real time assessment of regional myocardial perfusion. *J Am Coll Cardiol* 7: 189A.

35. Lim Y-J, Nanto S, Masuyama T, Kodama K,Ikeda T, Kitabatake A, Kamadi T (1989) Visualization of subedocardial myocardial ischemia with myocardial contrast echocardiography in humans. *Circulation* 79: 233–244.

36. Kaul S, Gillam LD, Weyman AE (1985) Contrast echocardiography in acute myocardial ischemia. II. The effect of site of injection of contrast agent on the estimation of area at risk for necrosis after coronary occlusion. *J Am Coll Cardiol* 6: 825–830.

37. Armstrong WF, West SR, Dillon JC, Feigenbaum H (1984) Assessment of location and size of myocardial infarction with contrast enhanced echocardiography. II Application of digital imaging techniques. *J Am Coll Cardiol* 4: 141–148.

38. Vandenberg BF, Feinstein SB, Kieso RA, Hunt M, Kerber RE (1988) Myocardial risk area and peak gray level measurement by contrast echocardiography: Effect of microbubble size and concentration, injection rate, and coronary vasodilation. *Am H Journal* 115: 733–739.

39. Armstrong WF, West SR, Dillon JC, Feigenbaum H (1984) Digital subtraction contrast echocardiography for quantification of myocardial infarction size. *Clin Res* 32: 149A.

40. Sakamaki T, Tei C, Meerbaum S, Shimaura K, Kondo S, Fishbein MC, Y-Rit J, Shah PM, Corday E (1984) Verification of myocardial contrast two-dimensional echocardiographic assessment of perfusion defects in ischemic myocardium. *J Am Coll Cardiol* 3: 34–38.

41. Kemper AJ, O'Boyle JE, Sharma S, Cohen CA, Kloner RA, Khuri SF, Parisi AF (1983) Hydrogen Peroxide contrast-enhanced two-dimensional echocardiography: Real-time in vivo delineation of regional myocardial perfusion. *Circulation* 68: 603–611.

42. West SR, Armstrong WF, Dillon JC, Feigenbaum H (1985) Digital subtraction contrast echocardiography: Superior prediction of infarct size than wall motion analysis. *J Am Coll Cardiol* 5: 475.

43. Kemper AJ, Force T, Perkins L, Gilfoil M, Parisi AF (1986) In vivo prediction of the transmural extent of experimental acute myocardial infarction using contrast echocardiography. *J Am Coll Cardiol* 8: 143–149.

44. Kemper AJ, O'Boyle JE, Cohen CA, Taylor A, Parisi AF (1984) Hydrogen peroxide contrast echocardiography: Quantification in vivo of myocardial risk area during coronary

occlusion and of the necrotic area remaining after myocardial reperfusion. *Circulation* 70: 309–317.

45. Gillam LA, Kaul S, Fallon JT, Levine RA, Hedley-Whyte T, Guerrero LJ, Wyman AE (1985) Functional and pathologic effects of multiple echocardiographic contrast injections on the myocardium, brain and kidney. *J Am Coll Cardiol* 6: 687–694.

46. Levine RA, Gillam LD, Guerro JL, Weyman AE (1985) Wall motion abnormalities following myocardial echo contrast injection are caused by microbubbles. *J Am Coll Cardiol* 5: 474.

47. Lang R, Borrow KM, Neuman A, Feinstein SB (1985) Echo contrast agents: Effect of sonicated microbubbles and carrier solutions on left ventricular contractility. *Circulation* 72: III–58.

48. Lang R, Borrow KM, Neumann A, Al-Sadir J, Feinstein S (1986) Effect of intracoronary injections of sonicated microbubbles on left ventricular contractility in humans. *J Am Coll Cardiol* 73: 189A.

49. Armstrong WF, Conley MJ, Dillon JC, Feigenbaum H (1984) Systolic expansion of infarcted myocardium expands the overestimation of infarct size by wall motion analyses. *J Am Coll Cardiol* 3: 513.

50. Force T, Kemper A, Perkins L, Gilfoil M, Cohen C, Parisi AF (1986) Overestimation of infarct size by quantitative two-dimensional echocardiography: The role of tethering and of analytic procedures. *Circulation* 73: 1360–1368.

51. Kaul S, Pandian BG, Gillam LD, Okada RD, Guerrero JL, Weyman AE (1984) The effect of altering coronary pressure in the non-occluded vessel on blood flow, wall motion and size of area at risk following acute coronary occlusion. *Circulation* 70: II–393.

52. Force T, Kemper A, Cohen C, Parisi A (1984) Response of contrast 2-D echo-defined ischemic and border zones to postextrasystolic potentiation (PESP). *Circulation* 70: II–183.

53. Vasey CG, De Santo JA, Armstrong WF (1986) Effect of intravenous metoprolol on infarct size following reperfusion evaluation using contrast echocardiography. *J Am Coll Cardiol* 7: 133A.

54. Feinstein SR, Lang R, Neuman A, Al-Sadir J, Chua KG, Carroll JD, Keller MW, Powsner SM, Borrow KM (1985) Intracoronary contrast echocardiography in humans: Reperfusion and anatomic correlates. *Circulation* 72: III–57.

55. Moore CA, Smucker ML, Kaul S (1986) Myocardial contrast echocardiography in humans: I. Safety-a comparison with routine coronary arteriography. *J Am Coll Cardiol* 8: 1066–1072.

56. Armstrong WF, Dillon JC, Feigenbaum H (1985) Assessment of myocardial perfusion using contrast enhanced echocardiography: Initial human experiment. *Clin Res* 33: 166A.

57. Lang RM, Feinstein SB, Feldman T, Neumann A, Chua KG, Borrow KM (1986) Contrast echocardiography for evaluation of myocardial perfusion: Effects of coronary angioplasty. *J Am Coll Cardiol* 8: 232–235.

58. Armstrong WF (1988) Assessment of myocardial perfusion with contrast-enhanced echocardiography, in: Kerber RE (ed), *Echocardiography in Coronary Artery Disease*, Chapter 19. Futura Publishing, Mount Kisco, New York.

59. Goldman ME, Mindich BP (1984) Intraoperative cardioplegic contrast echocardiography for assessing myocardial perfusion during open heart surgery. *J Am Coll Cardiol* 4: 1029–1034.

60. DePasquale EE, Nody AC, Depuey EG, Garcia EV, Pilcher G, Bredlau C, Roubin G, Gober A, Gruentzig A, D'Amato P, Berger HJ (1988) Quantitative rotational thallium-201 tomography for identifying and localizing coronary artery disease. *Circulation* 77: 316–327.

61. Bungo MW, Leland OS (1983) Disordance of exercise thallium testing with coronary arteriography in patient with atypical presentations. *Chest* 83: 112–116.

62. Schwartz RS, Jackson WG, Celio PV, Hickman JR (1988) Exercise thallium-201 scin-

tigraphy for detecting coronary artery disease in asymptomatic young men. *J Am Coll Cardiol* 76: 80A.

63. Gould KL (1988) Identifying and measuring severity of coronary artery stenosis: Quantitative Coronary Arteriography and Positron Emission Tomography. *Circulation* 78: 237–245.

64. Marcus ML, Rumberger JA, Stark CA, Weiss RM, Reiter SJ, Feiring AJ, Stanford W (1988) Cardiac Applications of Ultrafast Computed Tomography. *Am J Card Imaging* 2: 116–121.

65. Rumberger JA, Feiring AJ, Lipton MJ, Higgins CB, Ells R, Marcus ML (1987) Use of ultrafast computed tomography to quantitate regional myocardial perfusion: A preliminary report. *J Am Coll Cardiol* 9: 59–69.

66. Wang T, Ritman EL (1987) Regional myocardial perfusion quantitation with high speed volume scanning, CT. *Circulation* 76: IV–5.

67. Gould KL, Lipscomb K, Hamilton GW (1974) Physiologic basis for assessing critical coronary stenosis. *Am J Cardiol* 33: 87–94.

68. Marcus ML (1983) Metabolic regulation of coronary blood flow, in: *The Coronary Circulation in Health and Disease*, Chapter 3, McGraw-Hill, New York.

69. Hintze TH, Vatner SF (1984) Reactive dilation of large coronary arteries in conscious dogs. *Circ Res* 54: 50–57.

70. Wilson RF, Laughlin DE, Ackell PG, Armstrong ML, Marcus ML, White CW (1985) Transluminal subselective measurement of coronary artery blood flow velocity and vasodilator reserve in man. Circulation 72: 82–92.

71. White CW, Wright CB, Doty DB, Hiratzka LF, Eastham CL, Harrison DG, Marcus ML (1984) Does visual interpretation of the coronary arteriogram predict the physiologic importance of a coronary stenosis. *N Engl J Med* 310: 819–824.

72. Harrison DG, White CW, Hiratzka LF, Doty DB, Barnes DH, Eastham A, Marcus ML (1984) The value of lesion cross-sectional area determined by quantitative coronary angiography in assessing the physiologic significant of proximal left anterior descending coronary arterial stenoses. *Circulation* 69: 1111–1119.

73. McPherson DD, Hiratzka LF, Brandt B, Lamberth WC, Hunt M, Hartnett J, Clothier J, Eastham C, Kerber RE (1986) Relationship of echo demonstrated coronary atherosclerosis to reactive hyperemia. *Circulation* 74: II–85.

74. Wilson RF, Johnson MR, Marcus ML, Aylword PEG, Skorton DJ, Collins S, White CW (1988) The effect of coronary angioplasty on coronary flow reserve. *Circulation* 77: 873–885.

28. Contrast agents for myocardial perfusion studies
Mechanisms, state of the art and future prospects

RICHARD S. MELTZER, ANTONIO F. AMICO,
SHIMON A. REISNER and JANINE R. SHAPIRO

Introduction

Twenty years after Gramiak and Shah at the University of Rochester reported the echocardiographic contrast effect [1], the uses and applications of contrast echocardiography are still growing. The need for new and more standardized contrast agents with superior reproducibility and capillary transmission capability has been felt for years [2]. Meltzer et al. [3] and Armstrong et al. [4] reported on commercially prepared contrast agents in the early 1980s. Feinstein et al. [5] introduced the use of ultrasonic energy (sonication) to create smaller microbubbles. Current knowledge and future prospects about mechanisms of the ultrasound contrast effect and the new contrast agents are summarized in this chapter.

The source of ultrasonic contrast effect

During the late 1960s and early 1970s the ultrasound contrast effect was noted in different and unrelated solutions. A mechanical explanation was suggested: air microbubbles produced at the catheter tip by cavitation [6–8] or caused by a small amount of gas trapped at junctions within the injecting apparatus [9] were the proposed mechanisms. Although most authorities now agree that air microbubbles, produced by any of those mechanisms, are the source of contrast effect, some early studies proposed that particulate matter, such as platelets and fibrin in patients with prosthetic valve can cause intracavitary echoes [10].

Meltzer et al. [11–12] focused attention on the fluid inside the syringe rather than the injection technique. Different solutions (indocyanine green, water, carbonated water and commercially prepared microbubbles in gelatin) were assessed in both in vitro and in vivo models by direct visualization, light microscopy, A-mode and M-mode echocardiography. It was concluded that:

S. Iliceto et al. (eds.), Ultrasound in Coronary Artery Disease, 351–365.
© 1991 *Kluwer Academic Publishers.*

- Solutions allowed to stand overnight exposed to air ('degassing') contained no apparent microbubbles.
- Solutions exhibit bubbles in various quantity, size and stability. Solutions with low surface-tension properties created an increased number of smaller and more stable microbubbles.
- Cavitation occurred at a flow rate of 10 cc/sec through a 19-gauge needle. This rate was at the upper limit of maximum hand injection using 10 cc and 20 cc plastic syringes. The force of injection necessary to cause cavitation was higher than that used clinically through peripheral needles.
- There was a relationship between the content of microbubbles and the magnitude of contrast effect.
- The amount of gas needed to give a striking contrast effect was very small.

Physical influences on ultrasonic contrast effect: Viscosity, surface tension, and ph

Viscosity

Koenig and Meltzer [13] studied the relative viscosity of four potential contrast agents: cold (5°) and room temperature 70% Sorbitol, Renografin-76 and 50% dextrose. The microbubbles were generated by sonication of 6 cc of each solution and measured under light microscopy. Microbubble size in microns (means $\pm$ 1 S.D) and the relative viscosity are summarized in Table 1. As shown in Table 1, there was an inverse correlation between microbubble size and viscosity ($r = 0.92$, $p < 0.05$). A potential mechanism to explain these data is that a 'shell' of viscous material surrounds the bubble and protects it from coalescence. Other investigators have suggested that the half life time of microbubbles can be increased by reducing the temperature or by adding a viscosity increasing additive [14].

Table 1. Average size of microbubbles generated by sonication of four test liquids and their viscosities relative to 50% dextrose.

Liquid	MB Size (microns)	Relative viscosity
50% Dextrose	24 ± 12	1.0
Renografin-76 (R)	24 ± 9	2.3
Sorbitol	12 ± 4	24.0
Cold sorbitol	9 ± 3	57.0

MB – Microbubbles size (mirons, Mean ± 1 SD).

Reproduced with permission from: Koenig K and Meltzer RS (1986). Effect of viscosity on the size of microbubbles generated for use as echocardiographic contrast agents. *J Cardiovasc Ultrason*, 5: 3–4.

Surfactant properties

An important quality for a good ultrasound contrast agent is that the liquid phase must have good surfactant properties. Meltzer et al. [11] noted that, indocayanine green and gelatin were able to stabilized stabilize small micro-bubbles because both are good surfactants.

Coalescence may result from bringing gas bubbles into contact with each other. Coalescence leads to a reduction in total surface are and ultimately in total free energy for the system [15]. The gas in the smaller microbubbles is a higher pressure than in the larger microbubbles. Surfactants can be classified by their chemical structure or by the ionic activity [16]. Gelatin, which is composed of a complex mixture of charged peptide chains, is an example of an ionic surfactant. Other surfactants are uncharged and are capable of stabilizing small microbubbles for a long time [16].

Bommer et al. [17] studied the effect of surface-active agents in vitro and in dogs. Small amounts of 13 different surfactants (licithin, glycerin etc.) were added to water and blood (1 : 1000 dilution). The surface tension reduced between 29–62% in water and 13–37% in blood. Higher concentrations (1 : 100) were even more effective. The agents that produced the greatest in vitro reduction of surface tension also produced the brightest left heart and myocardial perfusion images by contrast echo videodensitometry. The authors concluded that pulmonary and systemic transmission of standard contrast-echo injections can be achieved by adding surfactants.

Keller et al. [18] sonicated 70% dextrose with the surfactant levo-alpha-phosphotydilcholine. The number of bubbles was larger and the decay rate (T 1/2) of the bubbles with surfactant was significantly slower than without surfactant.

The influence of pH

Air bubbles in a liquid acquire different charges depending on the composition of the solution in the fluid phase around them [19]. Air bubbles exhibit negative charges in pure water. Cationic surfactants produce positively charged bubbles. Anionic surfactants produce negatively charged bubbles in the alkaline ph range and positively charged bubbles in the acidic ph range. The pH also plays an important role in the charging mechanisms of bubbles produced with ionic surfactants [19].

Specific agents reported as echocardiographic contrast agents

The greatest stimulus for the search for new contrast agents is the desire to create an agent that can pass the pulmonary capillaries and yield contrast on the left side of the heart [20–23]. Such a contrast agent would enable better delineation of the left atrium and the left ventricle, detection of left-to-right shunt, myocardial perfusion imaging, and possibly yield information about the perfusion of other organs (kidney, brain, etc.).

Carbon dioxide

There was a large experience with intravascular injection of carbon dioxide in radiology, especially for the diagnosis of pericardial effusion, in the pre-echo-cardiographic era [24]. Since carbon dioxide is absorbed very rapidly, it is safer than other gases and doses as large as 7.5 cc/kg of carbon dioxide have been rapidly injected into the left ventricle experimentally with minimal cardiorespiratory effects [25]. Smaller doses have also been injected into the carotid artery experimentally.

Meltzer et al. [26] used 1–3 cc of medically pure carbon dioxide as an echocardiographic contrast agent and found it safe and efficacious in human subjects. Klicpera et al. [27] assessed the usefulness of carbon dioxide enriched saline (0.2 ml CO2/10 ml saline) as a contrast agent for myocardial contrast echocardiography in an animal model. They found good opacification of the myocardium that allowed an estimation of the distribution of flow. There were no serious side effects on hemodynamics or heart rhythm. Carbon dioxide has even been injected intra-coronary in humans without reported adverse effects [28]. Unfortunately, since carbon dioxide, like other gases, does not pass pulmonary capillaries [21] it has only limited prospects as a future contrast medium.

Hydrogen peroxide

In 1970, Merin, Neal and Gramiak used 0.3% hydrogen peroxide to obtain ultrasound contrast in an experimental model [29]. Wang et al. reported on animal [30] and human [31] studies with intravenous hydrogen peroxide in 1979, noting good right heart contrast effect, no left heart contrast, and transient but quite frequent toxicity. In 1980, Meltzer et al. in Rotterdam [22] used high doses of hydrogen peroxide in animal models. Injected into a peripheral vein, a high dose of hydrogen peroxide did pass the lungs but caused significant hemodynamic toxicity. Gaffney et al. [32] used 0.3% hydrogen peroxide passed through a millipore filter and diluted with heparinized saline solution and with a drop of blood in the syringe before injection. Studies in dogs, normal adults, and 36 patients with various cardiac disorders produced dense, sustained contrast with no complications.

Kemper et al. [33–34] in Parisi's laboratory in Boston have been using hydrogen peroxide as a contrast agent for myocardial perfusion imaging in experimental animals. They mixed 1.0 cc of blood with 1.0–2.0 cc of 0.3% hydrogen peroxide and injected it into the aortic root or coronary arteries. They found this method to be safe and consistently associated with good myocardial enhancement.

Hydrogen peroxide, when injected into the blood, splits with the aid of the catalytic action from the peroxidase in leukocytes, resulting in the liberation of free oxygen in sufficient quantities that local gas bubbles form. Low doses might be non-toxic, though higher doses clearly can cause air embolism [35]. Creation of oxygen bubbles in blood is related also to the availability of hydrogen peroxidase, located in white blood cells.

In vivo generation of contrast

Another approach to creating ultrasound contrast was to inject a mixture of substances so that their chemical reaction in vivo will produce the contrast material. Jiang et al. [36] have reported in a preliminary study the use of a mixture consisting of 4 ml of 5% sodium bicarbonate and 2 ml of 5% ascorbic acid injected into the left ventricle. This mixture is mixed and directly injected and it generated carbon dioxide immediately. They reported that injections yielded contrast in all 9 patients studied and that there were no adverse symptomatic or hemodynamic effects.

Contrast formed by bubbles in gelatin or Haemaccel®

Gelatin in a substance which for many years was available for intravenous use as a plasma expander, but has been removed from the market in the U.S. by the FDA due to occasional allergic reactions. It is a surfactant and stabilizes microbubbles to the point that they can be densely packed and centrifuged without causing coalescence. A preparation manufactured by Rasor Associates, Sunnyvale, CA, of these bubbles was studied by Meltzer et al. [3, 11], Carroll et al. [37], and Armstrong et al. [38]. Though these microbubbles seemed promising, Rasor stopped production and this contrast agent could not be further studied. Meltzer et al. [39] have shown that precision microbubbles can be generated for experimental echocardiographic use in commercially available gelatin.

Haemaccel®, the trade name of a gelatin-based solution produced by Hoechst and available commercially in Europe and most of the developing countries as plasma expander, is a surfactant and stabilizes small microbubbles. In a study by Ernst and Cikes [40], Haemaccel® was found to be a more effective contrast agent than 5% glucose in 70 of 100 peripheral injections in humans. Further, Santoso et al. [41] from Jakarta, Indonesia, reported the use of direct intra-coronary injections of Haemaccel® in 25 patients undergoing cardiac catheterization. Six patients had non-agitated and a subsequent 19 patients had hand-agitated solution. The bubble size was 12 ± 10 microns and the volume injected was 5.0 cc. Myocardial contrast was seen in 19/19 of the patients injected with the agitated solution, but only 3/6 patients after the non-agitated Haemaccel®. The contrast effect lasted 15 to 60 sec and caused mild and always transient adverse effects.

Bommer et al. [42] reported that microbubbles coated with gelatin or albumin can yield better left heart contrast after distal pulmonary artery injection in experimental animals than the standard contrast media.

Saccharide particles as ultrasound contrast agents

Sugar encapsulated microbubbles were developed by Rasor Associates (Sunnyvale, CA) and the rights to them were acquired by the German firm Schering (Berlin). For the past several years they have been developing contrast agents for commercial introduction. One of these agents, SHU-454, has been compared with the traditional agents for right heart contrast echocardiography and was found in Dr. DeMaria's laboratory to have a superior intensity, to be reproducible and non-toxic [43]. Other reports using Schering's polysaccharide contrast agent have also been published [44–48]. However, the chemical and physical properties and the mechanism by which this agent causes bubbles to form is currently not in the public domain.

Currently, Schering is actively pursuing the commercial introduction of this polysaccharide contrast agent. SHU 454 has been renamed Echovist® and is undergoing trials for intravenous injection as a right heart contrast agent. A smaller particle size polysaccharide agent is also undergoing tests for possible pulmonary transmission and left heart contrast after intravenous injections. It has been given the trade name 'Levocon®.' Note that this development is being performed by Schering, Berlin, which is not connected with Schering in the US – the American subsidiary of Schering, Berlin is Berlex. Most of the development of these agents is currently taking place in Europe.

Heavy liquids – fluorochemicals and fat emulsions

Matsuda et al. [49] reported the appearance of contrast in the right heart after injection of perfluorochemical emulsion (Fluosol®) into the inferior vena cava in dogs. Of the 18 dogs studied, 16 had 'clear' left heart contrast following the right heart injections. When 95% oxygen was mixed with the Fluosol®, left heart contrast intensity was reported to be greater. The myocardial wall echoes were also reported enhanced by the intravenous Fluosol® injections.

Valdes-Cruz and Sahn [50] have reported on left heart opacification after intravenous injection of 20% oxypherol, a synthetic oxygen carrying fluorocarbon, gasified separately with oxygen and carbon dioxide. They found fairly weak contrast compared to other agents tested. Mattrey and Andre [51] reported on ultrasonic enhancement of the infarcted area by perfluorocarbon in 9 dogs. Initial studies suggested that the mechanism of this enhancement was related to perfluorocarbon accumulation in macrophages within the infarcted zone. Several authors have noted that *Intralipid®* and other *fat emulsions* when infused intravenously can yield contrast of the right heart and can even pass through the lungs to enhance the left side of the heart [50–52].

This effect, as in fluorocarbons, is fairly weak and we feel that it will not be sufficient for clinical applications. An interesting theoretical question, however, relates to the mechanism of the contrast effect observed with this liquids: is it due to acoustic impedence mismatch with the surrounding blood? This is perhaps why those liquids yield contrast without the necessity to be associated with gas, and why their distribution in the body may be related to the reticuloendothelial system. Since the heart has very little if any reticuloendothelial system, enhancement due to macrophage uptake is quite weak.

Highly viscous solutions

Microbubbles created in a viscous solution such as Renografin-76®, 50% or 70% sorbitol, or 70% dextrose, are relatively small and stable compared to those created in 5% dextrose or saline [5]. The probable mechanism for this difference is that a 'shell' is produced by the viscous material around the microbubble, protecting it from shrinking or coalescence. In a study of Feinstein et al. [5], sonicated 70% sorbitol, sonicated 50% dextrose and sonicated Renografin-76® yielded microbubbles with diameters of 6 ± 2, 11 ± 5, and 10 ± 4 microns, respectively. The size of the microbubbles is proportional to the relative viscosity as noted in reference 13 and Table 1. In the same study, the most viscous solution − 70% sorbitol − has also the smallest range of bubble size and the longest persistence. The effect of dilution is demonstrated by the difference between 70% dextrose and 50% dextrose. The mean size of the microbubbles in 50% dextrose was 8 ± 3 microns as compared with 11 ± 5 microns for the microbubbles in 50% dextrose.

It is important to note that intracoronary injection of most of the echo contrast agents produce transient changes in coronary flow, left ventricular function and hemodynamics [53–55]. The viscous and usually high osmolarity solutions have been found to be responsible for those adverse effects [56, 57]. Due to its known intrinsic myocardial depression, therefore, Renografin®, the most widely used contrast agent in human studies [58, 59], is far from being the ideal contrast agent for myocardial contrast imaging.

Sonicated albumin microbubble suspensions

In 1979 Bommer reasoned that albumin was a surfactant and used it to coat microbubbles and attempt to stabilize small microbubbles for use as a contrast agent [42]. However, it remained for the group headed by Feinstein at the University of Chicago to apply their high intensity sonication method (see section 5 below) to albumin solutions to develop what is probably the most promising agent for myocardial perfusion imaging currently available [60, 61]. Sonicated albumin has been used by several groups for studies in experimental animals and seems to be a promising agent from several points of view. The microbubbles are smaller than those in sonicated Renografin® and therefore pass through capillary beds without 'hangup', with a more physiologic halftime [62, 63].

Sonicated albumin has most recently also been used in humans. In our laboratory we have used it after intracoronary injections in 14 patients, receiving a total of 38 injections. In a subgroup of 9 patients, sonicated albumin and sonicated Renografin® were injected using the same technique. One patient with unstable angina noted transient angina. No other patient experienced chest pain or subjective symptoms during intracoronary injection. No arrhythmias or changes in hemodynamics were observed. An excellent myocardial contrast effect was observed, with a shorter contrast washout halftime than for paired intracoronary injections of sonicated Renografin® in the same patients [64]. We concluded that sonicated albumin is an easily prepared, safe, and effective contrast agent for myocardial perfusion imaging.

Dr. Feinstein has assigned his patients regarding sonicated albumin [61] to Molecular Biosystems, Inc., of San Diego, CA. They are in the process of bringing a commercial preparation onto the market under the trade name of Albunex®. Several laboratories, including the University of Rochester, have examined this commercial preparation in experimental animals for the purpose of myocardial perfusion imaging. Most recently, Feinstein reported on initial human trials of intravenous injections of Albunex®, noting transpulmonary transmission and lack of significant toxicity [65].

The use of high intensity sonication for microbubble creation

Background

The group headed by Dr. Steven Feinstein, formerly in Dr. Elliot Corday's laboratory at Cedars-Sinai Hospital and currently in Chicago, has introduced the use of ultrasonic energy for microbubbles preparation. A lead zirconate-titanate electrostricture (piezoelectric) crystal was initially used as the source of controlled ultrasonic energy [5]. Introduction of the tip of the sonicator horn into a solution results in the production of surface agitation and cavitation. As a result of this energy, microcavities are created in the liquid. A second generation of bubbles from the released cavitation gas bubbles [66]. Microbubbles produced by sonication are significantly smaller than those produced by hand agitation [5].

Animal studies using sonicated albumin

Drs. Keller and Feinstein in Chicago, and subsequently Keller and Kaul in Virginia, have performed an elegant series of experiments using sonicated albumin in animals. In one series, 3–5 cc of sonicated albumin were injected intravenously in dogs [63]. Contrast appeared in the right ventricle in 56/72 attempts (91%) and in the left ventricle in 56/72 attempts (78%). The myo-

cardium was enhanced only in 9/72 injections (12.5%). There were no alteration in blood pressure, heart rate, or blood gases after repeated injections and
no organ damage revealed by histologic examination. In another series of
intracoronary injections in dogs Keller found no significant hemodynamic
effects or reactive hyperemia and noted that sonicated albumin has many of
the desired qualities of an ideal contrast agent [62].

Human studies using sonicated albumin

After the initial reports from Chicago about sonicated albumin as a contrast
agent, we and other investigators noted some difficulty in reproducibly and
reliably obtaining small microbubbles in 5% human albumin solutions after
sonication. We therefore modified the Chicago method by adding a capability
for direct injection of small amounts of air below the active sonication horn.
In our laboratory, this yields more reliable and reproducible results.

The method we use to prepare albumin as an echocardiographic contrast
agent is as follows: a 'sonication chamber' (Figures 1, 2) was built from readily
available, disposable supplies [66]. It allows precise injections of air into the
bottom of the chamber, with sampling of the echocontrast agent through a
side port. The resulting microbubbles are small and suitable for myocardial
perfusion studies and the number and size of microbubbles is related to the
volume of air injected, sonication protocol, and carrier fluid.

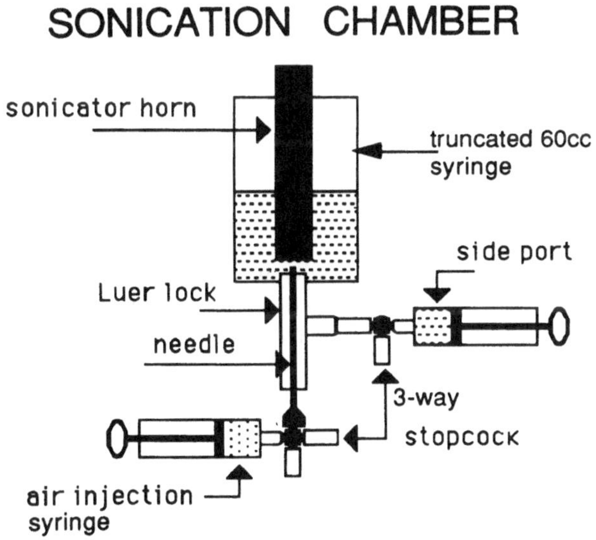

SONICATION CHAMBER

Figure 1. Diagram of sonication chamber designed to allow injection of small quantities of air
directly below an active sonication horn during sonication of a contrast agent. The sonication
chamber is a cut-off 60 cc syringe, with a Luer lock below and a needle inserted retrograde
through the barrel of the truncated 60 cc syringe, for air injection. After sonication, the contrast
agent with microbubble suspension is withdrawn through the side port. (See text and reference
[67] for discussion.)

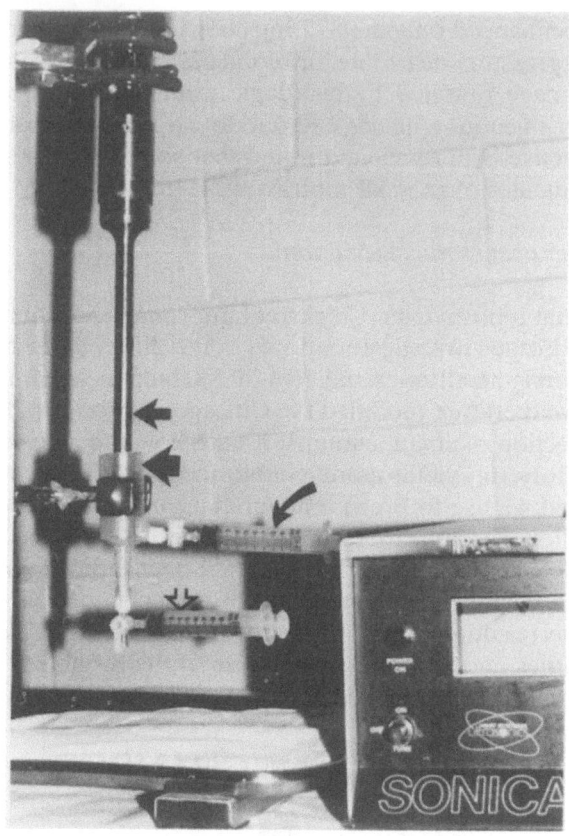

Figure 2. Photograph of the sonication chamber diagrammed in Figure 1, with the sonicator horn (small horizontal arrow) inserted into the syringe barrel (large horizontal arrow). Air is injected using the lower syringe (open vertical arrow) and withdrawn after sonication using the upper horizontal syringe (curved arrow).

Since there has been some difficulty in creating adequate contrast agents for human use by this method, we will describe in detail our method of preparation, using the sonicating chamber to sonicate 5% human albumin. A 1/2 inch horn of a Heat System (Farmingdale, NY) W-375 sonicator was placed 3 mm from the tip of the needle inserted retrograde into the bottom of the syringe used as sonicating chamber. To sonicate 10 cc of human albumin with the sonicator output setting on 8, two steps were needed:
- sonication for 60 sec to heat the solution, and
- infusion of 5 cc of air through the needle (3 mm below the activated horn) over 15 sec.

Within 3 min after completion of sonication, this resulted in separation of the human albumin into 2 layers: a lower clear layer with microbubble size of 1.9 ± 0.4 microns (mean ± 1 SD, by Coulter Counter) and an upper foamy layer with microbubble size of 4–9 microns. The mixture of both layers dilut-

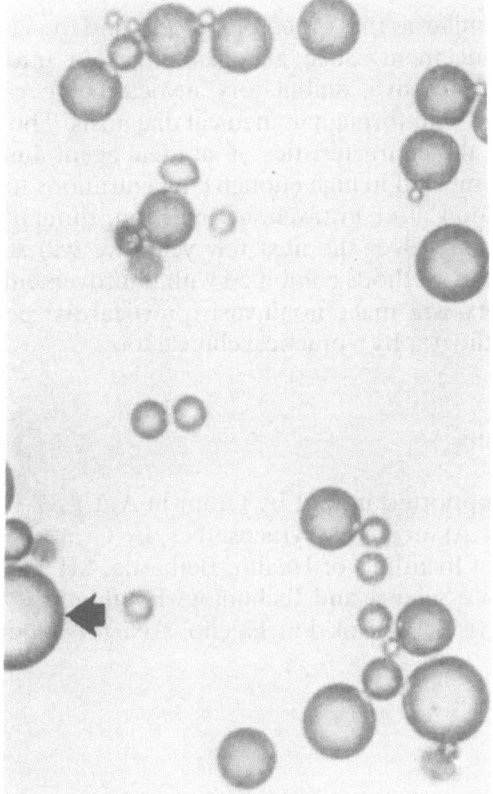

Figure 3. Photomicrograph of sonicated 5% human albumin. The mixture of the foamy and the fluid layers resulted in two populations of microbubbles (see text for the details). The microbubbles in the lower left corner (arrow) is 9 microns in size.

ed with 10 cc nonsonicated human albumin resulted in microbubble size of 5.2 ± 2.6 microns. The mixture of these two layers (Figure 3) is used in our laboratory as a contrast agent for myocardial perfusion imaging after intra-coronary injection [64] and also for transpulmonary left heart opacification after intravenous injection.

Conclusion

The large number of contrast agents that have been studied is probably relat-ed to the fact that none of them is ideal. The ideal echocardiographic contrast agent should contain extremely small microbubbles – less than 10 microns and preferably even smaller, which are uniform and stable, and non-toxic. This contrast agent has to be able to traverse the microcirculation in a manner physiologically similar to that of red blood cells and then to produce adequate myocardial enhancement. Such an agent, injected into a peripheral vein would allow non-invasive, ambulatory myocardial perfusion imaging and would be a major breakthrough in medical diagnosis. Though sonicated albumin has many of the characteristics of an ideal agent, initial impressions are that it cannot be injected in high enough concentrations to achieve good myocardial opacification after intravenous injection, though undoubtedly some opacification occurs. Over the next few years we will see if more sensitive computer detection methods combined with improvements in contrast agents and bolus delivery will make noninvasive myocardial perfusion imaging by contrast echocardiography a practical clinical tool.

Acknowledgements

This work was supported in part by Grant-in-Aid #87-018G from the New York State Heart Association, Syracuse NY, by Grant PHS S7RR05403-26 from the National Institutes of Health, Bethesda, MD, and by a Grant from the New York State Science and Technology Foundation, Albany, NY.

The authors wish to thank Pat Faiello, RN, for expert secretarial assistance.

References

1. Gramiak R, Shah PM (1968) Echocardiography of the aortic root. *Invest Radiol* 3: 356–366.
2. Meerbaum S (1986) Promise and status of myocardial contrast-enhanced two dimensional echocardiography: Delineation of ischemic risk zone and quantitation of myocardial perfusion defects. *J Am Coll Cardiol* 7: 395–396.
3. Meltzer RS, Vermeulen HW, Valk N, Verdow R, Lancee CT, Roelandt J (1982) New echocardiographic contrast agents: Transmission through the lungs and myocardial perfusion imaging. *J Cardiovasc Ultrason* 1: 277–282.
4. Armstrong WF, Mueller TM, Kinney EL, Tickner EG, Dillon JC, Feigenbaum H (1982) Assessment of myocardial perfusion abnormalities with contrast-enhanced two-dimensional echocardiography. *Circulation* 66: 166–173.
5. Feinstein SB, Ten Cate KJ, Zwehl W, Ong K, Maurer G, Tei C, Shah PM, Meerbaum S, Corday E (1984) Two-dimensional contrast echocardiography. I. In vitro development and quantitative analysis of echo contrast agents. *J Am Coll Cardiol* 3: 14–20.
6. Kremkau FW, Gramiak R, Carstensen EL, Shah PM, Kramer DH (1970) Ultrasonic detection of cavitation at catheter tips. *Am J Roentgenol* 110: 177–183.
7. Bove AA, Adams DF, Hugh AE, Lynch PR (1968) Cavitation at catheter tips. A possible cause of air embolus. *Invest Radiol* 3: 159–164.
8. Bove AA, Ziskin MC, Mulchin WL (1969) Ultrasonic detection of in vivo cavitation and pressure effects of high-speed injections through catheters. *Invest Radiol* 4: 236–240.
9. Barrera JG, Fulkerson PK, Rittgers SE, Nerem RM (1978) The nature of contrast echocardiographic 'targets'. *Circulation* 58 (suppl II): 233 (abstracts).
10. Schuchman H, Feigenbaum H, Dillon JC (1975) Intracavitary echoes in patients with mitral prosthetic valves. *J Clin Ultras* 3: 107–110.

11. Meltzer RS, Tickner EG, Popp RL (1980) The source of ultrasound contrast effect. *J Clin Ultras* 8: 121–127.

12. Meltzer RS, Tickner EG, Popp RL (1982) The source of echocardiographic contrast, in: Meltzer RS, Roelandt J (eds), *Contrast Echocardiography*, pp 7–16. The Hague: Martinus Nijhoff.

13. Koenig K, Meltzer RS (1986) Effect of viscosity on the size of microbubbles generated for use as echocardiographic contrast agents. *J Cardiovasc Ultrason* 5: 3–4.

14. Sebba F (1971) Microfoams – An unexploited colloid system. *J Colloid Interface Sci* 35: 643–646.

15. Yount DE (1983) A model for microbubble fission in surfactant solutions. *J Colloid Interface Sci* 91: 349–360.

16. D'Arrigo (1983) Biological surfactants stabilizing natural microbubbles in aqueous media. *Advances in Colloid and Interface Science*, 19: 253–307. Elsevier Science Publishers BV Amsterdam.

17. Bommer WJ, Miller L, Takeda P, Mason DT, DeMaria AN (1981) Contrast echocardiography: Pulmonary transmission and myocardial perfusion imaging using surfactant stabilized microbubbles. *Circulation* (suppl IV): IV–303 (abstracts).

18. Keller MW, Feinstein SB, Briller RA, Powsner SM (1986) Automated production and analysis of echo contrast agents. *J Ultrasound Med.* 5: 493–498.

19. Yoon RH, Yordan JL (1986) Zeta-potential measurements on microbubbles generated using various surfactants. *J Colloid Interface Sci* 113: 430–438.

20. Bommer WJ, Mason DT, DeMaria AN (1979) Studies in contrast echocardiography: Development of new agents with superior reproducibility and transmission through the lungs. *Circulation* 59–60 (suppl II): II–17.

21. Meltzer RS, Tickner EG, Popp RL (1980) Why do the lungs clear ultrasonic contrast? *Ultrasound in Med & Biol* 6: 263–269.

22. Meltzer RS, Sartorius OEH, Lancee CT, Serruys PW, Verdouw PD, Essed C, Roelandt J (1981) Transmission of ultrasonic contrast through the lungs. *Ultrasound in Med & Biol* 7: 377–384.

23. Meltzer RS, Vermulen HWJ, Valk NK, Verdouw PD, Lancee CT, Roelandt J (1982) New echocardiographic contrast agents: Transmission through the lungs and myocardial perfusion imaging. *J Cardiovasc Ultrason* 1: 277–282.

24. Phillips JH, Burch GE, Hellinger R (1961) The use of intracardiac carbon dioxide in the diagnosis of pericardial disease. *Am Heart J* 61: 748–755.

25. Oppenheismer MJ, Durant TM, Stauffer HM, Stewart GH, Lynch PR, Barrera F (1956) In vivo visualization of intracardiac structures with gaseous carbon dioxide. *Am J Physiol* 186: 325–334.

26. Meltzer RS, Serruys PW, Hugenholtz PG, Roelandt J (1981) Intravenous carbon dioxide as an echocardiographic contrast agent. *J Clin Ultrasound* 9: 127–131.

27. Klicpera M, Glogar D, Mayr H, Mohl W, Losert U, Kaindl F (1982) Myocardial perfusion evaluated by contrast echocardiography. *Chest* 82: 751–755.

28. Tambe A, McLaughlin WR, Zimmerman HA (1968) Double contrast medium technique for coronary blood flow studies. *Am J Cardiol* 21: 117 (abstracts).

29. Gramiak R (1982) Contrast agents for diagnostic ultrasound, in: Meltzer RS, Roelandt J (eds), *Contrast Echocardiography*. The Hague: Martinus Nijhoff.

30. Wang X, Wand J, Huang Y, Cai C (1979) Contrast echocardiography with hydrogen peroxide. I. Experimental study. *Chinese Med J* 92: 595–599.

31. Wang X, Wand J, Hanrong C, Lu C (1979) Contrast echocardiography with hydrogen peroxide. II. Clinical application. *Chinese Med J* 92: 693–702.

32. Gaffney FA, Lin JC, Peshock RM, Bush L, Buja LM (1983) Hydrogen peroxide contrast echocardiography. *Am J Cardiol* 52: 607–609.

33. Kemper AJ, O'Boyle JE, Sharma S, Cohen CA, Kloner RA, Khuri SR, Parisi AF (1983) Hydrogen peroxide contrast-enhanced two-dimensional echocardiography: Real-time in vivo delineation of regional myocardial perfusion. *Circulation* 68: 603–611.

34. Kemper AJ, O'Boyle BS, Cohen CA, Taylor A, Parisi AF (1984) Hydrogen peroxyde contrast echocardiography: Quantification in vivo of myocardial risk area during coronary occlusion and of the necrotic area remaining after myocardial reperfusion. *Circulation* 70: 309–317.

35. Finney JW, Jay BE, Race GJ, Urschel HC, Mallams JT, Balla GA (1966) Removal of cholesterol and other lipids from experimental animal and human atheromatous arteries by dilute hydrogen peroxide. *Angiology* 17: 223–228.

36. Jiang L, Pu SY, Yang MZ, Lu YZ, Chen HZ (1984) Left heart contrast echocardiography using a carbon dioxide producing agent. *Circulation* 70 (suppl II): II–5 (abstracts).

37. Carroll BA, Turner RJ, Tickner EG, Boyle DB, Young SW (1980) Gelatin encapsulated nitrogen microbubbles as ultrasonic contrast agents. *Invest Radiol* 15: 260–266.

38. Armstrong WF, Mueller TM, Kinney EL, Tickner EG, Dillon JC, Feigenbaum H (1982) Assessment of myocardial perfusion abnormalities with contrast-enhanced two-dimensional echocardiography. *Circulation* 66: 166–173.

39. Meltzer RS, Klig V, Teichholz LE (1985) Generating precision microbubbles for use as an echocardiographic contrast agent. *J Am Coll Cardiol* 5: 978–982.

40. Ernst A, Cikes I, Cistovic F (1984) Polygelin colloid solution as an echocardiographic contrast agent. *J Cardiovasc Ultrason* 3: 143–145.

41. Santoso T, Roelandt J, Mansyoer H, Abdurahman N, Meltzer RS, Hugenholtz PG (1985) Myocardial perfusion imaging in humans by contrast echocardiography using polygelin colloid solution. *J Am Coll Cardiol* 6: 612–620.

42. Bommer WJ, Mason DT, DeMaria AN (1979) Studies in contrast echocardiography: development of new agents with superior reproducibility and transmission through the lungs. *Circulation* 60 (suppl II): II–17.

43. Smith MD, Kwan OL, Reiser HJ, DeMaria AN (1984) Superior intensity and reproducibility of SHU-454, a new right heart contrast agent. *J Am Coll Cardiol* 3: 992–998.

44. Schartl M, Fritzsch T, Friedman W, Lange L (1984) Quantitative myocardial perfusion studies with a new safe echo contrast agent. *J Am Coll Cardiol* 3: 563 (abstracts).

45. Miszalok V, Fritzsch R, Schartl M (1986) Myocardial perfusion defects in contrast echocardiography: Spatial and temporal localization. *Ultrasound in Med & Biol* 12: 581–586.

46. Rovai D, Lombardi M, Ferdeghini EM, Marzilli M, Distante A, Taddei L, Benassi A, DeMaria AN, L'Abbate A (1987) Color-coded functional imaging of myocardial perfusion by contrast echocardiography. *Circulation* 76 (suppl IV): IV–504 (abstracts).

47. Rovai D, Lombardi M, DE Pieri G, Mazzarisi A, Taddei L, Distante A, Benassi A, L'Abbate A (1988) Accurate flow quantitation by radiofrequency analysis of contrast echo. *Circulation* 78 (suppl II): II–566 (abstracts).

48. Rovai D, Lombardi M, Ferdeghini EM, Marzilli M, Distante A, Taddei L, Landini L, Benassi A, L'Abbate A (1988) Detection of regional myocardial underperfusion by contrast-echo functional imaging. *J Am Coll Cardiol* 11: 76A (abstracts).

49. Matsuda M, Kuwako K, Sugishita Y, Ito I, Akatsuka T (1983) Contrast echocardiography of the left heart by intravenous injections of perfluorochemical emulsion. *J Cardiography* 13: 1021–1028.

50. Valdes-Cruz LM, Sahn DJ (1984) Ultrasonic contrast studies for the detection of cardiac shunts. *J Am Coll Cardiol* 3: 978–985.

51. Mattrey RF, Andre MP (1984) Ultrasonic enhancement of myocardial infarction with perfluorocarbon compounds in dogs. *Am J Cardiol* 206–210.

52. Valdes-Cruz LM, Sahn DJ, Horowitz S (1982) Left ventricular opacification by intravenous injection of safe echo contrast agents: Comparative studies in animals and initial human trials. *Circulation* 66: II–28 (abstracts).

53. Lang R, Borrow KM, Neuman A, Feinstein SB (1985) Echo contrast agents: Effects of sonicated microbubbles and carrier solutions on left ventricular contractility. *Circulation* 72: III–227 (abstracts).

54. Holt G, Reeves W, Rieder M, Daley L, Murthy M, Christensen C (1985) Negative inotropic effects of intracoronary echo-contrast agents. *J Am Coll Cardiol* 5: 474 (abstracts).

55. Kondo S, Tei C, Meerbaum S, Corday E, Shah P (1984) Hyperemic response of intracoronary contrast agents during two-dimentional echographic delineation of regional myocardium. *J Am Coll Cardiol* 4: 149–156.

56. Hayward R, Dawson P (1984) Contrast agents and angiocardiography. *Br Heart J* 52: 361–368.

57. Hajduczki I, Rajagopalan RE, Meerbaum S, Drury JK, Corday E (1987) Effects of intracoronary administered echo-contrast agents on epicardial coronary flow, ECG, and global and regional hemodynamics. *J Cardiovasc Ultrason* 6: 85–93.

58. Moore CA, Smucker MC, Kaul S (1986) Myocardial contrast echocardiography in humans: I. Safety comparison with routine coronary arteriography. *J Am Coll Cardiol* 8: 1066–1072.

59. Lang R, Borow KM, Neuman A, Al-Sadir J, Feinstein S (1986) Effect of intracoronary injections of sonicated microbubbles on left ventricular contractility in humans. *J Am Coll Cardiol* 7: 189A (abstracts).

60. Keller MW, Feinstein SB (1986) Successful transpulmonary contrast echocardiography for quantitation of myocardial perfusion. *Clin Res* 34 (2): 313A.

61. Feinstein SB Contrast agents for ultrasonic imaging. US Patent No 4,572,203, Feb 25, 1986 and No 4,718,433, Jan 12, 1988.

62. Keller MW, Glasheen W, Kuldeep T, Gear A, Kaul S (1988) Myocardial contrast echocardiography without significant hemodynamic effects or reactive hyperemia: A major advantage in the imaging of regional myocardial perfusion. *J Am Coll Cardiol* 12: 1039–1047.

63. Keller MW, Feinstein SB, Watson DD (1987) Successful left ventricular opacification following peripheral venous injection of sonicated contrast agent: An experimental evaluation. *Am Heart J* 114: 570–575.

64. Reisner SA, Ong LS, Shapiro JR, Lichtenberg GS, Amico AF, Allen MN, Meltzer RS (1988) Efficacy and safety of myocardial perfusion imaging using intracoronary sonicated albumin in humans. *Circulation* 78 (suppl II): II–565 (abstracts).

65. Feinstein SB, Heidenreich PA, Dick CD, Schneider JM, Pastoret AF, Rubenstein WA, Appelbaum J, Brehm JL, Aronson S, Ellis J, Roizen M (1988) Albunex®: A new intravascular ultrasound contrast agent: Preliminary safety and efficacy results. *Circulation* 78 (suppl II): II–565 (abstracts).

66. Willard GW (1953) Ultrasonically induced cavitation in water: A step by step process. *J Acoust Soc Am* 25: 669–686.

67. Reisner SA, Shapiro JR, Schwarz KQ, Meltzer RS (1988) Sonication of echocontrast agents: A standardized and reproducible method. *J Cardiovasc Ultrasonography* 7: 273–276.

29. Coronary anatomy and myocardial perfusion: Role of contrast echocardiography

ANTONIO F. AMICO, SABINO ILICETO,
RICHARD S. MELTZER, GAETANO D'AMBROSIO,
VITO MARANGELLI, CATALDO MEMMOLA,
GIULIA DE MARTINO, LUCIA SUBLIMI SAPONETTI
and PAOLO RIZZON

Introduction

Coronary stenoses reduce coronary flow and, consequently, myocardial perfusion. This is the main cause of clinical symptoms of coronary artery disease. Though coronary arteriography is the most important diagnostic examination for evaluating this disease, it does have several limitations. It cannot, for example, estimate the actual 'haemodynamic' severity of the coronary stenoses and, therefore, its real significance in limiting myocardial perfusion. Interpretation of coronary angiograms is also affected by an intra- and inter-observer variability which cannot be overlooked [1, 2]. Furthermore, coronary arteriography as performed in most institutions gives only qualitative information on the distribution and characteristics of coronary stenoses. Myocardial perfusion is further influenced by many other factors which cannot be evaluated by coronary angiography (the microcirculation, heart muscle conditions, interstitial characteristics, wall stress, collateral circulation etc.).

Myocardial contrast echocardiography is a promising technique for assessing myocardial perfusion. As the microbubbles injected into the coronary circulation follow the blood flow in virtually the same way as do red blood cells [3] it has been suggested that this technique may be able to delineate a vascular perfusion bed downstream of the point of the injection. Thus, contrast echocardiography can be used experimentally for defining the physiological relationship between myocardial blood flow and epicardial coronary artery anatomy.

Using contrast echocardiography to identify perfusion

In 1982 the first experimental study using contrast echocardiography to identify myocardial perfusion defects was published [4]. By injecting microcapsules of air in gelatin into animals whose circumflex coronary artery had been occluded, it was possible to single out ischemic areas more accurately than waiting for the onset of wall motion abnormalities. What is more, this

S. Iliceto et al. (eds.), Ultrasound in Coronary Artery Disease, 367–375.
© 1991 *Kluwer Academic Publishers.*

way of identifying areas at risk of necrosis has proven to be highly reproducible [5]. Kemper et al. [6], Sakamaki et al. [7] and Armstrong et al. [8] have
all found a close correlation between the area not opacified by the echocontrast and the infarct area identified in the same section by means of histological colouring or intravital colouring with monastral blue. Armstrong et al.
applied digital techniques to the images during the contrast echocardiography.

Myocardial perfusion and coronary anatomy

In the light of the studies which have demonstrated the accuracy of the
method in delineating the vascular bed downstream of a coronary occlusion,
contrast echocardiography seems to be a good way of identifying areas of perfusion in the coronary circulation. Two preliminary studies have been carried
out to evaluate the safety of this method in humans [9, 10]. In the study done
by Moore et al. [9], performed on 10 subjects without coronary disease, the
intramyocardial distribution of the contrast was not analysed. The contrast
solution used was sonicated Renografin. The echocardiogram and the common haemodynamic indices of left ventricular function (aortic pressure, left
ventricular end-diastolic and pulmonary capillary wedge pressure) did not
show any significant differences with respect to the injection of iodate contrast agents. However, studies Gillam et al. have done on dogs [11] have shown
the onset of wall motion abnormalities during intracoronary injection of
agitated Renografin which virtually cover all the opacified area. Lang et al.
[12] and Shapiro et al. [13] have demonstrated that the extent of the haemodynamic and wall motion alterations can be correlated with the size of the
microbubbles injected into the coronary circulation.

Santoso et al. [10] have carried out selective intracoronary injections of
non-agitated and hand-agitated polygelin colloid solution in 25 patients
without significant coronary artery disease. They used the long and short axis
parasternal planes for analysing the echocardiograms, dividing the former
into 5 segments (base-septum, midseptum, apex, mid-posterior and base-
posterior) and the latter into 4 segments (anterior, inferior, anterolateral and
inferolateral). For each intracoronary injection, the percent circumferential
extent of the contrast effect was evaluated. In 22 patients whose myocardium
was opacified, the contrast effect after injection into the left coronary artery
was limited to the basal and mid-anterior interventricular septum, apex and
anterolateral segment whereas, after injection into the right coronary the inferoposterior segments, the inferior part of the septum and the posteromedial papillary muscle were opacified. The inferoposterior segment was
opacified after left intracoronary injection when the left coronary was dominant. In 14/22 patients, opacification of the lateral wall, though present, was
not uniform after left intracoronary injection; in the same way, in 15/18
patients who received right intracoronary injection, the opacification of the

inferoposterior wall and the inferior portion of the septum was not homogeneous. This may be explained if the areas which are not evenly opacified are situated in the peripheric portion of the visualized vascular bed where the myocardium is supplied by the overlaying of peripheric branches of two coronary beds. This hypothesis seems to be confirmed by the sum of the circumferential contrast effect distribution after right and left coronary injection: this sum, as a percentage, was very near the expected value of 100%, indicating that there were no significant overestimations of the right and left coronary vascular bed.

Feinstein et al. [14] studied the distribution of myocardial perfusion in 14 patients without coronary artery disease by the intracoronary injection of sonicated Renografin-76. The parasternal short axis plane was used at the papillary muscle level. The two-dimensional cross sectional view was divided into 10 regions: anterior, anterolateral, posterolateral, posterior, inferior, inferoseptal, midseptal, anteroseptal and the anterolateral and posteromedial papillary muscle. In the areas which proved to be supplied by both the right and left coronaries, the dominance of perfusion was established if more than 50% of the area was opacified after injecting into just one coronary. In the patients with a right dominant coronary artery system, the distribution of the perfusion varied less from patient to patient: in fact, left intracoronary injection always opacified the anterior, anterolateral, posterolateral and posterior segments as well as the anterolateral papillary muscle. However, the midseptum, the inferior and inferoseptal regions and the posteromedial papillary muscle also sometimes became opacified after left intracoronary injection even though this happened more often after right intracoronary injection. In two cases with a left dominant system both papillary muscles were supplied from the left system. However, the inferior and inferoseptal regions were supplied from the left coronary system in one patient and from the right coronary one in the other. This rather singular situation was pointed out in a case of ours in which the presence of a left dominant system was associated with an unusually wide perfusional bed (Figure 1). The site and extent of the opacified areas did not vary when two injections were done one after the other into the same coronary.

Griffin et al. [15] have studied the distribution of contrast in 28 patients with coronary artery disease. In their study, they used equal parts of Urografin and physiological solution mixed by injecting them back and forth into two syringes. Considering the study population, in which a greater prevalence of collateral circulations and the presence of coronary occlusions could be assumed, their results are partially comparable to those to Feinstein's. In general, they found that right intracoronary injections opacify the inferior septum and the inferior wall whereas left intracoronary injections show up perfusion in the rest of the ventricle. As in Santoso's study, they found that the opacification of the lateral wall was less dense in 16 patients: this analogy may perhaps be due to the similarity of the contrast agents used in that the bubbles produced were larger in the one which was hand-agitated. If, as it is reason-

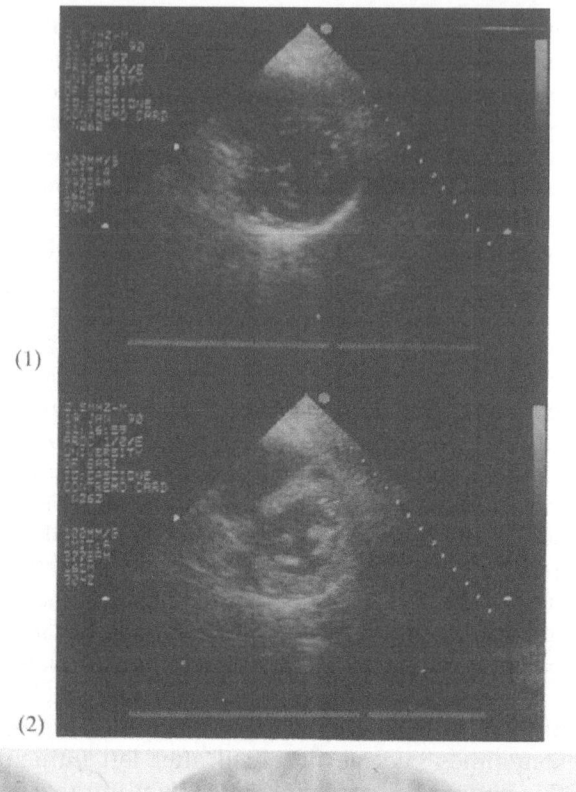

(1)

(2)

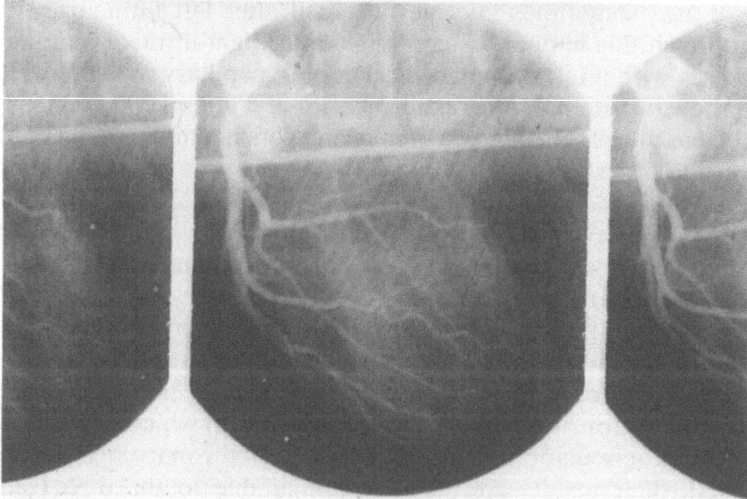

`  ` (3)

Figure 1. Delimitation of the perfusion bed by means of intracoronary injection of sonicated ioxglate (Hexabrix). Panel *(1)*: short axis view of the left ventricle at the papillary muscle level. Panel *(2)*: after injection into the left coronary widespread opacification of the left ventricle walls is observed except for the posterior portion of the interventricular septum and part of the inferior wall. Note the opacification of both the papillary muscles, of the trabecula and of part of the free wall of the right ventricle. Panel *(3)*: left coronary arteriography showing the large extension of the left vascular bed accounting for the perfusional findings.

able to suppose, these bubbles are trapped by the larger vessels, there would thus be fewer of them in the myocardial regions where the overlapping of two coronary circulations leads to a relative reduction of vessels of larger diameter coming from a single coronary. However this finding could be more easily explained by an artifact of imaging noted in all short axis views at the lateral edge of the sector. In fact, in conditions in which the resolution of the images is much better, as with the use of transesophageal probes, opacification of the lateral wall appears to be superimposable to that of the septum during injection in the left coronary (Figure 2). In Griffin's same study, 6 patients had a just slightly opacified inferior wall after left intracoronary injection even though angiography did not show up a collateral circulation in any of them.

The results of Feinstein and Griffin's studies show that while a general perfusion pattern can be expected by the epicardial distribution of the coronaries, there is a considerable variability in perfusion distribution among the individual patients. Thus contrast echocardiography gives information on myocardial perfusion which cannot be had from coronary angiography. It is likely that this information can help one to better understand the physiopathology of an individual's particular coronary disease and therefore help to guide therapeutic choices. Goldman and Mindich [16] used spontaneous opacification of the myocardium after infusion of cardioplegia solution to identify the areas most at risk of ischemia during open heart surgery. In 30 patients with coronary artery disease who underwent aorta-coronary by-pass surgery and in 12 patients who had open heart surgery for other reasons (the control group) an echocardiogram was recorded during infusion of the cardioplegia solution into the aortic root. In the patients without coronary stenosis in the short axis plane taken at the level of the papillary muscles, the myocardium opacified evenly. Dividing the short axis of the left ventricle into three regions corresponding to the areas of distribution of the three main coronary branches (anterolateral for the circumflex, septal for the anterior descending and inferior for the right coronary) showed, on the contrary, either no or poor echocardiographic opacification of myocardial areas where there were significant stenoses of the feeding coronaries. This information may have two important practical applications in:

- identifying the areas where the cardioplegia may be incomplete because not enough solution reaches it;
- guiding the heart surgeon in deciding on the priority of grafts.

However, we and others have been unable to reproduce Goldman's findings of consistent myocardial opacification with cardioplagia solution alone, and we feel addition of some further contrast agent is needed in order to reproducibly opacify the myocardium in the operating room. In a more recent study [17], the selective intracoronary injection of echocontrast made it possible to identify the area at risk of dyskinesia during angioplasty, thus demonstrating that in humans too the opacified areas do actually correspond to the regions perfused by the injected coronary. Figure 3 shows an example in

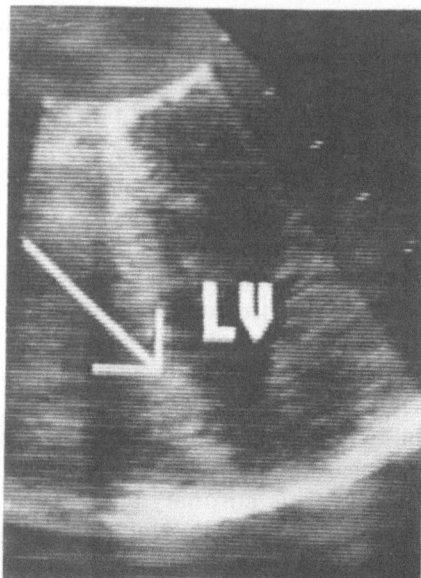
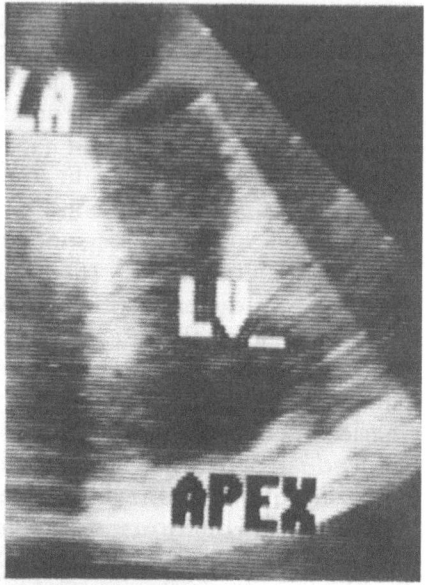
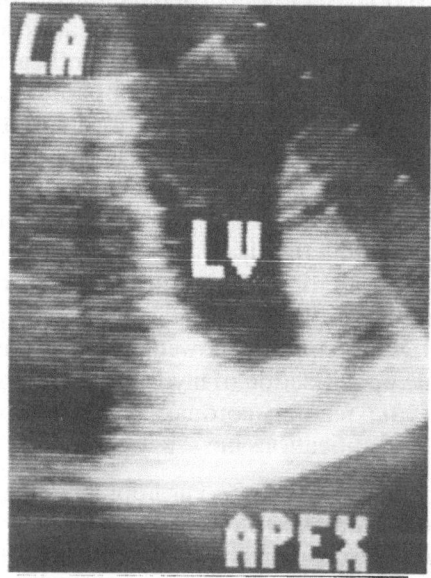

Figure 2. 3-Panel view of transesophageal echocardiogram in a dog subjected to transient occlusion of the LAD. Panel *(1)*: preocclusion. Injection of intracoronary sonicated Renografin contrast into the left coronary artery. The apex is indicated by an arrow. The brighter area within the outer sector represents an electronic 'area of interest' for tissue characterization studies. Panel *(2)*: several minutes after mid-Lad occlusion, after an injection of contrast into the left coronary orifice. Note opacification of the proximal interventricular septum (presumably from the proximal LAD). The apex is dyskinetic and shows a lack of perfusion. Panel *(3)*: several minutes after release of the mid-LAD occlusion, after an identical injection of contrast into the left coronary orifice. Note reactive hyperemia of the formerly non-perfused LV apex, which was also hypokinetic when viewed in real time.

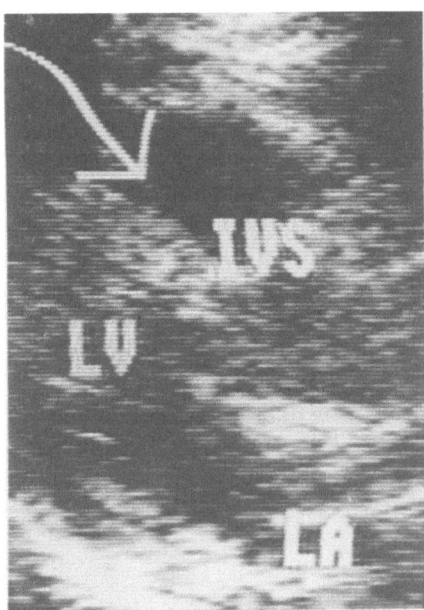 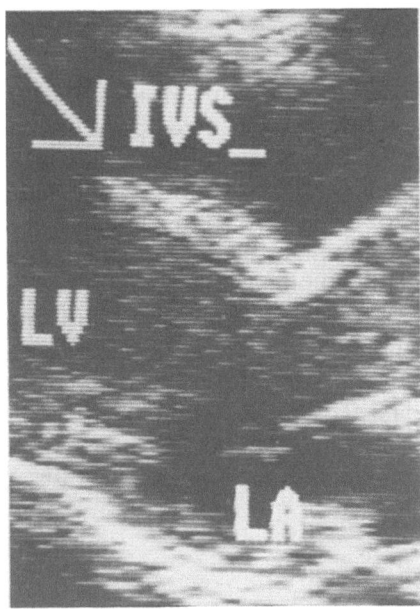

Figure 3. Stop-frame photographs performed in the catheterization laboratory in a patient pre- and post-angioplasty of a high grade proximal LAD lesion. Parasternal long axis view pre-angioplasty *(left panel)*: the proximal interventricular septum did not opacify after injection of sonicated 5% human albumin into the left coronary artery. Post-angioplasty *(right panel)*: after successful angioplasty, the proximal interventricular septum now opacifies with an identical injection of sonicated albumin into the left coronary orifice, implying better perfusion of the LAD perfusion bed.

which contrast echocardiography has enabled the LAD perfusional bed to be visualized and at the same time the efficacy of the angioplasty performed on the vessel to be assessed.

An important aspect of the physiopathology of coronary artery disease which contrast echocardiography helps study is the evaluation of collateral blood flow and myocardial microcirculation kinetics. Widimsky et al. [18] report two cases which are similar in their clinical characteristics but which have quite different perfusion conditions. Both patients had had an antero-septal infarction. In one coronary angiography showed two severe stenoses on the anterior descending with a collateral circulation between the distal portion of these stenoses and the right coronary. In the other patient, who had undergone angioplasty, the anterior descending was pervious. Injecting the echocontrast into the right coronary showed, in the former case, an opacification of the interventricular septum whereas, in the second case, the septum was not opacified either by left or by right intracoronary injection. Evidently, in the first case the tissue was vital and there was an active microcirculation around the interventricular septum whereas, in the second case, even though the coronaries were pervious there was no useful perfusion.

Conclusions

Myocardial perfusion is no longer just an interesting physiologic variable for those working in research laboratories. New pathophysiological entities in coronary artery disease such as myocardial stunning and hybernating myocardium [19] have moved the clinician's attention towards myocardial perfusion and the need to be able to discriminate between similar clinical situations which might be different in their anatomo-functional substrate. A method of assessing the significance of collateral circulation is needed. Myocardial contrast echocardiography gives information of myocardial perfusion, which, though it can be correlated with coronary anatomy, usefully complements the morphological data obtained by coronary angiography. Its relatively low cost and feasibility with respect to other more sophisticated methods may, in the future, help it to become more widely used in the overall evaluation of patients with coronary artery disease.

References

1. Zir LM, Miller SW, Dinsmore RE, Gilbert JP, Harthorne JW (1976) Interobserver variability in coronary angiography. *Circulation* 53: 627–632.
2. De Rouen TA, Murray JA, Owen W (1977) Variability in the analysis of coronary arteriograms. *Circulation* 55: 324–328.
3. Levine RA, Teichholz LE, Goldman ME, Steinmetz MY, Baker M, Meltzer RS (1984) Microbubbles have intracardiac velocities similar to those of red blood cells. *J Am Coll Cardiol* 3: 28–33.
4. Armstrong WF, Mueller TM, Kinney EL, Thickner EG, Dillon JC, Feigenbaum H (1982) Assessment of myocardial perfusion abnormalities with contrast enhanced two-dimensional echocardiography. *Circulation* 66: 166–173.
5. Tei C, Sakamaki T, Shah PM, Meerbaum S, Shimoura K, Kondo S, Corday E (1983) Myocardial contrast echocardiography: Reproducible technique of myocardial opacification for identifying regional perfusion deficits. *Circulation* 67: 585–592.
6. Kemper AJ, O'Boyle JE, Sharma S, Cohen CA, Kloner RA, Khuri SF, Parisi AF (1983) Hydrogen peroxide contrast-enhanced two-dimensional echocardiography: Real-time in vivo delineation of regional myocardial perfusion. *Circulation* 68: 603–611.
7. Sakamaki T, Tei C, Meerbaum S, Shimoura K, Kondo S, Fishbein MC, Y-Rit J, Shah PM, Corday E (1984) Verification of myocardial contrast two-dimensional echocardiography assessment of perfusion defects in ischemic myocardium. *J Am Coll Cardiol* 3: 34–38.
8. Armstrong WF, West SR, Dillon JC, Feigenbaum H (1984) Assessment of location and size of myocardial infarction with contrast enhanced echocardiography. II. Application of digital imaging techniques. *J Am Coll Card* 4: 141–148.
9. Moore CA, Smucker LM, Kaul S (1986) Myocardial contrast echocardiography in humans. I. Safety – A comparison with routine coronary arteriography. *J Am Coll Cardiol* 8: 1066–1072.
10. Santoso T, Roelandt J, Mansyoer H, Abdurahaman N, Meltzer RS (1985) Myocardial perfusion imaging in humans by contrast echocardiography using polygelin colloid solution. *J Am Coll Cardiol* 6: 612–620.
11. Gillam LD, Kaul S, Fallon JT, Levine RA, Hedley-White ET, Guerrero JL, Weyman AE (1985) Functional and pathologic effects of multiple echocardiographic contrast injections on the myocardium, brain and kidney. *J Am Coll Cardiol* 6: 687–694.

12. Lang RM, Borow KM, Neumann A, Feinstein SB (1987) Echocardiographic contrast agents: Effects of microbubbles and carrier solutions on left ventricular contractility. *J Am Coll Cardiol* 9: 910–919.

13. Shapiro JR, Xie F, Meltzer RS (1988) Myocardial contrast two-dimensional echocardiography: Dose-myocardial effect relations of intracoronary microbubbles. *J Am Coll Cardiol* 12: 765–771.

14. Feinstein SB, Lang RM, Dick C, Neumann A, Al-Sadir J, Chua KG, Carroll J, Feldman T, Borow KM (1988) Contrast echocardiography during coronary arteriography in humans: Perfusion and anatomic studies. *J Am Coll Cardiol* 11: 59–65.

15. Griffin B, Timmis AD, Sowton E (1987) Contrast perfusion echocardiography: Distribution and reproducibility of myocardial contrast enhancement in coronary artery disease. *Am J Cardiol* 60: 538–543.

16. Goldman ME, Mindich BP (1984) Intraoperative cardioplegic contrast echocardiography for assessing myocardial perfusion during open heart surgery. *J Am Coll Cardiol* 4: 1029–1034.

17. Griffin B, Timmis AB, Henderson RA, Sowton E (1987) Contrast perfusion echocardiography: Identification of area at risk of dyskinesia during percutaneous transluminal coronary angioplasty. *Am Heart J* 114: 497–502.

18. Widimsky P, Cornel JH, Ten Cate FJ (1988) Evaluation of collateral blood flow by myocardial contrast enhanced echocardiography. *Br Heart J* 59: 20–22.

19. Braunwald E, Rutherford JD (1986) Reversible ischemic left ventricular dysfunction: Evidence for 'hybernating myocardium'. *J Am Coll Cardiol* 6: 1467–1470.

30. Physiological heterogeneity of coronary blood flow in space and time by contrast echocardiography

DANIELE ROVAI, MASSIMO LOMBARDI,
STEVEN E. NISSEN, MARIO MARZILLI,
ALESSANDRO DISTANTE, LUIGI TADDEI,
ANTHONY N. DeMARIA and ANTONIO L'ABBATE

Introduction

Coronary blood flow and resistances

It is well recognized that blood flow at the inlet of the coronary system varies during the cardiac cycle, being higher during diastole than during systole. This is due to the generation of intramyocardial pressure during cardiac contraction, which limits coronary blood flow [1]. The flow, in fact, is inversely related to coronary resistance, an entity which in turn is comprised of 3 factors: viscous resistance, auto-regulatory resistance and compressive resistance [2]. The latter determinant is related to the compression of intramural vessels due to intramyocardial pressure and is characterized by both spatial and temporal heterogenity [3–5]. In fact, compressive resistance is three to four times higher during systole than in diastole, and it increases progressively from outer to the inner myocardial layers. As a result of compressive resistance, systolic perfusion would be anticipated to be predominantly subepicardial, and blood flow could even cease during systole in the inner portion of sub-endocardial layers [6, 7].

Myocardial perfusion and coronary resistances: The apparent contradiction

Experimental studies, based on radionuclide labelled microsphere techniques, have indicated that the blood flow per gram of subendocardial myocardium is equal to or slightly greater than blood flow per gram of subepicardial myocardium [8, 9]. The apparent contradiction between the equality of subendo and subepicardial blood flow despite greater compressive resistance on the inner myocardial layer may be related to reduced autoregulatory resistances or greater vasculatiry in the subendocardium [10–12] than in the subepicardium.

S. Iliceto et al. (eds.), Ultrasound in Coronary Artery Disease, 377–387.
© 1991 *Kluwer Academic Publishers.*

Radionuclyde labelled microspheres: Experimental models

In the animal models previously developed to study this issue by labelled microspheres, coronary perfusion was limited to the systolic phase by either creating acute aortic insufficiency [13], perfusing the coronary tree through the left ventricle [14], or limiting coronary perfusion to systole using ECG-triggered coronary occluders [15]. These unphysiological experimental models were designed in order to overcome the problem of integrated distribution of labelled microspheres over a relatively high number of cardiac cicles without possibility of distinguishing between systole and diastole [16]. The ability to conclude from such models on the systo-diastolic distribution of myocardial blood flow is questionable. In fact, limiting myocardial perfusion to either systole or diastole at the level of coronary arteries does not necessarily result in an exclusively systolic or diastolic microsphere distribution at the capillary level, due to the capacitance of the large epicardial coronary vessels.

Myocardial contrast echocardiography: The alternative tool

Several recent studies have demonstrated the ability to evaluate the spatial distribution of myocardial perfusion by contrast echocardiography. Specifically, the accuracy of contrast echocardiography in assessing the extent of at risk and necrotic myocardial areas following coronary occlusion is high [17–23], the intra- and interobserver variability of the measurements are low [19, 20, 22] and the findings are reproducible from injection to injection [19, 22]. Additionally, myocardial contrast echocardiography has been found to permit in vivo imaging of the transmural extent of myocardial infarction [24] and of the relative subendocardial underperfusion of pacing induced myocardial ischemia in men [25].

Myocardial contrast appearance: The working hipothesis

The approach used in this study to examine transmural myocardial blood flow is based on the analysis of the frames of initial myocardial contrast appearance. We have chosen to study contrast appearance, instead of contrast washout, to avoid the changes in coronary blood flow (reduction in flow and hyperemic effect) induced by echocardiographic contrast agents crossing the coronary microcirculation [26]. By chance, echocardiographic contrast agent can reach the myocardium in systole or in diastole. If the preceding end-diastolic or end-systolic frame is subtracted from the corresponding one at contrast appearance, resulting contrast distribution should reflect the diastolic or systolic distribution of myocardial perfusion, respectively, as schematically shown in Figure 1.

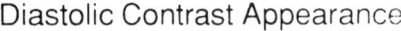

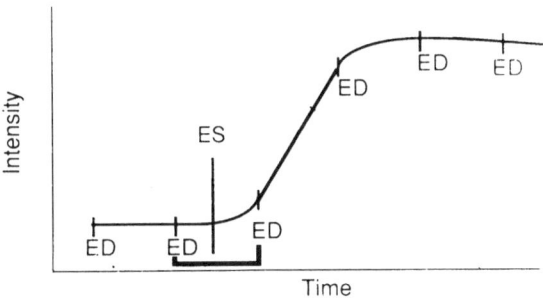

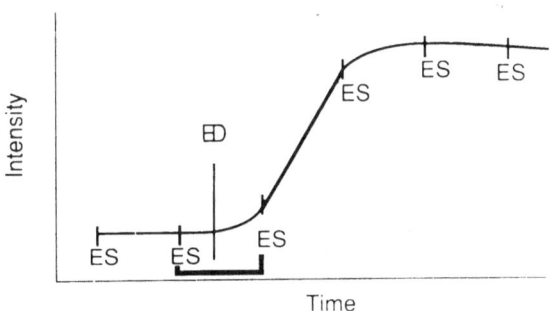

Figure 1. Schematic diagram of myocardial contrast appearance, occurring in diastole (ED) (upper panel) and in systole (ES) (lower panel). (With kind permission of *Circulation* 79: 185.)

Experimental animal preparation

The study was performed in 7 anesthetized mongrel dogs, intubated and ventilated. A left thoracotomy was performed and the pericardium excised. An electromagnetic flowmeter was implanted on the isolated left anterior descending (2 dogs) or circumflex (1 dog) coronary arteries. Via left carotid artery, a 5 F catheter was advanced to subselectively cannulate the isolated coronary artery and was used for contrast injection. To eliminate the possible influence of the intracoronary catheter on coronary perfusion pressure and blood flow, the echo contrast agent was injected into the aortic root by an 8 French pigtail catheter in 4 additional dogs. To measure aortic pressure, a Millar catheter (5 F) was advanced into the abdominal aorta. Before and during intracoronary injection of contrast, coronary blood flow, aortic pressure and an ECG lead were recorded on paper.

Echocardiographic examination

The dogs were studied in right lateral decubitus position on a table with a cutout corresponding to the heart region to facilitate echocardiographic examination. Two-dimensional echocardiograms were obtained utilyzing two electronic sector scanners (PASS I, General Electric or Hewlett Packard 77020) operating at 3.3 MHz and 3.5 MHz, respectively. The transducer was positioned on the right side of the chest, at the point of maximal cardiac pulsation and held in a fixed position of the optimal view by a mechanical sidearm. To minimize motion of the heart, the respirator was turned off immediately before injecting the echo contrast agent and restarted after a few seconds. Gain setting controls were adjusted on the basis of a subjective analysis, maintaining the amplification low enough to avoid the saturation during contrast effect. Once an optimal gain setting was chosen for each dog, it was unchanged during each study. Echocardiographic images were recorded on videotape-recorders for subsequent playback and analysis.

Echocardiographic contrast agent

The polysaccharide contrast agent SHU-454 was used in all experiments [27]. The agent consists of a milky solution containing microbubbles of a median diameter of 3.2 μm and microparticles of a median diameter of 3 μm [28]. In 3 dogs, this solution was injected into the cannulated coronary artery by an ECG-triggered injector apparatus (Angiomat 3000, Cordis). The injections began with the R wave of the electrocardiogram and lasted 1 sec at a flow rate of 2 ml/sec. In 4 dogs, 10 ml of contrast were injected into the aorta in one sec by a injector apparatus (Contrac, Conraves AG Zurich) without any ECG synchronization.

Analog to digital conversion

Echocardiographic images were digitized off-line by means of an array processor-based system for medical image processing: Mipron (Kontron, FRG). A 256×256 pixel matrix with 256 gray levels was used. Digitization included at least 4 beats preceding visual myocardial contrast appearance up to peak contrast intensity, for a total of at least 12 consecutive cardiac cycles. End-diastolic and end-systolic images were identified and were ordered in two separate temporal sequences. End-diastolic and end-systolic images were also digitally subtracted from the same frames of subsequent cardiac cycles to confirm the data regarding initial appearance and transmural distribution of contrast obtained by videodensitometry of unsubtracted images (vide infra).

Identification of contrast appearance

The two sequences of raw echocardiographic images, corresponding to end-systole and end-diastole, were reviewed in cine-loops and the ventricular wall which showed the best myocardial opacification was identified. In every end-diastolic and end-systolic image of each sequence a region of interest corresponding to this wall was traced. The same circumferential extension was maintained both in end-diastolic and in end-systolic images. Myocardial regions corresponding to the area of lateral drop-outs and to the posterior interface of the left ventricle with the lungs were not included in the measurements. When papillary muscles happened to be in the best opacified wall, they were included into the analysis. The mean videodensity inside the regions of interest was measured. Intensity values were plotted against time to obtain time-intensity curves. For each curve a mean background value and its 99% confidence limits were calculated for both diastole and systole on the basis of the initial four beats. The upper confidence limit was used as threshold and the first diastolic or systolic frame above threshold was identified and considered the one of contrast appearance.

Videodensitometry

The frame of initial contrast appearance (diastole or systole) and the immediately preceding one of the same phase of the cardiac cycle (diastole or systole) were sampled. In these frames, the region of interest was manually divided into 3 parallel layers of equal thickness, corresponding to the sub-endocardial, mid- and subepicardial myocardium. The mean intensity value of each layer was measured. The increment in videodensity for endo-, mid- and epicardial myocardium was calculated by subtracting, from the intensity values of the frame of contrast appearance, those of the previous frame of the same phase of the cardiac cycle. The increments were then normalized to the increment in videodensity of the entire wall and expressed as % change. The difference between increments in videodensity in the endo-, mid-, and epicardial myocardium in end-diastolic and end-systolic images was tested by the analysis of variance, multiple comparison procedure. Figure 2 shows the temporal sequence of changes in videodensity for the 3 myocardial layers in a case of systolic contrast appearance. For display purposes videodensity measurements were extended to several frames of the sequence.

Myocardial contrast effect: Feasibility

In the 7 dogs, injections of echo contrast agent were performed either intra-coronary (3 dogs) or into the aortic root (4 dogs). All intracoronary contrast injections produced obvious myocardial echo enhancement by visual examination. However, because of the possible influence of the contrast agent on myocardial blood flow distribution, only the first 2–3 injections in each dog made directly into the coronaries were analyzed, for a total of 7 injections in 3 dogs. Good myocardial opacification was also obtained in 17 aortic injections in 4 dogs. When a suboptimal contrast effect was produced, it was attributed

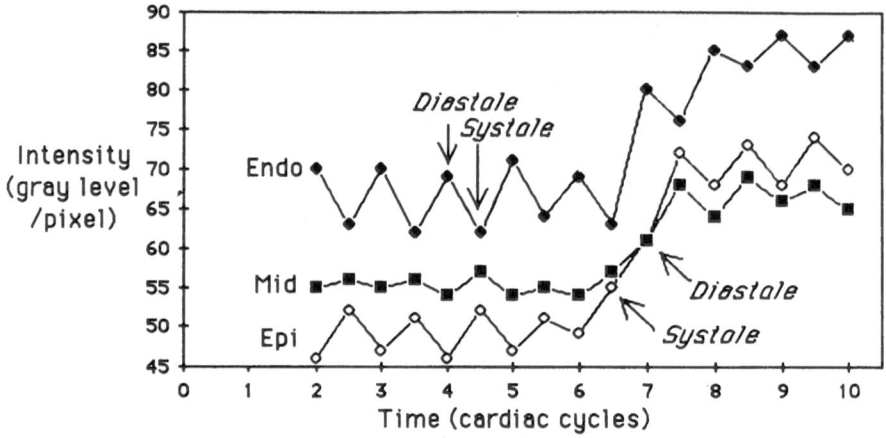

Figure 2. Time-Intensity curves of myocardial contrast appearance for the three myocardial layers. The echo contrast agent was injected into the left anterior descending coronary artery and the curve derived from the interventricular septum. The initial contrast effect appeared in systole (arrow) and was recorded in the subepicardium (EPI). In the following diastole (arrow) the videodensity of the subendocardium (ENDO) increased more than that of other myocardial layers. MID = midmyocardium. (With kind permission of *Circulation* 79: 183.)

to the position of the catheter, which was readjusted for the subsequent injections. These suboptimal injections were not considered in this study.

Contrast distribution to the ventricular walls

The myocardial distribution of echocardiographic contrast effect in the initial cardiac cycle of appearance varied according to the site of contrast injection. When the contrast was injected subselectively into the left anterior descending coronary artery (5 situations), the anteroseptal wall was the best opacified one; when injection was performed into the circumflex coronary artery (2 situations), the lateral wall was the best opacified one. Despite the site of injection, the echo contrast effect was distributed diffusely throughout the myocardium by the second cardiac cycle. This generalized distribution with intracoronary injections was attributed to the injection rate used (2 ml/sec), which probably exceeded the left anterior descending or circumflex coronary blood flow and caused reflux of contrast and enhancement of the myocardial areas perfused by the non-cannulated vessel. In the case of injections into the aortic root, the antero-septal and lateral wall were considered the best opacified walls in 9 and 3 situations, respectively, while the entire ventricular circumference was opacified uniformly in 5 injections. Initial opacification was identified during diastole in 12 injections and during systole in 12.

Transmural distribution of the contrast effect

At initial appearance, the transmural distribution of myocardial contrast

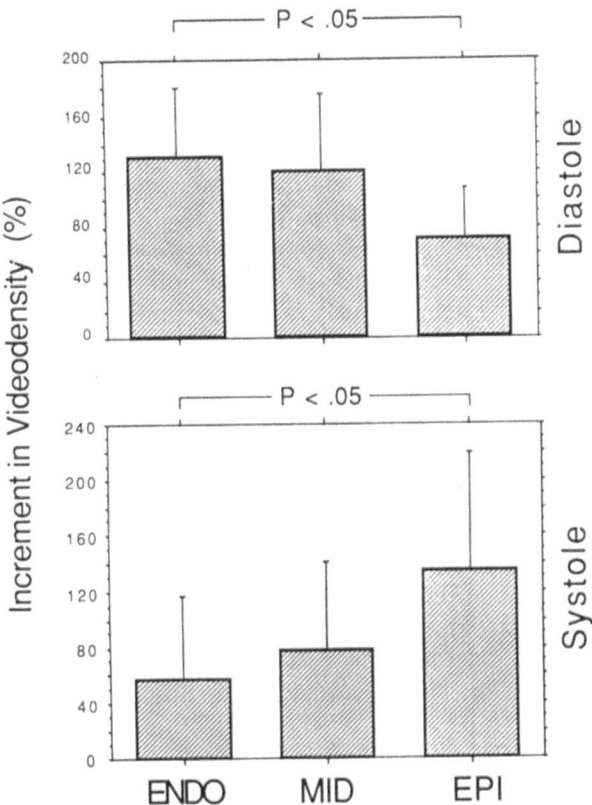

Figure 3. Transmural distribution of the increment in videointensity in the frames of first echo contrast appearance. Upper panel corresponds to the cases of diastolic contrast appearance, lower panel to the cases to systolic appearance. Each column represent the mean +1 standard deviation of the normalized increments in the subendocardium (ENDO), MID and subepicardium (EPI). (With kind permission of *Circulation* 79: 183.)

effect was different for the individual phases of the cardiac cycle. As shown in Figure 3 (upper panel) when the contrast initially appeared in diastole the increment in videodensity was significantly higher in the subendocardium $(131 \pm 48\%)$ than in the subepicardium $(71 \pm 37\%$ of the increment in videodensity of the entire wall), $p < 0.05$ by Anova. The increment in videodensity of the midmyocardium was intermediate in magnitude but was not significantly different from either of the other two layers $(119 \pm 56\%)$. In the injections in which the contrast initially appeared in systole (Figure 3 lower panel) the subepicardium exhibited a higher increment in videodensity $(136 \pm 83\%)$ than the subendocardium $(60 \pm 60\%$ of the increment in videodensity of the entire wall), $P < 0.05$ by Anova. For systolic frames too, the increment in videodensity of the midmyocardium was not significantly different from either of the other two layers (80 ± 61).

Limitations of the study

Recent studies have shown that the distribution of myocardial opacification by contrast echocardiography may be influenced by the site of injection of the contrast agent [29]. Thus, the area at risk was slightly but significantly larger when the contrast agent was injected into the occluded vessel ('positive risk area') than when it was injected proximally to the occlusion ('negative risk area'). Such variability was not a factor in the present study, however, since the same site of injection was used to evaluate both subendocardial and subepicardial perfusion which appeared as 'positive areas'.

A series of factors intrinsic to ultrasound imaging technique and unrelated to the anatomic distribution of contrast agent may influence gray level variability in contrast-enhanced echocardiographic images [30, 31]. Prominent among these is the attenuation of the transmitted ultrasound energy as it traverses tissue structures. Attenuation did not contribute to our findings, however, since the transmural distribution of contrast followed the same pattern regardless of the segment perfused (septal, anterior or lateral) and its spatial relationship with the ultrasound beam. Ultrasonic artifacts and riverberations could have confounded the findings of this study, particularly in regard to the lateral wall of the left ventricle. However, such artifacts would be expected to be both systolic and diastolic.

It is possible that the subepicardial contrast distribution, when appearing in systole at the first beat, might reflect opacification of large epicardial capacitance vessels [32]. Whenever contrast effect was observed in the shape of a streak of opacification – suggesting the opacification of a major coronary vessel – the image was not considered for densitometric analysis. However the possibility that phasic distribution of contrast appearance could reflect arterial intramiocardial capacitance distribution rather than capillary flow cannot be ruled out.

An open chest preparation, per se, might have partially influenced the transmural distribution of coronary blood flow during the cardiac cycle, because of the lack of normal intrapericardial or intrapleural pressure. The reported results, in addition, are relative to the studied section of the left ventricle, at the level of papillary muscles, and do not necessarily apply to different sections in the apex to base direction.

We considered the possibility that the intracoronary position of the catheter or the injection pressure may have influenced the results we observed. However, analysis of images derived by aortic injection confirms that the heterogeneous distribution – both spatial and temporal – of the contrast effect is purely physiologic and independent of the methodology.

The contrast agent utilized, SHU-454, was chosen since it is superior to the usually employed clinical agents in the production of contrast effect inside the cardiac chambers and has been shown to be more reproducible in contrast intensity created [27]. The agent itself may have been capable of influencing coronary flow by trapping of gas bubbles or microparticles. However, the latter effect would be expected to affect disappearance phenomena, but not the appearance characteristics catalogued in this study. A similar consideration applies to the stability of the agent. In previous studies the spontaneous disappearance of the contrast was studied in a closed, flowing, in vitro system and 90% of the peak contrast activity was present for 6 sec after injection [33]. The time interval in which myocardial blood flow distribution was evaluated in this study (one cardiac cycle) is therefore well within the time of contrast stability. Additionally, in each injection a new vial of agent was used and the solution was injected immediately after preparation. Finally, the difference in contrast effect between endo- and epicardial layers was relatively small, similar to findings by radionuclide techniques, and requires computer analysis of videointensity for accurate detection.

Contrast echocardiography versus radionuclyde labelled microspheres

Contrast-echocardiography has several advantages in the study of the transmural distribution of myocardial perfusion. In vivo imaging is possible, whereas with the labelled microsphere technique a post-mortem analysis must be carried out. In addition, the temporal resolution of contrast-echo imaging is high: 30 frames per sec at the depth setting utilized in this study. This high temporal resolution makes possible to study differences in the transmural distribution of coronary perfusion occurring within a cardiac cycle. Finally, as a tomographic imaging techniques, echocardiography is particularly well suited to study different characteristics of the various layers of myocardium, and is superior to the spatial resolution of in vivo nuclear medicine techniques.

Conclusions

This study demonstrates that the myocardial distribution of the echo contrast agent SHU-454 is heterogeneous both in time and space, being primarily subendocardial during diastole and primarily subepicardial during systole. Since previous studies have demonstrated that the distribution of the myocardial contrast effect reflects the distribution of myocardial perfusion [18–23], this study documents the physiological heterogeneity of coronary blood flow in the space and time domain during the cardiac cycle.

Acknowledgement

Supported by a CNR-NATO Fellowship and by a VA Merit Review. This is Grant Number 596-76-9148-001.

References

1. Sabiston DC Jr, Gregg DE (1957) Effect of cardiac contraction on coronary blood flow. *Circulation* 15: 14.
2. Klocke FJ (1976) Coronary blood flow in man. *Prog Cardiovas Dis* 19: 117.
3. Armour JA, Randall WC (1971) Canine left ventricular intramyocardial pressures. *Am J Physiol* 220: 1833.
4. Sestier FJ, Mildenberger RR, Klassen GA (1978) Role of autoregulation in spatial and temporal perfusion heterogeneity of canine myocardium. *Am J Physiol* 71: 235.
5. Stein PD, Marzilli M, Sabbah HN, Lee T (1980) Systolic and diastolic pressure gradients within the left ventricular wall. *Am J Physiol* 238: H625.
6. L'Abbate A, Marzilli M, Ballestra AM, Camici P (1978) Myocardial contraction: An additional determinant of transmural flow distribution, in: Maseri A, Klassen GA, Lesch M (eds), *Primary and Secondary Angina Pectoris*, p 21. New York: Grune & Stratton.
7. Marzilli M, Goldstein S, Sabbah HN, Lee T, Stein PD (1979) Modulating effect of regional myocardial performance on local myocardial perfusion in the dog. *Circ Res* 45: 634.
8. Moir TW (1972) Subendocardial distribution of coronary blood flow and the effect of antianginal drugs. *Circ Res* 30: 621.
9. Hoffman JIE, Buckberg GD (1976) Transmural variation in myocardial perfusion, in: Yu PN, Goodwin JF (eds), *Progress in Cardiology*, p 37. Philadelphia: Lea & Febiger.
10. Myers WW, Honig CR (1964) Number and distribution of capillaries as determinants of myocardial oxigen tension. *Am J Physiol* 207: 653.
11. Winbury MM, Weiss HR (1974) Nitroglicerin and Chromonar on small-vessel blood content of the ventricular walls. *Am J Physiol* 226: 838.
12. L'Abbate A, Marzilli M, Ballestra AM, Camici P, Trivella MG, Pelosi G, Klassen G (1980) Opposite transmural gradients of coronary resistance and extravascular pressure in the working dog's heart. *Cardiovas Res* 14: 21.
13. Rembert JC, Greenfield JC Jr, Alexander JA, Cobb FR (1978) Transmural distribution of systolic myocardial blood flow in the awake dog, in: Baan J. Noordergraaf A, Raines J (eds), *Cardiovascular System Dynamics*, p 40. Cambridge: Massachussets, The MIT Press.
14. Downey JM, Kirk ES (1974) Distribution of the coronary blood flow across the canine heart wall during systole. *Circ Res* 34: 251.
15. Hess DS, Bache RJ (1976) Transmural distribution of myocardial blood flow during systole in the awake dog. *Circ Res* 38: 5.
16. Heyman MA, Payne BD, Hoffman JIE, Rudolph AM (1977) Blood flow measurements with radionuclide-labelled particles. *Prog Cardiovasc Dis* 20: 55.
17. DeMaria AN, Bommer WJ, Riggs K, Dajee A, Keown M, Kwan OL, Mason DT (1980) Echocardiographic visualization of myocardial perfusion by left heart and intracoronary injections of echo contrast agents. *Circulation* 62 (suppl III): III–143.
18. Armstrong WF, Mueller TM, Kinney EL, Tickner EG, Dillon JC, Feigenbaum H (1982) Assessment of myocardial perfusion abnormalities with contrast-enhanced two-dimensional echocardiography. *Circulation* 66: 166.
19. Tei C, Sakamaki T, Shah PM, Meerbaum S, Shimoura K, Kondo S, Corday E (1983) Myocardial contrast echocardiography: A reproducible technique of myocardial opacification for identifying regional perfusion deficits. *Circulation* 67: 585.
20. Kemper AJ, O'Boyle JE, Sharma S, Cohen CA, Kloner RA, Khuri SF, Parisi AF (1983) Hydrogen peroxide contrast-enhanced Two-dimensional echocardiography real time in vivo delineation of regional myocardial perfusion. *Circulation* 68: 603.
21. Sakamaki T, Tei C, Meerbaum S, Shimour K, Kondo S, Fishbein MC, Y-Rit J, Shah PM, Corday E (1984) Verification of myocardial contrast two-dimensional echocardiographic assessment of perfusion defects in ischemic myocardium. *J Am Coll Cardiol* 3: 34.
22. Kaul S, Pandian NG, Okada RD, Pohost GM, Weyman AE (1984) Contrast echocardiography in acute myocardial ischemia. I. In vivo determination of total left ventricular 'area at risk'. *J Am Coll Cardiol* 4: 1272.

23. Armstrong WF, West SR, Dillon JC, Feigenbaum H (1984) Assessment of localization and size of myocardial infarction with contrast-enhanced echocardiography. II. Application of digital imaging techniques. *J Am Coll Cardiol* 4: 141.
24. Kemper AJ, Force T, Perkins L, Gilfoil M, Parisi AF (1986) In vivo prediction of the transmural extent of experimental acute myocardial infarction using contrast echocardiography. *J Am Coll Cardiol* 8: 143.
25. Lim YJ, Nanto S, Masuyama T, Kodama K, Ikeda T, Kitabatake A, Kamada T (1989) Visualization of subendocardial myocardial ischemia with myocardial contrast echocardiography in humans. *Circulation* 79: 233.
26. Kondo S, Tei C, Meerbaum S, Corday E, Shah PM (1984) Hyperemic response of intracoronary contrast agents during two-dimensional echographic delineation of regional myocardium. *J Amer Coll Cardiol* 4: 149.
27. Smith MD, Kwan OL, Reiser J, DeMaria AN (1984) Superior Intensity and reproducibility of SHU-454, a new right heart contrast agent. *J Am Coll Cardiol* 3: 992.
28. Schartl M, Fritsch T, Miszalok V (1986) Quantification of myocardial perfusion by contrast echocardiography. *Can J Cardiol* (suppl A): 25A.
29. Kaul S, Gillam LD, Weiman AE (1985) Contrast echocardiography in acute myocardial ischemia. II. The effect of site of injection of contrast agent on the estimation of area at risk for necrosis after coronary occlusion. *J Am Coll Cardiol* 6: 825.
30. Zwehl W, Areeda J, Schwartz G, Feinstein S, Ong K, Meerbaum S (1984) Physical factors influencing quantitation of two-dimensional contrast-echo amplitudes. *J Am Coll Cardiol* 4: 157.
31. Taylor AL, Collins SM, Skorton DJ, Kieso RA, Melton J, Kerber RE (1985) Artifactual regional gray level variability in contrast-enhanced two-dimensional echocardiographic images: Effect on measurement of the coronary perfusion bed. *J Am Coll Cardiol* 6: 831.
32. Goldman ME, Mindich BP (1984) Intraoperative cardioplegic contrast echocardiography for assessing myocardial perfusion during open heart surgery. *J Am Coll Cardiol* 4: 1029.
33. Rovai D, Nissen SE, Elion JE, Smith M, L'Abbate A, Kwan OL, DeMaria AN (1987) Contrast echo washout curves from the left ventricle: Application of basic principles of indicator-dilution theory and calculation of ejection fraction. *J Am Coll Cardiol* 10: 125.

31. Myocardial contrast echocardiography for the evaluation of coronary flow reserve
Potential and limitations

ANTONIO F. AMICO, SABINO ILICETO, LUCIA SUBLIMI
SAPONETTI, CATALDO MEMMOLA, PAOLO RIZZON

Introduction

Coronary angiography is the current 'gold standard' in the evaluation of the severity of coronary disease; the parameter usually adopted is the percent diameter of the visualized stenosis. The limitation of this approach is that it does not take into consideration other geometric features of the stenosis (such as the length and absolute value of the area of the lumen vessel at the point of the stenosis). In any case even an objective measurement of each of these parameters would not make it possible to predict the actual reduction in perfusion.

On the basis of the laws of hydrodynamics a physiological parameter has been suggested called 'coronary flow reserve' [1] which should be a sensitive indicator of the capacity of the coronary circulation to adapt to the oxygen requirements of the myocardium. By 'coronary flow reserve' is meant the difference between the coronary flow at rest and the maximal flow for a given perfusion pressure. Even though the coronary reserve can be reduced by numerous factors (blood viscosity, cardiac hypertrophy, heart frequency, increase in systolic pressure and myocardial contractility), the most immediate cause for its being altered is the presence of an obstacle to the coronary flow such as an atherosclerotic stenosis.

Evaluation of the coronary reserve in man

Unfortunately the quantitative evaluation of the coronary reserve pertains to experimental cardiology and is mostly carried out on animals. The methods so far put forward for the study of the coronary reserve in man have numerous disadvantages; digital subtraction angiography [2], even using intracoronary vasodilators like adenosine or papaverine have provided equivocal results [3, 4]; the Doppler technique with suction catheter can only be used during open heart surgery [5]; the intracoronary Doppler catheter is a highly invasive approach [6]. Both the Doppler techniques, moreover, can only

S. Iliceto et al. (eds.), Ultrasound in Coronary Artery Disease, 389–396.
© 1991 *Kluwer Academic Publishers.*

measure variations in velocity and not in actual flow, for which it is necessary to know the diameter of the vessel being explored.

A limitation of most of the measuring techniques for myocardial perfusion in man is the incapacity to evaluate separately the perfusion in the different layers of the myocardium. The alterations in transmural perfusion are very important for an understanding of the regulation of coronary circulation [7]. Moreover, the initial sign of an obstructive disease is the reduction exclusively in subendocardial perfusion [8]. Newer techniques which can make transmural perfusion evaluations are positron emission tomography [9] and single photon emission computed tomography (SPECT) [10]: the first still requires numerous technological improvements for it to be used extensively, though clinical studies have already been published [11]; the second requires even more sophisticated equipment and computers for processing the images than conventional myocardial scintigraphy; both are based on the use of radio-active materials.

Contrast echocardiography and myocardial perfusion quantitation

The visualization of myocardial perfusion with intracoronary injection of echocontrast agents has been reported since 1982 [12–14]. The large number of qualitative studies has, to some extent, supported the hypothesis that echocontrast agents can be used as myocardial perfusion indicators. The presence of an echocontrast agent inside the myocardium makes the image displayed by the echocardiographic equipment brighter. By plotting the intensity of this brightness versus time one obtains time-intensity curves which generally have a relatively steep upward slope followed by a peak and then a slower, less steep, downward part (Figure 1).

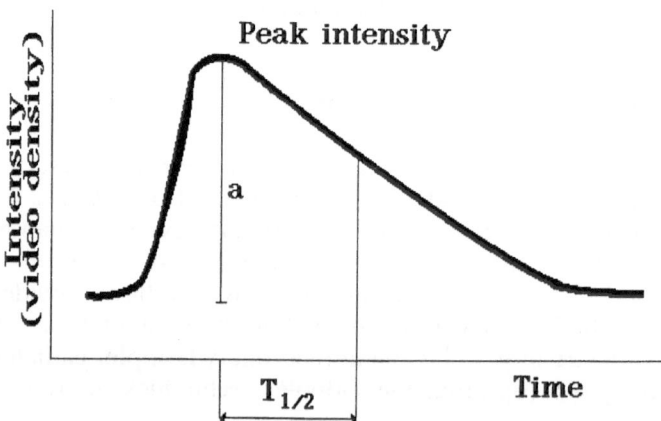

Fig. 1. Time-intensity curve obtained during a myocardial contrast perfusion study.

An initial attempt at correlating the brightness intensity peak (measured directly on the screen by a light meter) with absolute perfusion values obtained with radioactive microspheres was unsuccessful [12]. Subsequently, animal experiments done by Maurer et al. [15] enabled intensity-time curves to be obtained by digitizing the echocardiographic images and focusing their attention on the contrast wash-out phase. By assuming that the downward sloping part of the curve was monoexponential, it was possible to calculate the intensity half-life (t 1/2) by means of the formula:

$$t\,1/2 = \ln 2/k$$

where k is the coefficient of the curve obtained by logarithmically interpolating the downward slope. t 1/2 was calculated for normal flow conditions and also in the cases of an induced coronary stenosis of 85% and a coronary occlusion; in each condition, in order, t 1/2 was significantly greater. The authors concluded that this parameter can serve as an index for characterizing regional myocardial perfusion.

Tei et al. [16] obtained the same results in a similar experimental set-up. Ten Cate et al. [17] evaluated a series of parameters which can be obtained from the intensity-time curves in different conditions of coronary flow. They did not find any correlation between the peak of the curves and the coronary flow assessed by electromagnetic flow rate measurements. The other indices studied (time from the appearance of the contrast to the peak, t 1/2, total duration of the curve) were significantly modified by the changing coronary flow conditions. The only correlation coefficient they gave was between t 1/2 of the ischemic area and coronary flow: this coefficient had a very low ($r = 0.56$), even if significant, value.

Over the last few years there have been numerous scientific presentations on the subject. However, the data found in the literature are rather discordant. When the variations in the intensity-time curve peak have been compared with the variations in coronary flow, either positive correlations [18–23] or no correlation [17, 24–28] have been found. Similarly, both the area beneath the intensity-time curve and t 1/2 have not always given the same variations for different perfusion situations [19, 24, 29, 30–32]. A complex digital processing of the echocardiographic images has made it possible to diagnose myocardial hypoperfusion depending on the time it takes for the contrast to reach the inside of the myocardium [33, 34] but, at the same time, it has also revealed a spatial and temporal physiological heterogeneity of perfusion in the animal studied [35].

In conclusion, analysis of the intensity-time curve has not yet given satisfying results for the quantitation of myocardial perfusion by contrast echocardiography. There may be many different reasons for this: first of all, the parameters that have so far been adopted are based on the mathematical model behind the indicator dilution theory. Although this model has empirically proved to be efficient for calculating the left ventricular ejection fraction by means of contrast echocardiography [36], not enough is known about how echocontrast agents behave in the circulation and microcirculation to be able to state that this model is also valid for studying perfusion by means of this method. Even supposing that the indicator dilution theory holds for interpreting the intensity-time curves, some of the basic assumptions of this theory are not respected in most of the experimental situations (for example, the complete mixing of the indicator in the vascular compartment where the flow is to be calculated and the lack of influence of the indicator on the flow to be calculated). Finally, there is a series of technical problems due, in part, to the display of the echocardiographic images (non-linearity between the received and the displayed signal and the alterations of the image caused by smoothing, enhancement, etc.) and, in part, to the interaction between the echocontrast agent and the ultrasounds used to display them (like the absolute size and number of microbubbles injected) [37] which may seriously affect any quantitative parameter and the reproducibility of the video-densitometric data [38, 39].

Contrast echocardiography: Coronary reserve evaluation

The limitations regarding quantitation of myocardial perfusion by means of echocontrastography may not necessarily compromise a sufficient evaluation of the coronary reserve in clinical practice. To this end it is enough for an echocontrastographic parameter to present variations of the same size as the variations of the coronary flow in order to be able to discriminate those cases in which the incapacity of the coronary to vary within a wide range is indicative of a reduced coronary reserve. Cheirif et al. [40] have evaluated the variations of peak contrast intensity after intracoronary injection of papaverine in 40 patients and found that an increase in peak intensity not above 10 units was 80% sensitive and 92% specific for coronary artery disease. In the same study, however, the correlation between absolute change in peak intensity and the coronary angiographic cross sectional area and percent stenosis was only fair ($r = 0.58$).

Keller et al. [41] have carried out a quantitative analysis of the time-intensity curves, before and after papaverine intracoronary injection, obtained from the echocardiograms performed in dogs in which a critical stenosis had been created on a coronary branch. The area under the curve, peak contrast intensity and curve width did not correlate with absolute blood flows measured with radiolabelled microsphere. However, the ratios of the areas under the curves, derived from the 'normal' and 'hypoperfused' vascular bed, respectively, correlated well with the ratios of blood flows in the same myocardial region during each stage of the experiment.

A study conducted by Vandenberg et al. [28] highlighted the possibility of recognizing the areas with a 3.5 fold increase in coronary flow by using the maximal slope of the appearance curve of the contrast. This parameter showed excellent correlation with the percent changes of myocardial perfusion.

Cheirif et al. [42], in a model of critical coronary stenosis, have confirmed Keller's data, and found a significant correlation between percent change in myocardial flow and percent change in area under the curve. Likewise the ratios between area under the curves in the subendocardial and subepicardial halves correlated with the subendocardial and subepicardial flow ratios at baseline and after dipyridamole administration.

In conclusion myocardial contrast echocardiography seems to be able to differentiate the regions with normal increase in myocardial flow (obtainable with a powerful coronary vasodilator) from those supplied from a critically stenosed coronary in which there is no such increase. The accuracy of this evaluation still has to be tested: most experiments have been conducted on animals in whom it is possible to ascertain the increase of myocardial flow objectively. The lack of a true gold standard of measurement of the coronary reserve in humans makes it difficult to check the validity of the method in the clinical context. The presence of numerous variables which can affect the time intensity curve call for caution in analysing the experimental results: for example the time intensity curve is affected by the blood's velocity as well as by the intravascular volume; vasodilating agents can affect these two parameters differently and often not in a way that can be predicted [43].

The production of new and more 'physiological' contrast agents such as sonicated human albumin [44, 45] may be a step forward in the study of the coronary reserve with echocontrastography: the traditional agents cause coronary hyperemia and are formed of larger microbubbles and therefore can themselves affect the time intensity curve.

Conclusions

Even though numerous problems remain open as regards the quantitative evaluation of myocardial perfusion by echocardiography, the efforts being made in this direction are all quite justified. This method has the unique advantage of being able to visualize at same time the perfusion in tomographic sections in real time and the myocardial regional performance: these unique characteristics combine with the low cost and the practicality of echocardiography. Before deciding on the actual clinical use of this technique we can affirm in any case that the many studies in this sector have the merit of introducing the widely used technique of echocardiography to some fascinating aspects of physiology which have up to now been confined to pure research.

References

1. Gould KL, Lipscomb K, Hamilton GW (1974) Physiologic basis for assessing critical coronary stenosis. *Am J Cardiol* 33: 87–94.
2. Hodgson JM, LeGrand V, Bates ER, Mancini J, Aueron M, O'Neill WW, Simon SB, Beauman GJ, LeFree MT, Vogel RA (1985) Validation in dogs of a rapid digital angiographic technique to measure relative coronay blood flow during routine cardiac catheterization. *Am J Cardiol* 55: 188–193.
3. Nissen SE, Elion JL, Booth DC, Evans J, DeMaria AN (1986) Value and limitations of computer analysis of digital subtraction angiography in the assessment of coronary flow reserve. *Circulation* 73: 562–571.
4. Nishimura R, Togers PJ, Holmes DR, Gehring DG, Bove AA (1987) Assessment of myocardial perfusion by videodensitometry in the canine model. *J Am Coll Cardiol* 9: 891–897.
5. Marcus M, Wright C, Doty D, Eastham C, Laughlin D, Krumm P, Fastenow C, Brody M (1981) Measurements of coronary velocity and reactive hyperemia in the coronary circulation of humans. *Circ Res* 49: 877–891.
6. Wilson RF, Laughlin DE, Ackell PH, Chillian WM, Holida MD, Hartley CJ, Armstrong ML, Marcus ML, White CW (1985) Transluminal subselective measurement of coronary artery blood flow velocity and vasodilatory reserve in man. *Circulation* 72: 82.
7. Beyar R, Sideman S (1987) Time-dependent coronary blood flow distribution in left ventricular wall. *Am J Physiol* 252: H417–H433.
8. Marcus ML (1983) Transmural distribution of myocardial perfusion, in: The Coronary Circulation in Health and Disease. New York: Mc Graw Hill Book Company.
9. Bergmann SR, Fox KAA, Geltman EM, Sobel BE (1985) Positron emission tomography of the heart. *Prog Cardiovasc Dis* 28: 165.
10. Cerqueira MD, Harp GD, Ritchie JL (1987) Evaluation of myocardial perfusion and function by single photon emission computed tomography. *Seminars in Nuclear Medicine* 17: 200–213.
11. Gould KL, Goldstein RA, Mullani NA, Kirkeeide RL, Wong WH, Tewson TJ, Berridge MS, Bolomey LA, Hartz RK, Smalling WR, Fuentes F, Nishikawa A (1986) Non-invasive assessment of coronary stenoses by myocardial perfusion imaging during pharmacologic coronary vasodilation. VIII. Clinical feasibility of positron cardiac imaging without a cyclotron using generator-produced rubidium-82. *J Am Coll Cardiol* 7: 775–789.
12. Armstrong WF, Mueller TM, Kinney EL, Thickner EG, Dillon JC, Feigenbaum H (1982) Assessment of myocardial perfusion abnormalities with contrast enhanced two-dimensional echocardiography. *Circulation* 66: 166–173.
13. Tei C, Sakamaki T, Shah PM, Meerbaum S, Shimoura K, Kondo S, Corday E (1983) Myocardial contrast echocardiography: Reproducible technique of myocardial opacification for identifying regional perfusion deficits. *Circulation* 67: 585–592.
14. Kemper AJ, O'Boyle JE, Sharma S, Cohen CA, Kloner RA, Khuri SF, Parisi AF (1983) Hydrogen peroxide contrast-enhanced two-dimensional echocardiography: Real-time in vivo delineation of regional myocardial perfusion. *Circulation* 68: 603–611.
15. Maurer G, Ong K, Haendchen R, Torres M, Tei C, Wood F, Meerbaum S, Shah P, Corday E (1984) Myocardial contrast two-dimensional echocardiography: Comparison of contrast disappearance rate in normal and underperfused myocardium. *Circulation* 69: 418–429.
16. Tei C, Kondo S, Meerbaum S, Ong K, Maurer G, Wood F, Sakamaki T, Shimoura K, Corday E, Shah PM (1984) Correlation of myocardial echo contrast disappearance rate ('washout') and severity of experimental stenosis. *J Am Coll Cardiol* 3: 39–46.
17. Ten Cate FJ, Drury K, Meerbaum S, Noorsdy J, Feinstein S, Shah PM, Corday E (1984) Myocardial contrast two-dimensional echocardiography: Experimental examination at different coronary flow levels. *J Am Coll Cardiol* 3: 1219–1226.
18. Kondo S, Tei C, Meerbaum S, Corday E, Shah PM (1984) Hyperemic response of intracoronary contrast agents during two-dimensional echographic delineation of regional myocardium. *J Am Coll Cardiol* 4: 149–156.

19. Zotz RJ, Carls R, Erbel R, Clas W, Brenneke R, Meyer J (1986) A new method to quantify myocardial perfusion deficits in patients. *Circulation* 74 (II): 475.

20. Monaghan MJ, Quigley PJ, Metcalfe JM, Jevitt DE (1987) Assessment of myocardial perfusion by contrast enhanced digital subtraction echocardiography. *J Am Coll Cardiol* 9: 112A.

21. Cheirif J, Zoghbi WA, Zehler A, Winters WL, Bolli R, Lacy JL, Quinones MA (1987) Quantitative assessment of coronary reserve in critical stenosis by sonicated contrast echocardiography: Comparison with microspheres and Doppler flow probe. *J Am Coll Cardiol* 9: 112A.

22. Zotz RJ, Kann B, Brenneke R (1984) Evaluation of PTCA by video-intensitometric analysis of contrast echocardiograms. *Circulation* 76 (IV): 505.

23. Vandenberg BF, Kieso R, Fox-Eastham K, Chilian W, Kerber RE (1988) Demonstration of coronary flow reserve with contrast echocardiography. *J Am Coll Cardiol* 11: 75A.

24. Keller MW, Smucker M, Burwell M, Glasheen WP, Watson D, Kaul S (1987) Assessment of coronary blood flow reserve using myocardial contrast echocardiography. *Circulation* 76 (IV): 505.

25. Kaul S, Oliner JD, Kelly P, Watson DD (1987) Measurement of regional myocardial blood flow using myocardial contrast echocardiography. *J Am Coll Cardiol* 9: 2A.

26. Vandenberg BF, Feinstein SB, Kieso RA, Hunt M, Kerber RE (1988) Myocardial risk area and peak gray level measurement by contrast echocardiography: Effect of microbubble size and concentration, injection rate and coronary vasodilation. *Am Heart J* 115: 733–739.

27. Spotnitz WD, Keller MW, Nolan SP, Kaul S (1988) Success of internal mammary bypass grafting can be assessed intraoperatively using myocardial contrast echocardiography. *J Am Coll Cardiol* 11: 76A.

28. Vandenberg BF, Kieso R, Fox-Eastham K, Chilian W, Kerber RE (1989) Quantitation of myocardial perfusion by contrast echocardiography: Analysis of contrast gray level appearance variables and intracyclic variability. *J Am Coll Cardiol* 13: 200–206.

29. Cheirif J, Zoghbi WA, Bolli R, O'Neill PG, Winters WL, Quinones MA (1988) Contrast echocardiography: assessment of endocardial to epicardial blood flow relation during dypiridamole induced hyperemia in experimental coronary stenosis. *J Am Coll Cardiol* 11: 75A.

30. Ten Cate FJ, Cornel JH, Widimsky P, Serruys PW, Vletter WB, Mittertreiner WH (1987) Effect of papaverine administration on myocardial echocontrast distribution. *Am Heart J* 114: 1248–1249.

31. Ten Cate FJ, Cornell JH, Serruys PW, Vletter WB, Reiber JC (1987) Quantitative myocardial perfusion imaging using contrast two-dimensional echocardiography. *J Am Coll Cardiol* 9: 112A.

32. Segil LJ, Dicj CD, Feinstein SB, Silverman P, Reese M (1987) Contrast echocardiography – experimental validation of quantitation of regional intramyocardial coronary blood flow. *Circulation* 76 (IV): 504.

33. Rovai D, Lombardi M, Ferdeghini EM, Marzilli M, Distante A, Taddei L, Benassi A, DeMaria AN, L'Abbate A (1987) Colorcoded functional imaging of myocardial perfusion by contrast echocardiography. *Circulation* 76 (IV): 504.

34. Rovai D, Lombardini M, Ferdeghini EM, Marzilli M, Distante A, Taddei L, Landini L, Benassi A, L'Abbate A (1988) Detection of regional myocardial underperfusion by contrast-echo functional imaging. *J Am Coll Cardiol* 11: 76A.

35. Rovai D, Lombardi M, Nissen SE, Distante A, Marzilli M, DeMaria AN, L'Abbate A (1987) Spatial and temporal heterogeneity of coronary blood flow by myocardial contrast echocardiography. *J Am Coll Cardiol* 9: 112A.

36. Rovai D, Nissen SE, Elion J, Smith M, L'Abbate A, Kwan OL, DeMaria AN (1987) Contrast echo washout curves from the left ventricle: Application of basic principles of indicator-dilution theory and calculation of ejection fraction. *J Am Coll Cardiol* 10: 125–134.

37. Powsner SM, Feinstein SB (1987) Quantitative radiofrequency analysis of sonicated echo-

contrast agents, in: Roelandt J (ed), *Digital Techniques in Echocardiography*, pp 13–27. Dordrecht: Martinus Nijhoff Publishers.

38. Zwehl W, Areda J, Schwartz G, Feinstein S, Ong K, Meerbaum S (1984) Physical factors influencing quantitation of two-dimensional contrast echo amplitudes. *J Am Coll Cardiol* 4: 157–164.

39. Reisner SA, Shapiro JR, Amico AF, Meltzer RS (1989) Reproducibility of washout curves derived from myocardial contrast echo. *J Am Coll Cardiol* 13: 115A.

40. Cheirif J, Zoghbi WA, Raizner AE, Minor ST, Winters WL, Klein MS, DeBauche TL, Lewis JM, Roberts R, Quinones MA (1988) Assessment of myocardial perfusion in humans by contrast echocardiography. I. Evaluation of regional coronary reserve by peak contrast intensity. *J Am Coll Cardiol* 11: 735–743.

41. Keller MW, Glasheen W, Smucker ML, Burwell LR, Watson DD, Kaul S (1988) Myocardial contrast echocardiography in humans. II. Assessment of coronary blood flow reserve. *J Am Coll Cardiol* 12: 925–934.

42. Cheirif J, Zoghbi WA, Bolli R, O'Neill P, Hoyt BD, Quinones MA (1989) Assessment of regional myocardial perfusion by contrast echocardiography. II. Detection of changes in transmural and subendocardial perfusion during dypiridamole-induced hyperemia in a model of critical coronary stenosis. *J Am Coll Cardiol* 14: 1555–1565.

43. Reisner SA, Shapiro JR, Amico AF, Meltzer RS (1989) Myocardial contrast echo washout curves: The influence of ischemia and hyperemia. *J Am Coll Cardiol* 13: 115A.

44. Keller MW, Glasheen W, Teja K, Gear A, Kaul S (1988) Myocardial contrast echocardiography without significant hemodynamic effects or reactive hyperemia: A major advantage in the imaging of regional myocardial perfusion. *J Am Coll Cardiol* 12: 1039–1047.

45. Reisner SA, Ong SL, Lichtenberg GS, Amico AF, Shapiro JR, Allen MN, Meltzer RS (1989) Myocardial perfusion imaging by contrast echocardiography with use of intracoronary sonicated albumin in humans. *J Am Coll Cardiol* 14: 660–665.

Subject index

60. R.Th. van Dam and A. van Oosterom (eds.): *Electrocardiographic Body Surface Mapping*. Proceedings of the 3rd International Symposium on B.S.M., held in Nijmegen, The Netherlands (1985). 1986   ISBN 0-89838-834-1
61. M.P. Spencer (ed.): *Ultrasonic Diagnosis of Cerebrovascular Disease*. Doppler Techniques and Pulse Echo Imaging. 1987   ISBN 0-89838-836-8
62. M.J. Legato (ed.): *The Stressed Heart*. 1987   ISBN 0-89838-849-X
63. M.E. Safar (ed.): *Arterial and Venous Systems in Essential Hypertension*. With Assistance of G.M. London, A.Ch. Simon and Y.A. Weiss. 1987
                ISBN 0-89838-857-0
64. J. Roelandt (ed.): *Digital Techniques in Echocardiography*. 1987
                ISBN 0-89838-861-9
65. N.S. Dhalla, P.K. Singal and R.E. Beamish (eds.): *Pathology of Heart Disease*. Proceedings of the 8th Annual Meeting of the American Section of the I.S.H.R., held in Winnipeg, Canada, 1986 (Vol. 1). 1987   ISBN 0-89838-864-3
66. N.S. Dhalla, G.N. Pierce and R.E. Beamish (eds.): *Heart Function and Metabolism*. Proceedings of the 8th Annual Meeting of the American Section of the I.S.H.R., held in Winnipeg, Canada, 1986 (Vol. 2). 1987   ISBN 0-89838-865-1
67. N.S. Dhalla, I.R. Innes and R.E. Beamish (eds.): *Myocardial Ischemia*. Proceedings of a Satellite Symposium of the 30th International Physiological Congress, held in Winnipeg, Canada (1986). 1987   ISBN 0-89838-866-X
68. R.E. Beamish, V. Panagia and N.S. Dhalla (eds.): *Pharmacological Aspects of Heart Disease*. Proceedings of an International Symposium, held in Winnipeg, Canada (1986). 1987   ISBN 0-89838-867-8
69. H.E.D.J. ter Keurs and J.V. Tyberg (eds.): *Mechanics of the Circulation*. Proceedings of a Satellite Symposium of the 30th International Physiological Congress, held in Banff, Alberta, Canada (1986). 1987   ISBN 0-89838-870-8
70. S. Sideman and R. Beyar (eds.): *Activation, Metabolism and Perfusion of the Heart*. Simulation and Experimental Models. Proceedings of the 3rd Henry Goldberg Workshop, held in Piscataway, N.J., U.S.A. (1986). 1987   ISBN 0-89838-871-6
71. E. Aliot and R. Lazzara (eds.): *Ventricular Tachycardias*. From Mechanism to Therapy. 1987   ISBN 0-89838-881-3
72. A. Schneeweiss and G. Schettler: *Cardiovascular Drug Therapoy in the Elderly*. 1988
                ISBN 0-89838-883-X
73. J.V. Chapman and A. Sgalambro (eds.): *Basic Concepts in Doppler Echocardio-graphy*. Methods of Clinical Applications based on a Multi-modality Doppler Approach. 1987   ISBN 0-89838-888-0
74. S. Chien, J. Dormandy, E. Ernst and A. Matrai (eds.): *Clinical Hemorheology*. Applications in Cardiovascular and Hematological Disease, Diabetes, Surgery and Gynecology. 1987   ISBN 0-89838-807-4
75. J. Morganroth and E.N. Moore (eds.): *Congestive Heart Failure*. Proceedings of the 7th Annual Symposium on New Drugs and Devices, held in Philadelphia, Pa., U.S.A. (1986). 1987   ISBN 0-89838-955-0
76. F.H. Messerli (ed.): *Cardiovascular Disease in the Elderly*. 2nd ed. 1988
                ISBN 0-89838-962-3
77. P.H. Heintzen and J.H. Bürsch (eds.): *Progress in Digital Angiocardiography*. 1988
                ISBN 0-89838-965-8

Developments in Cardiovascular Medicine

100. J. Morganroth and E.N. Moore (eds.): *Risk/Benefit Analysis for the Use and Approval of Thrombolytic, Antiarrhythmic, and Hypolipidemic Agents.* Proceedings of the 9th Annual Symposium on New Drugs and Devices (1988). 1989   ISBN 0-7923-0294-X
101. P.W. Serruys, R. Simon and K.J. Beatt (eds.): *PTCA - An Investigational Tool and a Non-operative Treatment of Acute Ischemia.* 1990   ISBN 0-7923-0346-6
102. I.S. Anand, P.I. Wahi and N.S. Dhalla (eds.): *Pathophysiology and Pharmacology of Heart Disease.* 1989   ISBN 0-7923-0367-9
103. G.S. Abela (ed.): *Lasers in Cardiovascular Medicine and Surgery.* Fundamentals and Technique. 1990   ISBN 0-7923-0440-3
104. H.M. Piper (ed.): *Pathophysiology of Severe Ischemic Myocardial Injury.* 1990
    ISBN 0-7923-0459-4
105. S.M. Teague (ed.): *Stress Doppler Echocardiography.* 1990   ISBN 0-7923-0499-3
106. P.R. Saxena, D.I. Wallis, W. Wouters and P. Bevan (eds.): *Cardiovascular Pharmacology of 5-Hydroxytryptamine.* Prospective Therapeutic Applications. 1990
    ISBN 0-7923-0502-7
107. A.P. Shepherd and P.A. Öberg (eds.): *Laser-Doppler Blood Flowmetry.* 1990
    ISBN 0-7923-0508-6
108. J. Soler-Soler, G. Permanyer-Miralda and J. Sagristà-Sauleda (eds.): *Pericardial Disease.* New Insights and Old Dilemmas. Preface by Ralph Shabetai. 1990
    ISBN 0-7923-0510-8
109. J.P.M. Hamer: *Practical Echocardiography in the Adult.* With Doppler and Color-Doppler Flow Imaging. 1990   ISBN 0-7923-0670-8
110. A. Bayés de Luna, P. Brugada, J. Cosin Aguilar and F. Navarro Lopez (eds.): *Sudden Cardiac Death.* 1990   ISBN 0-7923-0716-X
111. E. Andries and R. Stroobandt (eds.): *Hemodynamics in Daily Practice.* 1990
    ISBN 0-7923-0725-9
112. J. Morganroth and E.N. Moore (eds.): *Use and Approval of Antihypertensive Agents and Surrogate Endpoints for the Approval of Drugs affecting Antiarrhythmic Heart Failure and Hypolipidemia.* Proceedings of the 10th Annual Symposium on New Drugs and Devices (1989). 1990   ISBN 0-7923-0756-9
113. S. Iliceto, P. Rizzon and J.R.T.C. Roelandt (eds.): *Ultrasound in Coronary Artery Disease.* Present Role and Future Perspectives. 1990   ISBN 0-7923-0784-4
114. J.V. Chapman and G.R. Sutherland (eds.): *The Noninvasive Evaluation of Hemodynamics in Congenital Heart Disease.* Doppler Ultrasound Applications in the Adult and Pediatric Patient with Congenital Heart Disease. 1990
    ISBN 0-7923-0836-0
115. G.T. Meester and F. Pinciroli (eds.): *Databases for Cardiology.* 1991 (forthcoming)
    ISBN 0-7923-0886-7
116. B. Korecky and N.S. Dhalla (eds.): *Subcellular Basis of Contractile Failure.* 1990
    ISBN 0-7923-0890-5
117. J.H.C. Reiber and P.W. Serruys (eds.): *Quantitative Coronary Arteriography.* 1991 (forthcoming)   ISBN 0-7923-0913-8
118. E. van der Wall and A. de Roos (eds.): *Magnetic Resonance Imaging in Coronary Artery Disease.* 1991 (forthcoming)   ISBN 0-7923-0940-5

Developments in Cardiovascular Medicine

Previous volumes are still available

KLUWER ACADEMIC PUBLISHERS – DORDRECHT / BOSTON / LONDON